ORTHOPEDIC BOARDS REVIEW

Orthopedic Boards Review

TIMOTHY S. LOTH, M.D.
Former Chief of Hand and Microsurgery
Former Assistant Professor of Orthopaedic Surgery
Department of Orthopaedic Surgery
St. Louis University
St. Louis, Missouri

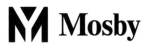

Mosby

St. Louis Baltimore Boston Chicago London Philadelphia Sydney Toronto

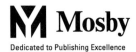

Sponsoring Editor: James D. Ryan
Assistant Editor: Karyn Fell
Associate Managing Editor, Manuscript Services: Deborah Thorp
Production Manager: Carol A. Reynolds
Proofroom Manager: Barbara M. Kelly

Mosby-Year Book, Inc.
11830 Westline Industrial Drive
St. Louis, MO 63416

3   4   5   6   7   8   9   0   UG   MA   97   96   95   94

Library of Congress Cataloging-in-Publication Data

Orthopaedic board review / [edited by] Timothy S. Loth.
    p.   cm.
    Includes bibliographical references and index.
    ISBN 0-8016-2740-0
    1. Orthopedics—Examinations, questions, etc.
2. Orthopedics—
    Outlines, syllabi, etc.   I. Loth, Timothy S.
    [DNLM: 1. Orthopedics—examination questions.   WE 18
0765]
    RD732.6.O77   1992
    617.3′0076—dc20   92-22708
    DNLM/DLC   CIP
    for Library of Congress

To my wife, Lisa,
and my children, Renée and Karl.

CONTRIBUTORS

ROBERT E. BURDGE, M.D.

Professor and Chairman
Department of Orthopaedic Surgery
St. Louis University
St. Louis, Missouri

J. KENNETH BURKUS, M.D.

Associate Professor
Department of Orthopaedic Surgery
St. Louis, University
St. Louis, Missouri

KEITH GABRIEL, M.D.

Assistant Professor
Department of Orthopaedic Surgery
St. Louis University
St. Louis, Missouri

TIMOTHY S. LOTH, M.D.

Former Chief of Hand and Microsurgery
Former Assistant Professor of Orthopaedic Surgery
Department of Orthopaedic Surgery
St. Louis University
St. Lous, Missouri

STEVEN MARDJETKO, M.D.

Former Assistant Professor
Department of Orthopaedic Surgery
St. Louis University
St. Louis, Missouri

DOUGLAS McDONALD, M.D.

Associate Professor
Department of Orthopaedic Surgery
St. Louis University
St. Louis, Missouri

THOMAS OTTO, M.D.

Assistant Professor
Department of Orthopaedic Surgery
St. Louis University
St. Louis, Missouri

ROBERT PIERRON, M.D.

Assistant Professor
Department of Orthopaedic Surgery
St. Louis University
St. Louis, Missouri

DAVID W. STREGE, M.D.

Assistant Professor
Department of Orthopaedic Surgery
St. Louis University
St. Louis, Missouri

FOREWORD

Preparing for the Orthopaedic Board Examinations (written or oral) is one of life's most stressful experiences. This apprehension is compounded by the frustration of trying to determine which journals and texts to review in order to best prepare for the questions that will be asked on the test. During the preboard preparation the student is forced to prioritize his or her efforts in an attempt to achieve a comprehensive review of a vast spectrum of orthopedic knowledge. While the review discipline may achieve its goal of retrieving and reinforcing preexisting information and supplementing that wisdom with new intelligence, it often fails to adequately prepare the applicant to utilize that information most effectively during an examination. Too often students readying themselves for the Boards fail to subject themselves to the disciplines of intellectual inquiry that are crucial to the preparation for such a rigorous inquisition. There can be no question that a test preparation instrument that poses numerous challenging questions covering the entire field of orthopedics and provides thorough and up-to-date answers to those questions would be of enormous benefit. Fortunately, that need has now been addressed by the excellent text, *Orthopedic Boards Review*, by Timothy S. Loth, M.D.

Dr. Loth's volume is indeed a unique effort to provide an exhaustive review of the most timely and pertinent information in orthopedics in question-and-answer form. Together with his excellent co-authors, Dr. Loth has integrated the important elements of basic science, patient care (including diagnosis), nonsurgical and surgical treatment, and postoperative care into chapters dealing with general orthopedics, pediatric orthopedics, pediatric trauma, metabolic disease, the spine, the upper extremity, the hand and wrist, the lower extremity, total joint reconstruction, the foot and ankle, biomechanics, and tumors. Each chapter is carefully designed to stimulate the thought processes of the reader and force him or her to draw on considerable knowledge to arrive at the appropriate answers. Even when the student's fund of knowledge is insufficient to adequately respond to a particular interrogatory, the book allows for a rapid satisfaction of that void by providing a complete explanation of each answer. The intellectual rewards of this format are immediate and long-lasting. The student is not only more likely to retain the information gleaned from this question-answer approach, but he or she will also benefit considerably from the test-taking discipline that this text requires.

While the advantages of using this volume as one nears the end of the Orthopaedic Board Examination review process would seem obvious, it might be equally beneficial to read through it at the beginning of test preparation to identify areas of weakness so as to best prioritize the study effort and to decide how much time to devote to each area and which books or articles to read. Further, the individual chapters of the book provide an excellent "spot check" of the adequacy of preparation as the student completes the review of each subject. This tripartite use of the text—at the beginning of study, after each topic, and when the review is nearly complete—would seem to offer the student tremendous assistance in work allocation, an opportunity to rapidly evaluate the adequacy of preparation on each subject, and a final assessment of the thoroughness of the entire study effort with a chance to determine any remaining "holes of knowledge." Along the way students will have familiarized themselves with the process of interrogation and response and will most assuredly be more comfortable with the mechanics and rigors of the Board examination process.

Orthopedic Boards Review is an innovative and much-needed adjunct to the study armamentarium of the Board candidate. It should greatly enhance the ability to assess the adequacy of preparation including specific areas of weakness and, unlike any previous study instruments, should give the student a chance to strengthen his or her test-taking skills, which are of paramount importance to the successful completion of the Board Examination process. Moreover, this text could have great value to those orthopedists not involved in Board or recertification review but who are desirous of updating their knowledge and expertise in an effort to remain current in all areas of the specialty.

Dr. Loth and his co-authors are to be commended on an innovative, thorough, and scholarly effort that can be of great value to both Orthopaedic Board applicants and nonapplicants wishing to review and update their general level of knowledge.

James W. Strickland
Clinical Professor of Orthopaedic Surgery
Indiana University School of Medicine
Past President
American Society for Surgery of the Hand
Bloomington, Indiana

PREFACE

When I began preparing for the "boards" in 1985, I sought a good review book in a question/answer format from which I could both learn and review orthopedic surgery. My search was fruitless. With a vivid recollection of this deficiency, I embarked on this project to improve the review process by writing a book that I hoped would be challenging, stimulating, and applicable to all of the orthopedic examinations: the Orthopaedic In-Training Examination (OITE), Parts I and II of the Board Exams, and recertification. It is with empathy for those who will be confronting these hurdles of competency that I completed this work.

TIMOTHY S. LOTH, M.D.

ACKNOWLEDGMENTS

I am grateful to many individuals who contributed to the completion of this book. Without the help of my colleagues at St. Louis University, who took time from their busy schedules to write and review chapters, this book would have remained partially completed, collecting dust in my office. Their enthusiasm for the project and their valuable contributions are deeply appreciated. My thanks to our residents for perceptive criticisms and suggestions regarding content and format.

I also thank Jim Ryan, Executive Editor, Mosby-Year Book, for his encouragement and enthusiasm regarding the project; Melanie Richardson, my secretary, who typed the text and its countless revisions; and my mentors, Drs. James W. Strickland, William W. Eversmann, Jr., Hill Hastings II, and Mr. A. Graham Apley, outstanding physician role-models and brilliant educators.

TIMOTHY S. LOTH, M.D.

HOW TO USE THIS BOOK

The goal of this book is to better prepare orthopedic surgeons and residents for their Orthopaedic Board Exams, OITE, and recertification examinations. The book's essay-question format simulates the oral examination of the Orthopaedic Board Exams and provides more rigorous test preparation than the multiple-choice format adapted in most other reviews. In addition to identifying deficiencies in knowledge and conceptualization, our format provides short discussions of grouped topics, which better prepares the reviewer for both the written and oral examinations.

Although some will think it an undesirable omission, I have deleted references from this text. A text peppered with references can be distracting. They are not in this book because most of the information in these questions and answers represents "common" knowledge found in standard orthopedic texts. Anyone preparing for boards, recertification, or the in-training exam, should be familiar with and have access to appropriate texts (which have tremendous reference lists), thereby eliminating the need for references in this one.

No attempt has been made to comprehensively review all of orthopedic surgery in this book. This would clearly be impossible. We have, however, attempted to discuss many current clinical topics as well as some of the esoteric ones that are recurrently encountered during examinations. We attempted to present "accepted" approaches to orthopedic problems and have not sought to present every option for treatment. We have not avoided controversial areas, and instead have attempted to identify these and give short explanations for each advocated approach. All

of the questions and answers contained within this text have been verified through multiple resident, peer, and editor reviews.

I would suggest that this book be used in the following ways: first, to review and reinforce concepts and information, and second, to determine areas of deficiency or vague concept development. To be most efficient in your review I suggest that the book be used in close proximity to your personal or your departmental library. If expansion of topics or concepts is needed you can easily look up these sections in appropriate orthopedic surgery texts.

Please allocate enough time to go through the book at least twice before your exams. On the first time through, identify those questions that were answered incorrectly or in which your concept development was weak. I would then recommend going through the same section with attention to the incorrectly answered questions several days later to assure that the information has been retained. Finally, I would review everything once again just prior to the exam to assure that the information is reinforced and easily retrievable.

I invite you to send me your impressions (positive or negative) regarding this book. I shall use these suggestions to improve subsequent editions.

I believe that mastering this book will give you a core of knowledge that will serve you well in your short-term goals of board certification and success on the in-training exams, as well as the more important pursuit of excellence in patient care. Best of luck.

TIMOTHY S. LOTH, M.D.

CONTENTS

CHAPTER 1

General Orthopedics

Robert Pierron, M.D.

Timothy S. Loth, M.D.

QUESTIONS

1. What are the three phases of fracture healing?

2. Describe key events in the inflammatory phase.

3. Describe the reparative phase.

4. What are the components of a fracture callus?

5. Describe the remodeling phase.

6. What findings in debridement of muscle were considered significant in determining viability?

7. Frequently the shot cloud in a close-range shotgun wound comes to lie against the fascia on the far side of the injured extremity. The wadding is often found in it. How should it be approached surgically?

8. In an emergency situation, what type blood can be given?

ANSWERS

1. (1) The inflammatory phase, (2) reparative phase, and (3) remodeling phase.

2. Local necrotic material elicits an immediate and intense acute inflammatory response. Vasodilation and plasma exudation occur. Polymorphonuclear neutrophils (PMNs) enter the region followed by macrophages.

3. The hematoma becomes organized. The pH is acidic. Electronegativity is found in the region of a fresh fracture, which is nonstress-generated. Mesenchymal cells (which are pleuripotential) repair the fracture damage; they enter the fracture site with granulation tissue and surrounding vessels. Callus forms. The cartilage in callus is replaced through endochondral ossification. Decreased oxygen tension favors cartilage formation. Reabsorption of necrotic bone fragments is performed by osteoclasts.

4. Fibrous tissue, cartilage, and immature fiber bone.

5. Osteoclastic resorption of poorly organized trabeculae occurs and new bone is laid down in response to lines of force.

6. The four C's (*c*onsistency, *c*apacity to bleed, *c*ontractility, and *c*olor) were frequently cited as helpful signs in assessing muscle viability. Contractility is significant, if present, but not all noncontractile muscle is necessarily nonvital. Color is the least reliable indicator of viability.

7. A counterincision opposite the entry wound is often the easiest access to the shot cloud and the associated wadding.

8. In an emergency, major grouping and Rh typing can be done in 10 minutes and is 99% safe. The use of universal donor (O, negative) blood is no quicker and somewhat less safe than type-specific blood and should be abandoned. A fully matched transfusion takes 1½ hours to prepare.

QUESTIONS

9. What are the basic colloid replacement fluids? Why are they better than crystalloid replacement fluid?

10. Under what circumstances is supplemental albumin contraindicated?

11. What essential tests should be monitored when treating a patient who is in shock?

12. What is the normal adult urine output per hour?

13. How long after cardiac arrest does irreversible central nervous system (CNS) damage occur?

14. What are the fundamental principles for managing any cardiac arrest?

15. Which clotting system does prothrombin time (PT) evaluate? How about partial thromboplastin time (PTT)?

16. Describe the normal hemostatic mechanisms in clot formation.

17. What is the rate of deep vein thrombosis (DVT) in patients with lower extremity joint replacements or fractures?

18. How many of the patients with DVT have pulmonary emboli?

19. What is the most accurate method of detecting a pulmonary embolus?

ANSWERS

9. The basic colloid replacement fluids are 5% albumin, plasma protein fraction (Plasmanate), and dextran 40. Ninety percent of the crystalloid volume leaks into the interstitial water compartment, whereas colloids do not.

10. In hypovolemic shock because albumin impairs coagulation, decreases pulmonary function, increases interstitial pulmonary water from trapped albumin, and impairs left ventricular function.

11. Arterial blood pressure, pulse, central venous pressure, and urinary output.

12. 20–40 mL/hr.

13. 4 minutes.

14. Maintain the airway; ventilate the patient if needed; ensure adequate cardiac output. Maintain F_{IO_2} at 100%. Maintain intravascular volume, correct acidosis that occurs secondary to respiratory insufficiency, and correct underlying disorders in electrolytes or rhythm.

15. PT evaluates the extrinsic clotting system, PTT the intrinsic.

16. Platelets adhere to the site of injury to form a hemostatic plug. Activation of the coagulation system results in fibrin formation.

17. 50%.

18. 10%.

19. Pulmonary angiography.

QUESTIONS

20. What are the indications for ventilator assistance in fat embolism?

21. What is the mechanism of gas gangrene in clostridial infections?

22. What is the incubation period for clostridial gas gangrene?

23. What are the key clinical features of clostridial myonecrosis?

24. What is the most important measure in preventing clostridial myonecrosis?

25. How is gas gangrene treated?

26. What is the routine prophylaxis dose of tetanus immunoglobulin?

27. What is the recommended tetanus prophylaxis for clean, minor wounds?

28. What are the recommendations for tetanus prophylaxis for severe, neglected, or old (>24 hours) tetanus-prone wounds?

29. How is tetanus treated?

30. When are bone changes demonstrated on radiograph in osteomyelitis?

ANSWERS

20. Tachypnea with carbon dioxide tension (Pco_2) >50 mm Hg, and oxygen pressure (Po_2) <60 mm Hg. Arterial Po_2 should be maintained at >70 mm Hg. Some authors (Gustillo) advocate industrial-strength steroids—methylprednisone sodium succinate, 600 to 1,200 mg intravenously (IV) in divided doses over 24 hours.

21. The release of histotoxins such as alpha toxin.

ANSWERS

22. 12–24 hours.

23. Severe local pain and swelling associated with severe tissue destruction and systemic toxemia. Gas formation is not pathognomonic and in some instances may be scant.

24. Complete debridement of all necrotic tissue from a wound.

25. (1) Surgery. Multiple incisions and fasciotomies for decompression and drainage of the fascial compartments, excision of the involved muscles, and open amputation constitute appropriate operative management. (2) Penicillin, 3 million units q.3h., and often an aminoglycoside is added because of the common presence of other *Clostridia* species. (3) Hyperbaric O_2 has been helpful as well: 3 atm for 60 to 90 min q.8h. for four to six exposures. If the diagnosis is made early in the course of the disease, thorough debridement, antibiotics, and hyperbaric O_2 (if available) can save the patient without need for complete amputation.

26. 250 units.

27. 0.5 cc of tetanus toxoid for immunized and hemi-immunized patients.

28. For patients immunized within the last 10 years, 0.5 cc of tetanus toxoid is given unless the last booster dose was given within 1 year. For patients immunized over 10 years ago and patients never immunized, 0.5 cc of tetanus toxoid plus 250 units of tetanus immunoglobulin are administered (also consider tetracycline or penicillin).

29. The wound is debrided. Penicillin, 2 million units q.6h. plus streptomycin 0.5 g intramuscularly (IM) q.12h., is administered. Tetanus immunoglobulin, 500 to 1,000 units to a total dosage of 6,000 to 10,000 units, is given. The patient is supported with sedation.

30. After 10 to 21 days.

QUESTIONS

31. How much bone substance must be removed to demonstrate radiographic change?

32. What are the clinical features of reflex sympathetic dystrophy (RSD)?

33. What are the three stages of RSD?

34. What causes the hand-shoulder syndrome?

35. How long does irreversible muscle and nerve damage occur after the onset of a compartmental syndrome?

36. What are the recommended factor activity levels for hemophilic patients with hemarthrosis and joint aspiration, serious muscle bleeds, serious neural bleed, and surgical procedures?

37. How are muscular bleeds treated in hemophilia?

38. How should you evaluate a potential compartmental syndrome in a hemophilia IM bleed?

ANSWERS

31. 40%.

32. Pain, hyperesthesia, and tenderness, usually much greater than expected for the level of injury; swelling; decreased range of motion; skin color, texture, and temperature changes. Early signs are increased sweating, redness, warmth, and swelling. Late signs are pallor; dry, shiny skin; and coolness.

33. (1) Early—constant, burning or aching, pain out of proportion to the injury; (2) dystrophic (3 months)—cold, glossy skin, decreased range of motion, osteoporosis demonstrated on radiograph; (3) atrophic—atrophy of skin and muscle; decreased range of motion with joint contractures.

ANSWERS

34. It may follow cervical spondylitis, all types of fractures, and trauma, cerebrovascular accident, or myocardial infarction. Treatment is gradual restoration of range of motion and reduction of pain through a coordinated program of therapy, medical intervention (antidepressants, etc.), and interruption of excessive sympathetic activity (stellate ganglion blocks or other injections).

35. Muscle damage occurs in 4 to 12 hours; nerve damage in 12 to 24 hours.

36. Hemarthrosis—30% to 40%; serious muscle bleeds—40% to 50%; serious neural bleed—80% to 100%; surgery—100%.

37. (1) Factor replacement to levels of 40% to 50%; (2) ice to the area; (3) immobilization in a position of comfort for 1 to 7 days; (4) when pain and spasm have subsided, active and passive range of motion exercises may be reinitiated.

38. (1) Raise the factor level immediately to 40%; (2) measure compartment pressures; (3) if compartment pressures are elevated to a level requiring surgical decompression, factor levels should be increased to 100% before proceeding with surgery.

QUESTIONS

39. How should fractures in hemophilia be treated?

40. What is the most common infective organism in elective surgery without perioperative antibiotics?

41. What are the features of toxic shock syndrome?

42. What is the agent of choice for treating *Staphylococcus epidermidis* infection which is resistant to penicillin and penicillinase-resistant penicillins?

43. What is the most frequently identified causative organism in pseudomembranous enterocolitis?

44. What is the most common complication after lower extremity surgery in adults?

45. What percentage of thrombophlebitis is detected by clinical examination alone?

46. What is the mechanism through which low-dose heparin works?

47. What are aspirin's antithrombotic effects attributed to?

ANSWERS

39. Increase factor levels-stable fractures to 30% to 40% for 2 to 4 days up to 1 week, and unstable fractures to 30% to 50% for 1 to 3 weeks. Once hemostasis is achieved, treat using standard fracture management. Avoid traction pins because of potential bleeding. Open reduction with internal fixation can be performed when indicated with a 100% factor level at surgery and no less than 30% for the next 14 days.

40. *Staphylococcus aureus.*

41. Fever, profound multisystem dysfunction, desquamative erythroderma, and minimal infection or colonization with *S. aureus.* Enterotoxin F may be responsible for the marked reaction in susceptible patients.

42. Vancomycin.

43. *Clostridium difficile.*

44. Thrombophlebitis occurs in 40% to 60% of patients over 40 years old undergoing surgery about the knee or hips.

45. From 5% to 30%. (*Note:* Measurements of venous flow obstruction include pneumatic plethysmography, cuff impedance phlebography, and Doppler ultrasound techniques. These methods are unreliable for clots in small veins. They are more reliable for clots in major veins.)

46. It increases the rate at which antithrombin III inhibits activated factor X and thrombin.

47. Inhibition of prostaglandins, thromboxane, and prostacyclin.

QUESTIONS

48. What are the stages of osteonecrosis described by Arlet and Ficat?

49. How are stage I and II osteonecrosis treated?

50. How are stage III and IV osteonecrosis treated?

51. How should osteonecrosis of the femoral condyle be treated? Describe early and late-stage treatment.

52. How should nontraumatic osteonecrosis of the humeral head be treated?

53. What is the proposed mechanism of fat embolism syndrome?

54. What factors are associated with fat embolism syndrome?

55. What are the key factors in preventing the clinical manifestation of fat embolism syndrome?

56. What complications are more frequent in those patients with sickle cell anemia who undergo major operations such as total hip arthroplasty?

57. What is the average age at which sickle cell dactylitis occurs? How long does it last?

ANSWERS

48. *Stage I*—Normal radiographs; diagnosis is based on magnetic resonance imaging (MRI) or biopsy. *Stage II*—Radiographic changes are present, but may not be typical for ischemic necrosis; no osteochondral fracture is present. *Stage III*—Radiographic changes of avascular necrosis (AVN) consisting of wedge-shaped increased density and mottled osteoporosis are demonstrated. A subchondral lucent line is visible; the head is no longer spherical. *Stage IV*—There are marked changes in the femoral head with secondary degenerative joint disease of the hips.

ANSWERS

49. The use of vascularized fibular bone graft has been popular, as well as protected weightbearing and range-of-motion exercises, surgical decompression of the femoral head, or electromagnetic field application.

50. Once osteochondral fracture and collapse occur in the femoral head, most patients require arthroplasty or arthrodesis.

51. Early treatment consists of nonweightbearing, immobilization, or realignment osteotomy. Late treatment (osteochondral fractures and collapse) consists of realignment osteotomy, removal of loose bodies, arthrodesis, or prosthetic reconstruction.

52. Limitation of activity to decrease forces across the joint, and range-of-motion exercises. With severe symptoms, prosthetic replacement without glenoid replacement is done.

53. Both platelets and erythrocytes adhere to fat globules resulting in emboli which lodge in the lungs. These fat emboli are metabolized into free fatty acids which have a toxic action on the lung parenchyma and produce respiratory distress and chemical pneumonitis.

54. Multiple long-bone fractures, open fractures, fractures caused by high-energy trauma (vehicular accidents), hypovolemia, and poor oxygenation.

55. Maintenance of normal blood volume; proper oxygenation (30%–40% F_{IO_2}) via mask may suffice for some patients. Some will require positive pressure breathing or ventilation.

56. Pulmonary problems and infection.

57. Sickle cell dactylitis occurs at an average age of 18 months. It is self-limited to a few days to a few weeks.

QUESTIONS

58. What are the radiographic findings in sickle cell dactylitis?

59. What hematologic abnormality is associated with radial clubhand?

60. How is this associated platelet deficiency best treated?

61. What is the inheritance pattern for malignant hyperthermia?

62. What musculoskeletal abnormalities are associated with malignant hyperthermia?

63. Which anesthetic agents are associated with malignant hyperthermia?

64. What are the first signs of malignant hyperthermia?

65. What is the pathogenesis of malignant hyperthermia?

66. What is the best method of preoperative evaluation for malignant hyperthermia?

67. How should one treat malignant hyperthermia?

68. What is the recommended prophylaxis for a patient with a strong family history of malignant hyperthermia?

69. What is a common gastrointestinal (GI) complication following multiple trauma?

ANSWERS

58. Soft tissue swelling may be the only finding for 1 to 2 weeks. Then the films show subperiosteal bone formation in a rectangular shape along the phalanges, cortical thinning, and irregular medullary densities. Radiographic changes usually disappear after several months.

ANSWERS

59. Platelet deficiency.

60. Transfusion of platelets from tissue-matched donors.

61. Autosomal dominant.

62. Myopathy, recurrent dislocation of joints, scoliosis, kyphosis.

63. Halothane and succinylcholine.

64. Rapidly rising temperature and tachycardia.

65. Abnormal calcium transport which leads to recurrent sarcomere contraction with increased metabolic rate, increased temperature, increased CO_2, increased O_2 use, and cyanosis. The mortality rate is related to the severity of the fever.

66. Thorough family and personal history; sometimes serologic testing reveals increased serum creatine phosphokinase (CPK).

67. Terminate the surgical procedure. Discontinue muscle relaxants and anesthesia. Hyperventilate the patient with oxygen. Administer dantrolene sodium, 1.5 mg/kg initial dose (dantrolene is an inhibitor of calcium release from the sarcotubular system) followed by incremented doses of 1 mg/kg up to a total dose of 10 mg/kg until a clinical response is seen. Administer-$NaHCO_3$ for acidosis, furosemide and mannitol for urine output. Cool the patient in an ice bath with fans, if needed.

68. Dantrolene sodium, 1.0 to 1.5 mg/kg po 4 to 12 hours prior to surgery. Avoid halothane and succinylcholine.

69. GI bleeds.

QUESTIONS

70. What is the prophylaxis for GI bleeds?

71. What is the prime energy source in each of the following? (1) 100-yard dash, (2) intermediate activity (e.g., middle-distance running), (3) endurance activity (e.g., aerobic system, bicycle riding for 1 hour).

72. What does the myofibril consist of?

73. What is a sarcomere?

74. Draw a sarcomere and the associated bands.

75. The I band consists of what protein?

76. What does the A band consist of?

77. What is the H zone?

78. What is a motor unit?

ANSWERS

70. Antacids or H_2 blockers, or both, are given to keep the gastric pH above 3.5.

71. (1) Phosphagen system (phosphocreatinine energy source). (2) Muscle glycogen is the prime energy source for intermediate activity. (3) The energy source for endurance activity is 75% muscle glycogen and triglycerides and 25% blood-borne fuels.

72. Actin and myosin.

73. The area from one Z line to another.

ANSWERS

74.

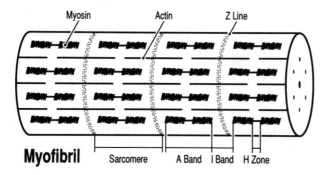

75. Actin.

76. Interdigitating fibers of actin and myosin.

77. An area that consists of myosin fibers only.

78. A motor nerve and the muscle fibers it innervates.

QUESTIONS

79. Can the ratio of slow-twitch to fast-twitch fibers be altered by specific training?

80. What are the five types of collagen and in what tissues are they found?

81. What is the collagen molecule composed of?

82. What are three mechanisms through which organisms can inoculate joints and lead to septic arthritis?

83. In which age groups are infected joints seen most commonly? What percentage of septic joints are monarticular in presentation?

84. Which joint is most commonly infected?

85. What diagnostic procedures should be done in evaluating a suspected septic arthritis?

86. Describe the treatment for septic joints.

87. Describe the clinical characteristics of gonococcal arthritis.

88. Describe tuberculous (TB) arthritis.

ANSWERS

79. No. This is genetically determined.

80. *Type I* is found in skin, bone, and tendon; *type II* in cartilage; *type III* in blood vessels, skin, and spleen; *type IV* in basement membrane; and *type V* in placenta and smooth muscle.

81. Three polypeptide alpha chains of about a thousand amino acids each.

ANSWERS

82. (1) Hematogenous spread; (2) extension from preexisting infection in adjacent soft tissue or bone; (3) direct introduction into the joint through a puncture wound.

83. Infected joints are most common in the very young and the elderly, especially in those with preexisting chronic debilitating disease (e.g., rheumatoid arthritis), or with deficient host defense mechanisms (alcoholics or patients on immunosuppressive drugs). Eighty-three percent are monarticular.

84. The knee.

85. Blood cultures and joint aspiration.

86. Parental antibiotics in moderately high doses are given for 1 to 2 weeks. After *S. aureus* infection, oral antibiotic treatment should be continued for another 4 to 6 weeks. The joint is flushed or drained as needed to prevent tense joint swelling. Formal irrigation and drainage, arthroscopy, and serial needle aspirations are options. Physical measures are initial splinting, followed by a program of physical therapy after inflammation subsides.

87. Gonococcal arthritis is found mostly in young women, is often polyarticular (hematogenous spread), with milder joint involvement in contrast to most other types of septic arthritis. Tenosynovitis may be present, as well as macular and vesicular skin lesions on the extremities. The diagnosis is made by isolating the gonococcus from the genitourinary (GU) tract, since it is difficult to isolate from the joint. Perform joint aspiration and obtain synovial fluid for analysis and culture.

88. Chronic, insidious joint involvement; monarticular arthritis with pain and swelling but often no warmth. X-ray findings are bone and cartilage destruction. The chest film may show signs of TB. Synovial biopsy is often necessary to make the diagnosis; granuloma and acid-fast bacteria are present. Conventional treatment for pulmonary TB is given. The patient often comes to surgery for reconstruction.

QUESTIONS

89. Which viruses can cause polyarticular arthritis?

90. What fungi may be recovered on joint aspiration?

91. What is the mechanism for arthritis in acute rheumatic fever?

93. What three distinct forms of rheumatic disease are associated with hepatitis B?

94. In pelvic fractures, unrecognized blood loss can lead to life-threatening hypovolemia and shock. What does a pulse rate greater than 100 bpm indicate regarding the percentage of blood loss? What does a systolic blood pressure of less than 100 mm Hg indicate?

95. In pelvic fractures, where is hemorrhage usually demonstrated during angiographic evaluation for massive bleeding?

96. What are effective methods of controlling hemorrhage in pelvic fractures?

97. If significant bleeding continues after angiographic arterial embolization, what should be done next?

98. Hematuria secondary to pelvic fractures requires immediate radiologic investigation. What three studies visualize the entire urinary tract?

ANSWERS

89. Rubella, rubella vaccine, mumps, varicella, and infectious mononucleosis may have arthritis as one of the acute clinical manifestations, presumably due to invasion of the joint space by the virus.

90. Blastomycetes, *Coccidioides immitis*, *Histoplasma species*, and *Sporothrix schenkii* are the fungi most frequently isolated.

ANSWERS

91. It is thought to be an inflammatory or immune response.

93. (1) A serum sickness–like syndrome in the prodromal phase of acute hepatitis associated with urticarial rash, detectable circulating hepatitis B antigen, and low serum complement levels. (2) Posthepatitic periarteritis nodosa with acute necrotizing inflammation of small and medium-sized arteries of the skin, heart, kidney, lung, GI tract, and peripheral nervous system. Complexes of hepatitis B antigen and specific antibody are detectable in involved blood vessel walls. (3) Essential mixed cryoglobulinemia in chronic active hepatitis.

94. A pulse rate >100 bpm indicates a blood volume deficit of 20%. Systolic blood pressure <100 mm Hg indicates blood volume deficit of 30%.

95. In branches of the hypogastric artery.

96. Ligation of vessels, use of the G-suit, external fixation, skeletal traction, massive fluid and blood replacement, and therapeutic embolization of bleeding vessels.

97. Venography to attempt to localize big venous bleeders. Bleeding can be stopped with intravascular balloons. Patients should later be repaired surgically or ligated. Sometimes skeletal stabilization can markedly decrease hemorrhage.

98. Retrograde urethrogram, cystogram, and intravenous pyelography (IVP).

QUESTIONS

99. What are the indications for a retrograde urethrogram prior to Foley catheter insertion?

100. What should be done if the urethrogram is normal?

101. What should be done if the cystogram is abnormal?

102. How are bladder ruptures treated?

103. Describe the Garden classification of femoral neck fractures.

104. When does the scapula migrate from C5 to T5 in utero?

105. When does the epiphysis of the humeral head fuse to the shaft?

106. When does the coracoid process unite to the body of the scapula ossification center?

107. How many ossification centers does the acromion arise from and when do they fuse?

108. What are the associated skeletal anomalies in Sprengel's deformity?

109. How often is the omovertebral body present in Sprengel's deformity?

ANSWERS

99. Blood in the urethral meatus, penile or scrotal trauma, a "high-riding" prostate on rectal examination, wide diastasis of the symphysis, or straddle fractures of the pelvis.

100. If the urethrogram is normal, then a Foley catheter can be inserted and a cystogram can be done.

ANSWERS

101. An IVP is done to rule out the presence of upper GU injury. Call the urologist.

102. Surgical repair as soon as possible. Divert urinary flow via suprapubic cystostomy.

103. *Grade I* is an incomplete or impacted fracture. *Grade II* is a complete fracture without displacement. *Grade III* is a complete fracture with partial displacement. The retinaculum (capsule) remains attached to the distal and proximal fragments. The trabecular pattern of the femoral head does not line up with that of the acetabulum, demonstrating incomplete displacement between the femoral fragments. *Grade IV* is a complete fracture with complete displacement. The trabecular patterns of the acetabulum and femoral head align, indicating complete separation of the femoral fracture fragments.

104. 5–8 weeks.

105. Age 19 years.

106. Age 15 years.

107. Two. They fuse at age 22 years.

108. Scoliosis; cervical ribs; anomalies of rib and vertebral segmentation (Klipped-Feil syndrome); torticollis; hypoplasia of the pectoralis major (Poland's syndrome), rhomboids, serratus anterior, latissimus dorsi, and most commonly the trapezius. Renal anomalies are also seen.

109. The omovertebral body is an attachment between the scapula and vertebral column and consists of bone, fibrous tissue, or cartilage. It is present in 30% of patients with Sprengel's deformity.

QUESTIONS

110. How should Sprengel's deformity be treated and when?

111. What congenital deformity causes elevation and winging of the scapula when the arm is adducted and disappearance of the scapula when the arm is raised above the horizontal?

112. How should congenital fibrotic bands of the deltoid be treated?

113. What is the most common birth brachial plexus injury?

114. What muscles are affected in Erb's palsy?

115. What is the second most common birth plexus injury?

116. How should birth brachial plexus injuries be worked up?

117. What is the distribution of weakness in Klumpke's disease?

118. How are brachial plexus injuries treated for the first 18 to 24 months?

119. How often in juvenile rheumatoid arthritis (JRA) is progressive severe joint destruction seen?

ANSWERS

110. Observation for mild deformities. Operative treatment is the Woodward procedure, carried out at age 3 to 7 years. Resect the supraspinous portion of the scapula, release the vertebral attachments of the muscles. Relocate the scapula inferiorly; derotate. Reattach the vertebral muscles inferiorly. Perform osteotomy of the clavicle to avoid neurovascular problems at the thoracic outlet. Over age 8 years or when the deformity is not severe, excision of the superior angle of the scapula and any vertebral connections can give improved function and cosmesis. This can also be done for patients of any age with a minor deformity.

111. Congenital fibrotic bands of the deltoid. This is also seen in iatrogenic bands from IM injections (especially tetracycline).

112. Surgical excision of the scar.

113. Erb's palsy due to a lesion of the roots of the C5–6 nerves.

114. The deltoid, biceps, brachialis, supinator, supraspinatus, infraspinatus, and subscapularis.

115. Total plexus involvement. The extremity is limp; there is loss of tendon reflexes; loss of the Moro reflex; and Horner's syndrome is present.

116. Radiographs of the neck and both upper extremities should be obtained to rule out fracture, as well as electromyelogram (EMG) to document recovery and identify the muscles available for transfer. The usefulness of myelography is controversial. Thermography has also been used to evaluate nerve damage.

117. The wrist and finger flexors and intrinsics.

118. Prevention of contractures and observation for neurologic recovery; range of motion exercises; and intermittent static splinting. Some advocate exploration and repair if there has been no improvement after 3 months of observation.

119. In 5% of patients.

QUESTION

120. What are the stabilizing ligaments of the lateral side of the ankle joint?

ANSWER

120. The anterior talofibular ligament, calcaneal fibular ligament, anterior and posterior tibial fibular ligaments, and interosseus membrane.

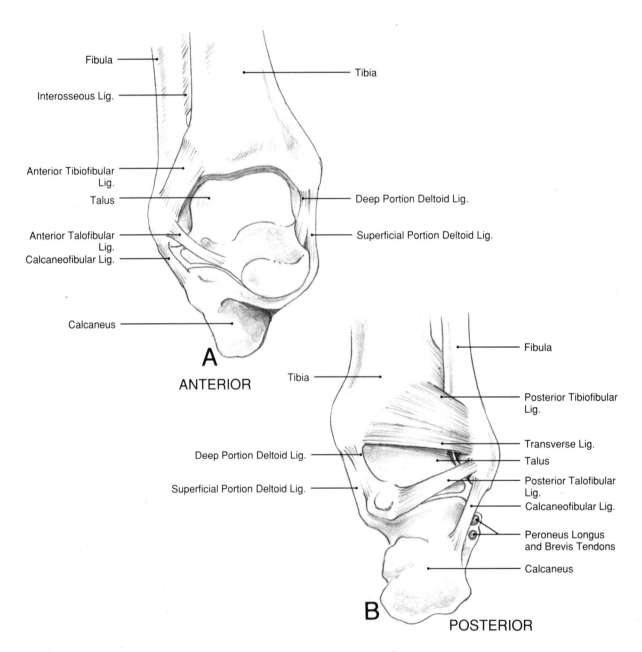

Ligamentous structures of the ankle and hindfoot. **A,** anterior view. **B,** posterior view.

ANSWER

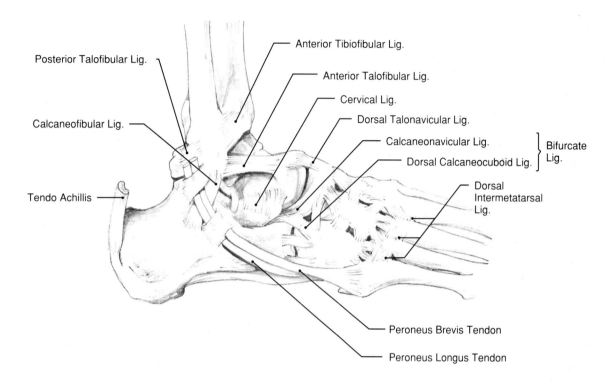

Ligaments of the ankle and foot (lateral view).

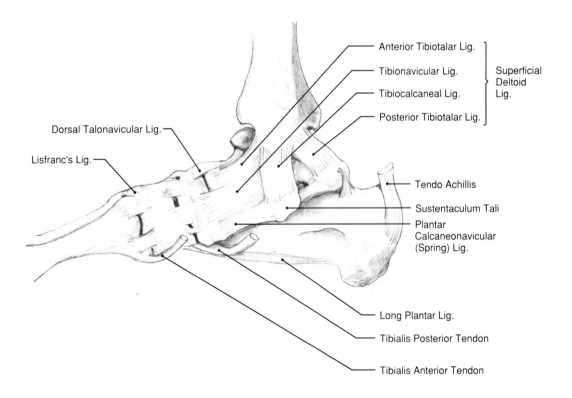

Ligaments of the ankle and foot (medial view).

QUESTIONS

121. In an inversion ankle sprain, what tests evaluate joint stability?

122. What is the preferred treatment for monarticular end-stage arthritis of the ankle joint in a 35-year-old laborer?

123. What is the best position for ankle fusion?

124. What is the most likely diagnosis of a patient who presents with shoulder pain of gradual onset starting the day following "spring cleaning" demonstrating pain in all planes of motion with abduction severely limited but also limitation of rotation of motion at 0 degrees of abduction?

125. What is the most likely diagnosis in a patient who presents with shoulder pain of sudden onset at the time of a fall with severe pain at attempts of both forward flexion and abduction and night pain on a daily basis 6 weeks post injury but with normal strength at neutral abduction and flexion?

126. What is the most likely cause of longstanding problems in a patient with pain distributed diffusely across the anterior knee, no instability on clinical testing, increase of parapatellar pain during resisted knee extension, and localized tenderness on palpation of the borders of the patella?

127. A patient presents with a history of sudden pain when twisting on his flexed knee. He "felt a pop" and experienced swelling that occurred overnight after the injury. He demonstrates local joint line tenderness on clinical examination. What is the most likely diagnosis?

128. What further tests are confirmatory?

129. A patient presents with a history of hyperextension injury during running. He "felt a pop" and experienced immediate swelling. On initial evaluation in the emergency room, joint aspiration reveals hemarthrosis. The most likely diagnosis is

ANSWERS

121. (1) The anterior drawer test in plantar flexion evaluates the anterior talofibular ligament. (2) The inversion or varus stress test ("talar tilt"): 15 degrees of tilt or 10 degrees of tilt greater than the opposite side indicates both anterior talofibular and calcaneal fibular ligament disruption. (3) An arthrogram or peroneal tendon sheath injection that demonstrates a communication between the ankle joint and peroneal tendon sheath indicates calcaneofibular ligament disruption.

122. Tibiotalar arthrodesis.

123. Neutral flexion (slight plantar flexion in a female who wishes to wear heels), in 0 to 5 degrees of valgus, and 5 to 10 degrees of external rotation.

124. Tendinitis or bursitis.

125. Rotator cuff tear.

126. Patellofemoral dysfunction. The patient should be evaluated for patellar alignment or patellar tracking problems and muscle imbalance in the quadriceps and hamstrings.

127. Torn meniscus.

128. A positive McMurray test, an Apley grind test demonstrating pain during compression and relief during distraction, radiographic studies, MRI or an arthrogram, and arthroscopy (indicated urgently only if mechanical locking of the knee is present).

129. Anterior cruciate ligament rupture. Associated pathologic findings such as a torn meniscus may be present in a significant percentage of cases.

QUESTIONS

130. What further tests are indicated before the patient is given a medical release to return to sports activities?

131. The best test to clinically evaluate for instability due to anterior cruciate ligament rupture is

132. Functional anterior cruciate ligament insufficiency in an athletically active 20-year-old with symptoms persisting after rehabilitation is best treated by

133. The best treatment for a peripheral one-third tear of the medial meniscus extending greater than 1 cm in length that can be displaced into the joint when probed in a 20-year-old athlete with no other injury is

134. What is the most sensitive diagnostic study to evaluate for possible stress fracture in an extremity painful during activity for 2 weeks?

135. What is the most sensitive diagnostic study to evaluate for possible chronic compartmental syndrome?

136. How should one test for possible neurologic injury associated with shoulder dislocation?

137. How should one evaluate possible neurologic injury in hip dislocation?

138. How should one evaluate possible neurologic injury in distal humeral fractures?

ANSWERS

130. Clinical evaluation for instability by the Lachman test, and the pivot shift test. Consider arthroscopy, particularly if the patient's age and activity level suggests he will need further intervention. Most patients require rehabilitation and bracing or cruciate ligament reconstruction to safely resume a competitive level of sports if complete rupture of the anterior cruciate is diagnosed.

ANSWERS

131. The Lachman test. In longstanding insufficiency the anterior drawer and pivot shift test are also positive.

132. Reconstruction of the anterior cruciate ligament using autologous material such as bone-patellar tendon or bone-hamstring tendon grafts. Repair of intersubstance tears of the anterior cruciate have shown unreliable results. Patient with lower-level expectations may return to asymptomatic daily activities with a rehabilitation program and brace support for noncompetitive sports.

133. Arthroscopic repair. There is a high success rate of repair in this type of lesion and total meniscectomy increases the risk of degenerative joint disease.

134. Technetium 99m bone scan.

135. Compartment pressure testing with activity stress. The resting pressure is measured both before and after active exercise.

136. Sensation should be tested in the "lateral shoulder patch" area overlying the deltoid. Evaluate for deltoid strength because of the high risk or axillary nerve injury with shoulder dislocation.

137. Evaluate for sensation in the lateral calf and dorsal foot and dorsiflexion strength of the foot and toes since sciatic nerve injury, especially the peroneal branch, is at highest risk in hip dislocation.

138. Check sensation on the dorsoradial hand and evaluate the strength of wrist and finger extension on account of the high risk of radial nerve injury.

QUESTIONS

139. In a patient with hemodynamic instability associated with pelvic fracture, emergency treatment should consist of

140. In a patient with pelvic fracture who has demonstrated hemodynamic instability prior to initial resuscitation and whose x-ray films demonstrate an anterior diastasis, treatment should consist of

141. If pneumatic antishock garments are used for emergency transportation in a multi-injured patient, what pressure limits should be used if transport is expected to take more than 1 hour?

142. In the multiple trauma patient, what treatments are helpful in preventing adult respiratory distress syndrome (ARDS)?

143. Which knee problems are most accurately diagnosed by MRI?

144. What radiologic tests are useful for diagnosing a torn meniscus?

145. What internal derangements of the knee are not seen well by MRI?

146. The best treatment for isolated acute tear of the medial collateral ligament is

147. In pelvic fractures the leading causes of mortality are

148. Because of the high incidence of GU injury associated with pelvic fractures, evaluation before placement of an indwelling catheter should include

ANSWERS

139. Stabilization for transport, possibly with use of a pneumatic anti-shock garment, and rapid fluid infusion and planning for massive blood transfusion.

140. Application of an external fixator as soon as possible. Add skeletal traction if vertical displacement is evident by radiographic or clinical examination.

141. About 20 mm Hg. Pressures >30 mm Hg have been shown to cause tissue damage in as little as 90 minutes.

142. Splinting fractures before moving or transporting the patient; early internal fixation within the first 24 hours, if possible; treatments which allow the patient to be mobilized early so that change of position and sitting up for pulmonary care can be accomplished as soon as possible; fluid replacement to correct hypovolemic shock.

143. Torn meniscus; AVN about the knee; tumor; torn cruciate ligament (some false negatives have been reported). MR scan does not ''see'' articular cartilage surfaces well.

144. The MR scan shows the highest correlation in diagnosing both medial and lateral meniscus tears, but will show degenerative changes when a full-thickness tear is not present. An arthrogram is not as reliable in diagnosing cruciate tears as MRI.

145. Articular cartilage chondromalacia, plica, and loss of functional integrity of the anterior cruciate ligament, although a complete rupture can usually be diagnosed in a high percentage of cases.

146. A cast brace with early protected range of motion.

147. Blood loss, CNS injury, and the complications of multiple trauma (e.g., ARDS).

148. A retrograde cystourethrogram, especially if inspection of the penile meatus reveals blood.

QUESTIONS

149. Describe the steps for emergency resuscitation in pelvic fractures.

150. What is the indication for emergency placement of an external fixator in fractures of the pelvis?

151. What radiographic studies are used to evaluate a posterior wall fracture of the acetabulum?

152. After closed reduction of a hip dislocation associated with a posterior wall fracture of the acetabulum, what radiographic findings would indicate the need for open surgical intervention?

153. What are the advantages and disadvantages of the shoulder arthrogram in evaluating a patient with persistent shoulder pain for possible rotator cuff tear?

154. What are the advantages and disadvantages of ultrasound in evaluating a patient with persistent shoulder pain for rotator cuff tear?

155. What are the advantages and disadvantages of MRI in evaluating a patient with persistent shoulder pain for rotator cuff tear?

156. A full-thickness rotator cuff tear persistently painful longer than 6 weeks in a 40-year-old laborer is best treated by

157. How can you clinically differentiate acromioclavicular joint pain from other causes of shoulder pain?

158. What are some common sources of referred pain to the shoulder?

ANSWERS

149. (1) Massive blood and fluid replacement; (2) evaluation for CNS injury; (3) evaluation for intraabdominal injury; (4) splinting of long-bone fractures; and (5) stabilization of the pelvis by external fixator or traction if indicated.

ANSWERS

150. An "open book"–type injury with diastasis of the symphysis pubis, anterior diastasis of the sacroiliac joint, and hemodynamic instability.

151. A computed tomography (CT) scan and Judet x-ray views (obturator oblique and iliac oblique).

152. Intraarticular fracture fragments trapped within the joint space, greater than 40% loss of the posterior acetabular wall, and instability of the hip.

153. The arthrogram best demonstrates a full-thickness rotator cuff tear but shows poor resolution of the glenoid labrum and requires invasive technique.

154. Ultrasound offers a noninvasive technique but is somewhat operator-dependent and may miss a full-thickness tear that only involves a portion of one tendon muscle group.

155. MRI offers a noninvasive technique that will demonstrate both tendinitis and partial rotator cuff tears. It is very reliable in evaluating complete tear of muscle tendon groups and may reveal other pathologic changes such as tears of the glenoid labrum. There may be false positives or difficulty in evaluating the "thickness" of partial tears.

156. Open surgical repair. Arthroscopic techniques are being refined for use in selected patients and tear patterns. In older age groups debridement can offer pain relief in tears that are not repairable.

157. By localized tenderness, reproduction of pain by anteroposterior stress on the clavicle, and by a trial of local anesthetic block of the joint.

158. The cervical spine (radiculopathy), heart (myocardial infarction), lung (pneumonia, pancoast tumor), gallbladder, and periscapular muscle spasm (tension fibrositis).

QUESTIONS

159. In athletes with a slipping or "dead arm" sensation on overhead throwing, symptoms are most likely due to

160. What anatomic abnormalities would most likely be present in clinical glenohumeral instability?

161. In athletes who throw, shoulder pain without antecedent trauma may be due to

162. What nonoperative measures may be helpful in treating an athlete with clinical shoulder instability without dislocation?

163. What potential complications accompany estrogen replacement therapy for prevention of osteoporosis?

164. What nonhormonal treatments have proved effective in reducing the severity of postmenopausal osteoporosis?

165. What serum and urine studies correlate with activity in Paget's disease?

166. Surgical treatment of fractures in patients with Paget's disease is complicated by

167. What problems can be approached for diagnosis and treatment by ankle arthroscopy?

168. What medical treatment should be discontinued during fracture care in patients with Paget's disease?

169. In the acute postoperative period the combination of fever, macular rash, hypotension, or acute multiorgan failure in the face of a benign-appearing wound is suspicious of

170. Toxic shock syndrome has been reported in orthopedic patients postoperatively. What is the best treatment?

ANSWERS

159. Instability of the glenohumeral joint.

160. Anterior glenoid labrum detachment from prior dislocation, and a lax anterior capsule associated with straight anterior or multidirectional instability.

161. Tendinitis, instability, or poor training techniques.

162. Strengthening exercises for the rotator cuff, especially the anterior rotator cuff; flexibility exercises for the shoulder, especially the posterior rotator cuff; modification of training emphasizing a warm-up period, proper follow-through in throwing mechanics, and a training program that incorporates gradual progression of force in throwing.

163. Postmenopausal bleeding, thrombophlebitis, and acceleration of hormone-sensitive tumors such as breast or uterine cancer.

164. Adequate calcium intake, and maintaining a high activity level.

165. Elevated serum alkaline phosphatase due to increased osteoblast new bone formation, and elevated urinary hydroxyproline.

166. Increased bleeding from hypervascular bone.

167. Osteochondral fracture of the talus, persistent post–sprained ankle joint pain, synovitis, and posttraumatic ankle arthritis.

168. Diphosphonate therapy may slow fracture healing by inhibition of calcification. Calcitonin should be continued and may decrease blood loss, if open reduction is necessary, by decreasing disease activity.

169. Toxic shock syndrome.

170. Fluid volume replacement, antibiotics, and wound debridement.

QUESTIONS

171. What is the best treatment for an acute fracture of the patella in a patient with a preexisting total knee arthroplasty who demonstrates normal knee extension and shows no change of position of the patellar component by radiograph?

172. What is the best treatment for an acute patellar fracture in a patient with preexisting total knee arthroplasty who is unable to extend the leg and shows change of position of the patellar component compared with postoperative films?

173. An active 68-year-old patient with a late deep infection after total knee revision is best treated by

174. A 10-degree fixed varus deformity is best managed during total knee arthroplasty by

175. During total knee arthroplasty, proper component fit in full extension depends on which steps of the procedure?

176. The best treatment for monarticular, severe posttraumatic arthritis of the ankle in a laborer is

177. The most common cause of acute-onset severe flatfoot deformity in adult patients is

178. Treatment of ruptured posterior tibial tendon in adults is

179. What is the primary indication for total knee arthroplasty?

180. What are the contraindications to total knee arthroplasty?

181. What is the best method of preventing recurrent heterotopic ossification after surgical excision?

ANSWERS

171. Closed treatment with the leg supported in extension, such as a knee-immobilizing brace, and protected weightbearing until fracture healing.

172. Excision of the comminuted patellar fragments with repair of the extensor mechanism.

173. Removal of components and all cement with extensive debridement followed by knee fusion.

174. Medial soft tissue release.

175. On a distal femoral cut that is adequate to gain full extension, on release of any residual posterior capsular contractures, and on proper selection of components matching flexion and extension gaps.

176. Ankle fusion in neutral flexion, 5 degrees of valgus, and 10 degrees of external rotation.

177. Ruptured posterior tibial tendon.

178. Reconstruction with the flexor digitorum or flexor hallucis tendon.

179. Severe pain in a patient with multiple compartment arthritis in the sixth decade of life.

180. (1) A nonfunctioning extensor mechanism. (2) Active infection. Relative contraindications include younger age, high activity level requirement, and anticipated high loads (increased weight, increased activity). (3) A neuropathic (Charcot) joint.

181. Low-dose radiation. Nonsteroidals such as indomethacin (Indocin) have also shown some benefit in preventing heterotopic ossification.

QUESTIONS

182. What radiographic study best delineates AVN of the femoral head?

183. What is the primary indication for total hip surgery?

184. What are the most common complications following total hip arthroplasty?

185. What preoperative finding best correlates with postoperative range of motion after total hip replacement?

186. What factors contribute to the predictability of survival vs. amputation in a "mangled extremity?"

187. Which laser, used in arthroscopic surgery, requires a gas medium?

188. Which lasers are useful for arthroscopic surgery?

189. Which laser is used in arthroscopy by contact tips for cutting and coagulation?

190. Which material is more readily vaporized by CO_2 laser energy— bone or methylmethacrylate?

191. What risk does the use of lasers add to the operating room?

192. Pain on the plantar surface of the heel with no history of trauma in a 50-year-old woman is most likely due to

193. What clinical findings are indicative of Morton's neuroma?

ANSWERS

182. MR scan. Depending on the stage of disease, timed bone scans and plain radiographs may be helpful. Biopsy is the definitive diagnostic test.

ANSWERS

183. Severe pain unresponsive to nonoperative measures in a patient with severe hip arthritis. Limitation of motion and leg length inequality may also be secondarily improved.

184. Persistent pain, dislocation, leg length inequality, postoperative anemia, heterotopic ossification, deep venous thrombosis, aseptic loosening, infection.

185. Preoperative range of motion.

186. Patient age, limb ischemia, hemodynamic status, and energy of injury.

187. CO_2. CO_2 laser energy is completely absorbed by water.

188. CO_2 (requires a gas medium), holmium:yttrium-aluminum-garnet (YAG), neodymium:YAG, and excimer (experimental) lasers.

189. Neodymium:YAG.

190. Polymethylmethacrylate. A short burst of CO_2 laser energy will totally vaporize acrylic while only slightly increasing bone temperature.

191. Burns, eye injury, and fire from a misdirected or reflected laser; inhalation of toxins from laser plumes; fire from ignition of laser plumes.

192. Plantar fasciitis.

193. Tenderness in the third web space of the foot, pain with mediolateral compression of metatarsals, a history of pain with activity during shoe wear (typically improved by removing the shoes and rubbing the foot), and a history of snapping or intermittent numbness of the third and fourth toes.

QUESTIONS

194. What clinical findings are indicative of Reiter's syndrome?

195. What skin changes on the feet may be associated with Reiter's syndrome?

196. A patient with sacroiliac arthritis and erosive arthritis of the distal interphalangeal joints of both hands would likely have what skin changes?

197. A 68-year-old woman with sudden onset of painful swelling in the knee is found on radiograph to have spur formation, slight narrowing of the medial joint, and fine white specks that seem to outline the menisci. What will joint aspiration likely show on microscopic examination?

198. A 45-year-old man with sudden painful swelling of the knee reports no trauma. He has had sudden onset of swelling, redness, and pain in the foot twice in the last 6 months that resolved over 2 to 3 days spontaneously. He started medical treatment for hypertension a month before his first episode. Knee aspiration would likely show

199. A 60-year-old woman has painful burning of both feet. Vibratory sense is decreased in the toes but intact at the knees. Pulses are present at the dorsalis pedis and posterior tibial arteries. The most likely abnormality on screening blood chemistry is

200. What is the most common fatal complication following total hip arthroplasty?

201. What is the best treatment for flexible pes planovalgus in a 3-year-old?

202. What is the best treatment for internal tibial torsion in a 12-month-old infant?

203. What treatment should be offered a 6-week-old infant with a subluxatable hip and no other abnormalities?

ANSWERS

194. Monarticular arthritis or heel pain in the young adult male with a history of conjunctivitis and penile discharge.

195. Keratoderma blennorrhagicum.

196. Psoriasis.

197. Calcium pyrophosphate crystals—pseudogout.

198. Uric acid crystals.

199. Increased blood glucose. The patient's symptoms suggest polyneuropathy and diabetes is the most common cause.

200. Pulmonary embolism.

201. Observation. Anticipate spontaneous improvement over the next 3 years.

202. Observation. Anticipate spontaneous improvement over the next 6 to 12 months.

203. An abduction splint such as a Pavlik harness.

QUESTIONS

204. A 4-year-old child whose feet were normal since birth is brought in for evaluation of intoeing. Clinical examination reveals inversion of both feet with high arches. The examination is otherwise normal except for a small hair patch over the lumbar spine. Further evaluation should include

205. A 7-year-old girl is brought in for evaluation of "tripping and clumsiness." Clinical examination shows inversion of the left foot and decreased dorsiflexion of the ankle compared with the right ankle. When the patient runs, she "postures" the left arm with flexion of the elbow. What is the most likely cause of her problems?

206. A 12-year-old boy is brought in for evaluation of a limp. He rubs his anterolateral thigh while describing intermittent right "leg" pain. On clinical examination he is overweight and although he has full range and motion of the knee, the entire lower extremity does not externally rotate on the right as it does on the left during hip and knee flexion. What further diagnostic studies are indicated?

207. A 5-year-old boy is brought in for evaluation of a limp. He gives no history of pain but the clinical examination shows decreased abduction of the left hip compared with the right. The parents give no history of current or recent illness. He is afebrile and shows no other abnormalities during the examination. What will an AP pelvis film likely show?

208. You are consulted on an infant in the newborn nursery who is found to have talipes equinovarus. What treatment do you recommend for the foot deformity?

209. A 40-year-old man with a fracture at the base of the right femoral neck and no other injuries should be treated by

210. What are the indications for surgical treatment of a herniated lumbar disc?

211. What are the contraindications to lumbar disc excision by percutaneous techniques?

ANSWERS

204. Radiograph of the lumbar spine to evaluate for spinal dysraphism, and an MR scan of the spine, especially to look for tethered spinal cord or diastematomyelia.

205. Cerebral palsy due to perinatal distress.

206. An anteroposterior (AP) film of the pelvis, and a lateral film of the right hip to evaluate for slipped capital femoral epiphysis.

207. AVN due to Legg-Perthes disease.

208. Start manipulation and casting immediately.

209. Urgent closed reduction and pinning.

210. Urgent surgery if cauda equina syndrome develops; elective surgery if persistent pain or neurologic deficit coinciding with a radiographically proven herniated disc is unresponsive to nonsurgical treatment for greater than 6 weeks.

211. Absence of indications for surgical intervention; an extruded or sequestered disc fragment demonstrated by radiographic studies; coexistent spinal abnormalities such as facet arthritis, severe spondylosis, or spinal stenosis (relative).

QUESTIONS

212. A 6-year-old boy with intoeing is found to have femoral anteversion with external rotation to 45 degrees and internal rotation to 80 degrees from neutral. Treatment at this time should be

213. An 8-year-old boy is treated by immediate spica cast for a midshaft femur fracture. Return for 3-week follow-up shows 25 degrees of varus angulation. How should you proceed?

214. A 13-year-old boy complains of pain in the right foot, which worsens with activity. Physical examination reveals flatfeet with reflex dorsiflexion and eversion on attempted passive inversion of the right foot. AP and lateral films were reported to be normal. What further tests are indicated?

215. A 7-year-old boy presents because of persistent nighttime pain in the right leg. He settles down after a leg rub and aspirin. Radiograph reveals a sclerotic area in the middle of the tibia. Further texts should include

216. A 2-year-old child has refused to walk and has become progressively more fussy in the last 24 hours. On examination any attempt to move the left hip from a flexed and externally rotated position causes the child to cry more loudly. What tests should be ordered at this time?

217. Aspiration of the hip of this child is easily accomplished and 2 cc of purulent material is sent for Gram stain and culture. Treatment should now be

218. An 11-year-old female gymnast has been having increasing low back pain for 6 weeks. The clinical examination is normal except for slight tightness in the hamstrings in an otherwise very flexible, athletic preadolescent girl. AP and lateral rediographs are normal. What further tests should be done prior to medical clearance for competitive gymnastics?

219. Radiograph in this girl shows elongation and a fracture line in the L5 pars interarticularis. The bone scan is positive at the same area. Treatment should be

ANSWERS

212. Observation. Anticipate improvement with growth.

213. Correct the angulation and recast.

214. Evaluate for tarsal coalition. Compare the forefoot and hindfoot inversion and eversion range of motion; obtain oblique and jumper's view radiographs to evaluate the subtalar joints; consider tomograms or CT scans to demonstrate tarsal coalition.

215. Bone scan and tomograms to evaluate for osteoid osteoma.

216. Complete blood count with white blood cell (WBC) differential, sedimentation rate, blood culture, radiograph, and aspiration of the left hip.

217. Parenteral antibiotics; open decompression and irrigation of the hip joint.

218. Oblique films to evaluate for elongation or fracture of the pars interarticularis; bone scan with oblique lumbar imaging to determine activity of possible stress reaction or spondylolysis.

219. Restriction of activities to decrease impact load and hyperextension of the lumbar spine. If pain persists, use a body shell back brace such as a Boston brace molded to decrease pelvic flexion.

QUESTIONS

220. A patient presents with radicular pain 6 months after lumbar disc excision. What imaging technique offers the highest sensitivity and specificity with the lowest radiation exposure to evaluate for possible recurrent disc herniation?

221. A patient with diffuse thigh pain developing 6 years after total hip replacement has equivocal findings on plain radiographs showing small and incomplete lucent lines. What diagnostic study has a high specificity for demonstrating femoral component loosening?

222. A bone scan may be useful in demonstrating sites of infection or prosthetic loosening after total joint arthroplasty. How soon after cemented total hip replacement does the bone scan return to normal in asymptomatic patients?

223. A 64-year-old patient, 8 years status post lumbar disc excision, shows lumbar spondylosis on plain radiographs. Clinical symptoms include radicular pain and decreased extensor hallucis longus strength. What is your differential diagnosis?

224. What radiographic studies would you order for this patient?

225. Which imaging techniques has greater sensitivity for detection of disc herniation—CT or myelogram?

226. What imaging technique is the best diagnostic procedure for suspected spinal neoplastic lesions causing myelopathy (both extradural and intramedullary)?

227. Discography has been used to evaluate the clinical significance of disc abnormality by reproducing symptoms and proving, by leakage of contrast, a communication of the fluid space from the nucleus through the annulus. Should discography be used to document placement of the needle for chemonucleolysis with chymopapain?

ANSWERS

220. Gadolinium-enhanced MRI.

221. Aspiration arthrography. This technique also offers the opportunity of recovering a culture specimen in case of infection. A bone scan may be positive but does not differentiate aseptic loosening from infection or stress reaction.

222. The area of the lesser trochanter to the midshaft of the prosthesis usually becomes normal in about 6 months. The area around the acetabulum, greater trochanter, and tip of the prosthesis may show increased activity for up to 2 years, but on average shows normal findings at about 1 year in the majority of patients.

223. (1) Spinal stenosis; (2) nerve root entrapment by facet hypertrophic arthropathy; (3) herniated nucleus pulposus, recurrent or new; (4) referred pain of degenerative spondylosis; (5) a residual neurologic deficit from a previous herniated nucleus pulposus.

224. A CT scan will identify bone changes or significant disc herniation, either new or recurrent. Also consider IV contrast enhancement to differentiate scar from recurrent disc, or myelogram-CT to evaluate spinal stenosis or nerve root encroachment.

225. CT.

226. MRI.

227. No. There is a suspected correlation of admixture of contrast material with the chymopapain enzyme escaping into the spinal canal causing one of the most serious complications of chemonucleolysis—transverse myelitis.

QUESTIONS

228. Epidural venography may be positive in the L5–S1 herniated disc when the myelogram is negative owing to the proximity of the venous plexus to the annulus in the large epidural space at that level. Which is more sensitive and specific for disc herniation at L5–S1—epidural venogram or MRI?

229. Which is more sensitive for lateral disc herniation—lumbar myelogram or CT scan?

230. Which imaging technique is most sensitive in demonstrating osteonecrosis of the femoral head?

231. A diffuse region of low signal intensity on T1-weighted MRI involving a large posterior portion of the femoral head in a multiple trauma patient most likely represents

232. If plain radiographs in AP, lateral, and oblique views fail to clearly identify solid union vs. nonunion at a fracture site, what studies may be useful?

233. A postmenopausal patient asks about calcium supplements to prevent osteoporosis. What dose of calcium do you recommend?

234. In spite of adequate intake of calcium and vitamin D, a postmenopausal patient with severe osteoporosis has severe pain associated with vertebral compression fracture. Workup for malignancy or endocrinopathy is negative. Owing to a history of thrombophlebitis, the patient is not a candidate for estrogen therapy. What do you recommend?

235. Osteopetrosis is due to a genetic defect resulting in disruption of osteoclast function. Treatment of the severe congenital form consists of

236. A college football player is treated for hamstring strain. Pain relief is excellent. What parameter will you evaluate during rehabilitation to determine an appropriate safe return to competitive-level sports?

ANSWERS

228. MRI.

229. CT scan.

230. MRI.

231. Synovitis or bone marrow edema. Classic osteonecrosis is not common in trauma without fracture or dislocation and usually is limited to the superior portion of the femoral head.

232. (1) Tomograms; (2) CT scan with multiplanar reconstruction; (3) single photon emission computed tomography (SPECT).

233. A dose adequate to assure daily intake of 1,500 mg/day of elemental calcium and 400 to 800 IU of vitamin D.

234. One treatment choice would be calcitonin, which can be given by injection of 50 units three times per week while continuing calcium supplement. Another option would be to consider sodium fluoride at a dose of 1 mg/kg/day although the bone formed with fluoride dosage may be more brittle than normal and the incidence of side effects, especially GI distress, is fairly high.

235. Bone marrow transplant at a young age, if an appropriate HLA-matched donor is available. Medical treatment with prednisone, dietary manipulation, and high doses of calcitriol may be partially effective.

236. Hamstring strength, especially the quadriceps-hamstring ratio, should be corrected to normal. The patient should be advised of the importance of maintaining balanced strength and flexibility when he returns to competitive sports.

QUESTIONS

237. During August preseason football practice, a high school player wanders toward the sideline and appears somewhat confused. He complains of headache and although it is 90°F his skin is dry. What would you check next?

238. On further evaluation, this patient is found to have an irregular pulse and a temperature of 40.5°C. What treatment should be initiated?

239. What is the leading cause of sudden death during exercise in adult athletes?

240. Reiter's syndrome or reactive arthritis may follow which infections?

241. Sexually acquired reactive arthritis (Reiter's syndrome) may present with one or all of the classic triad of symptoms. What are they?

242. Treatment of arthritis symptoms in Reiter's syndrome is best achieved with which nonsteroidal anti-inflammatory drug?

243. Reiter's syndrome is found frequently in young adult males with which immunodeficiency disorder?

244. In a patient with arthritis of the hands, a predominant involvement of the distal interphalangeal joints, and pitting of the fingernails, the most likely diagnosis is

245. What are the major manifestations (Jones's criteria) in rheumatic fever?

246. A 21-year-old woman complains of severe pain in the knee without injury. Although motion is limited there is no redness and little swelling. She reports a rash on the trunk during a shower, but has had no itching and no rashes are visible on clinical examination. Sedimentation rate is elevated. Streptozyme is positive at 1:200 dilution. What treatment do you prescribe?

ANSWERS

237. Body temperature. Hyperthermia characterized by confusion, increased core temperature $\geq 40°C$, headache, decreased sweating, and muscle cramps can lead to cardiac arrhythmia and death in up to 50% of patients if the temperature is allowed to increase to over 41°C.

238. Lower the body temperature as quickly as possible by removing clothing, applying ice, and providing hydration. Move the patient out of the sun and if he is not taking fluids well, start IV hydration.

239. Cardiovascular disease, especially arteriosclerosis.

240. (1) Nongonococcal urethritis (sexually acquired) caused by *Chlamydia trachomatis* or *Ureaplasma urealyticum;* (2) intestinal infection (enteric) caused by *Shigella flexneri* (dysentery), salmonella, *Yersinia,* and *Campylobacter* species.

241. (1) Arthritis, (2) urethritis, (3) conjunctivitis.

242. Indomethacin.

243. Acquired immunodeficiency syndrome (AIDS).

244. Psoriatic arthritis.

245. Carditis, polyarthritis, chorea, erythema marginatum, and subcutaneous nodules.

246. This patient's presentation is consistent with a diagnosis of rheumatic fever. Treatment should consist of: (1) evaluation for possible carditis and, if present, treatment with corticosteroids; (2) treatment with acetylsalicylic acid for arthritis or arthralgia symptoms; (3) prevention of recurrence with penicillin prophylaxis.

QUESTIONS

247. Secondary hypertrophic osteoarthropathy is associated with clubbing of the fingers and arthritis with noninflammatory synovial fluid. What is it most often "secondary" to?

248. In a patient with a history of gout, how likely is an acute attack following surgery if no prophylaxis is used?

249. Initial attacks of gouty arthritis are usually monarticular, occurring in the foot. As the disease progresses in untreated patients, how does the character of acute attacks change?

250. What laboratory finding has the highest specificity for gouty arthritis?

251. What is the most common site of hematogenous osteomyelitis in an adult?

252. Excluding *Neisseria gonorrhoeae*, what bacteria cause the majority of joint infections?

253. In septic arthritis, to what level is the fasting synovial fluid glucose reduced compared with blood glucose?

254. In nongonococcal bacterial arthritis in patients aged over 65 years, what is the prevalence of underlying joint disease?

255. How is septic arthritis different in a patient with longstanding rheumatoid arthritis?

256. IV drug abuse is associated with an increased risk of bone and joint infections by which bacterial pathogens?

257. Skeletal infections in IV drug users occur most frequently in which locations?

ANSWERS

247. Pulmonary disease. A neoplastic or suppurative process should be ruled out.

248. Very likely. In one series 86% of patients had an acute attack 3 to 5 days postoperatively.

249. (1) They increase in frequency; (2) have an increasing tendency to involve other joints and be polyarticular; (3) increase in severity; (4) are longer-lasting; and (5) are more often associated with fever.

250. Intercellular monosodium urate crystals in synovial fluid leukocytes.

251. Vertebral body.

252. *S. aureus.*

253. Less than or equal to 50%.

254. Greater than or equal to 50%.

255. It is more likely polyarticular (25%) and less likely to have fever (76%) or leukocytosis (56%); morbidity (50% poor outcome) and mortality (25%) are increased.

256. *Pseudomonas aeruginosa, S. aureus, Serratia,* and other gram-negative bacteria.

257. (1) In the vertebral column—the lumbar, cervical, and thoracic in order of decreasing frequency; (2) in the fibrocartilaginous articulations of the pelvis and sternum, including the sacroiliac, sternoclavicular, sternocostal, and symphysis pubis.

QUESTIONS

258. A cat bite may cause *Pasteurella multocida* septic arthritis with osteomyelitis in the hand. How is it best treated?

259. What is the most common cause of bacterial arthritis in young adults?

ANSWERS

258. Drainage of the infected joint, and penicillin.

259. *N. gonorrhoeae.*

CHAPTER 2

Pediatric Orthopedics

Keith Gabriel, M.D.

Steven Mardjetko, M.D.

QUESTIONS

1. Describe the diagnostic anatomic feature of congenital vertical talus (CVT).

2. What is the difference between type A and type B CVT?

3. Describe the characteristic findings on physical examination of CVT.

4. Describe the pathoanatomy of the medial side of the foot in CVT.

5. Discuss the principles of treatment of CVT.

6. In children over 3 years of age, what additional step should be considered at surgery?

7. What specific radiograph is frequently used to distinguish a true CVT from the flexible calcaneovalgus positional deformity?

ANSWERS

1. Dorsal dislocation of the tarsal navicular with respect to the head of the talus.

2. In type A, the calcaneocuboid joint remains in its normal anatomic alignment. The more severe type B deformity includes dislocation of the calcaneocuboid joint. If this is not recognized and corrected along with the talonavicular dislocation, a higher recurrence rate is likely.

3. There is a midfoot breech, such that the forefoot is positioned in relative calcaneus (dorsiflexion and abduction) while the hindfoot is held rigidly in equinus. The head of the talus is prominent at the medial sole of the foot.

4. The distal portion (head and neck) of the talus rotates downward and medially over the incompetent sustentaculum and spring ligament as the navicular dislocates dorsally. The posterior tibialis and flexor digitorum longus move anterior to the axis of the ankle joint to become functional dorsiflexors of the midfoot.

5. Nonoperative treatment is ineffective. Surgical procedures must address two aspects of the deformity: (1) the midfoot dislocation must be reduced and stabilized; and (2) the equinus position of the hindfoot must be corrected. This may be done in one or two stages.

6. Subtalar stabilization, usually by a technique similar to the Grice extraarticular arthrodesis.

7. The maximum plantar flexion lateral view of the foot.

QUESTIONS

8. How does this radiograph distinguish CVT from flexible deformities?

9. In the adolescent or adult, correction of the CVT usually requires what procedure?

10. What is the expected age range for Legg-Calvé Perthes disease (LCP)?

11. What is the expected sex ratio for LCP?

ANSWERS

8. Imagine a line projected through the longitudinal axis of the talus. In the normal (*A*), and in flexible situations, that line falls to the dorsal side of the tarsal navicular on the maximum plantar flexion lateral view. Since the navicular does not ossify until age 3 years or so, it may be better to say that that line should fall to the dorsal side of the cuboid. In CVT (*B*), the line through the talus is plantar to the navicular (cuboid) in both the resting lateral and plantar-flexed lateral views.

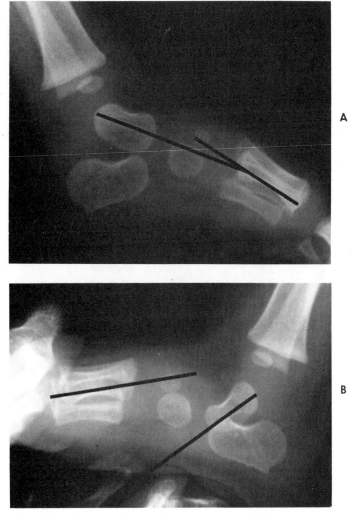

9. Triple arthrodesis.

10. Age 2 to 12 years, although most cases occur between 4 and 8 years.

11. Male. About 4:1.

QUESTIONS

12. How often is LCP bilateral?

13. In cases of bilateral symmetric LCP, what other radiographs should be obtained?

14. What other entities might present initially as bilateral LCP?

15. What constitutes the classic presentation of LCP?

16. What are the four stages of LCP?

17. Describe four radiographic findings which may be seen during the initial stage of LCP.

18. What is the "crescent sign" (Caffey's sign)?

19. Describe Salter's proposed sequence in the development of clinical LCP.

20. How long does it usually take for a patient to progress through the LCP sequence?

21. How long does it take for a hip to progress from clinical presentation to the fragmentation stage?

22. At what stage of LCP can the Catterall grouping be determined?

23. Briefly describe changes seen in Catterall group 1 LCP.

ANSWERS

12. In 10% to 12% of cases.

13. Other epiphyseal areas should be evaluated. Radiographs of wrists, knees, lateral skull, and lateral spine are helpful.

ANSWERS

14. Multiple epiphyseal dysplasia; spondyloepiphyseal dysplasia; endocrine disorders such as hypothyroidism; and various problems, such as sickle cell anemia, that cause avascular necrosis.

15. A painless limp (externally rotated) in a 4- to 8-year-old boy. Unexplained anterior knee pain is another very typical presentation.

16. (1) Initial (avascular), (2) fragmentation, (3) reossification (regrowth, regeneration), and (4) healed (residual).

17. (1) The ossific nucleus fails to grow and therefore looks smaller; (2) the surrounding bone may become osteopenic and therefore the ossific nucleus looks more dense; (3) cartilage of the femoral head continues to grow and therefore the medial joint space looks widened; (4) a "crescent sign" (Caffey's sign) may be seen.

18. A radiolucent line in the superior lateral periphery of the ossific nucleus. It represents a stress fracture or compression fracture in the subchondral bone.

19. One or more vascular insults occur, causing an avascular necrosis of the ossific nucleus. Without additional trauma, this remains subclinical. Superimposed trauma or repetitive microtrauma creates a stress or compression fracture of the avascular subchondral bone, which we see as the "crescent sign." The repair processes thus set in motion constitute clinical LCP.

20. This varies widely, but 18 to 24 months is a useful estimate.

21. This varies widely, but 6 to 8 months is a useful estimate.

22. The hip must be well into the fragmentation stage.

23. Anterior head involvement, no sequestrum, no metaphyseal changes. The lateral column is intact.

QUESTIONS

24. Briefly describe changes seen in Catterall group 2 LCP.

25. Briefly describe changes seen in Catterall group 3 LCP.

26. Briefly describe changes seen in Caterall group 4 LCP.

27. What are the Caterall "head at risk" radiographic signs in LCP?

28. What clinical finding is sometimes included as a head risk sign?

29. Briefly describe the Salter-Thompson classification of LCP.

30. Is there some advantage to using the Salter-Thompson rather than the Catterall groupings?

31. The Catterall 2½ subgroup has recently been suggested. Describe.

32. The reverse Caterall 3 subgroup has recently been suggested. Describe.

33. Suggest imaging modalities that may provide early diagnosis of LCP.

34. What is the most important single factor determining outcome in LCP?

ANSWERS

24. Anterolateral head involvement, with sequestrum, with clear space between the involved and uninvolved head, with anterolateral metaphyseal changes. The lateral column is intact.

25. Large sequestrum involves the anterolateral 75% of the head, specifically including the lateral column; metaphyseal changes are diffuse.

26. All of the femoral head is involved, specifically including the lateral column.

27. Lateral extrusion (subluxation) of the head, calcification lateral to the epiphysis, horizontal growth plate (as seen on the anteroposterior [AP] view), radiolucency in the lateral epiphysis and metaphysis (Gage's sign), and metaphyseal changes (widening and cysts).

28. Loss of range of motion.

29. In group A, the crescent sign extends over less than 50% of the femoral head, roughly corresponding to Catterall groups 1 and 2. In group B, the crescent sign extends over more than 50% of the femoral head, roughly corresponding to Catterall groups 3 and 4.

30. The crescent sign is seen very early in the clinical course of LCP, frequently even on the first radiograph.

31. This is basically a group 2 picture, but with some transient lucent changes in the lateral column. There is no actual collapse or sequestration of the lateral column.

32. About 75% of the head is sequestered, but it is the anteromedial portion. The lateral column is preserved.

33. Technitium 99m bone scan; magnetic resonance imaging (MRI).

34. Patient age. Eight years seems to be a watershed, with a much poorer prognosis for older children irrespective of the extent of head involvement.

QUESTIONS

35. Which patients require no active treatment?

36. Within the above guideline, what constitutes the "younger patient?"

37. What about a 4-year-old child who has one or more head at risk signs?

38. What is the first treatment goal for the newly diagnosed LCP patient?

39. How may hip motion be reestablished?

40. Once motion is regained, what is the usual treatment concept?

41. Suggest nonsurgical methods of containment in LCP.

42. When should nonsurgical containment devices be discontinued?

43. Suggest surgical methods for containment in LCP.

44. What radiographic criteria are useful in the long-term prognosis of healed LCP?

45. Describe a system for predicting long-term function which considers the relative contours of both femoral head and acetabulum after healing of LCP.

ANSWERS

35. Those already well into the reossification stage when first seen; Catterall groups 1 and 2 (Salter-Thompson Group A) having no head at risk signs; younger patients with no head at risk signs regardless of extent of involvement.

36. This remains controversial. Most would agree that patients below the age of 5 years do not require treatment.

37. Patients having head at risk signs should be treated.

38. Reestablish a normal range of hip motion.

39. Traction with physical therapy, or serial broomstick (Petrie) casts. Occasionally surgical release of the adductor longus is needed.

40. Containment of the involved portion of the femoral head within the acetabulum by nonsurgical or surgical means.

41. Petrie (broomstick) casts; orthoses such as the Newington brace or the Scottish rite brace.

42. When the lateral column of the femoral head reossifies.

43. Varus osteotomy of the proximal femur; innominate (Salter) osteotomy of the pelvis.

44. Sphericity of the femoral head and congruence of the head within the acetabulum.

45. Spherical congruence—no arthritis develops; aspherical congruence—mild to moderate arthritis develops late in life; aspherical incongruence—severe arthritis before age 50 (Stuhlberg, Cooperman, Wallensten, 1981).

QUESTIONS

46. What kinds of femoral head deformity result from LCP?

47. What is the characteristic presentation of osteochondritis dissecans following LCP?

48. What is "hinge abduction" with reference to the hip in LCP?

49. Suggest salvage procedures for the femoral head that has become uncontainable in LCP.

50. What must be considered following LCP when physeal arrest has occurred and the patient has a Trendelenburg gait?

51. What is the "sagging rope sign" (G. Apley)?

52. What is the most common single gene disorder in humans?

53. What are some features of each of the two types of NF?

ANSWERS

46. Coxa magna, physeal arrest, irregular femoral head, osteochondritis dissecans.

47. Usually in males; average of about 9 years after LCP; hip pain, loss of motion, locking sensations.

ANSWERS

48. If so much lateral extrusion occurs that the femoral head can no longer be contained in the acetabulum, then abduction takes place by hinging of the head against the lateral acetabular rim (see Figure).

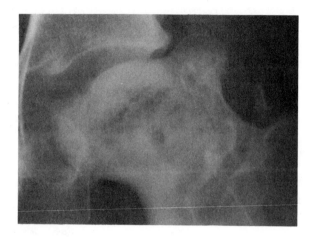

49. Cheilectomy may occasionally be helpful; acetabular augmentation by shelf or Chiari osteotomy; abduction (valgus-producing) osteotomy of the proximal femur.

50. Distal advancement of the greater trochanter may be indicated to correct trochanteric overgrowth in patients over 8 years. Trochanteric arrest should be considered in children younger than 8 years when the acetabulotrochanteric (articulotrochanteric) distance, usually 1 cm, starts to diminish.

51. This radiographic finding is often seen in LCP when the femoral head is deformed into a mushroom shape with coxa magna and coxa plana. An irregular curved sclerotic line is seen through the femoral neck. It represents the posterior articular margin of the deformed head.

52. Neurofibromatosis (NF). It is thought to occur in about 1 in 3,000 live births.

53. Type 1 (NF-1) includes cutaneous findings such as café-au-lait spots, axillary or inguinal freckling, nevi, dermal fibromas, plexiform neurofibromas, as well as Lisch nodules and optic glioma. Type 2 (NF-2) is bilateral acoustic neuroma.

QUESTIONS

54. What chromosomes have been identified as the gene loci for NF-1 and NF-2?

55. Orthopedic manifestations generally are restricted to those patients having which type of NF?

56. List some of the recognized orthopedic disorders associated with NF.

57. The dysplastic scoliosis associated with NF may be recognized by:

58. How should anterolateral bowing of the tibia be managed in the young NF patient?

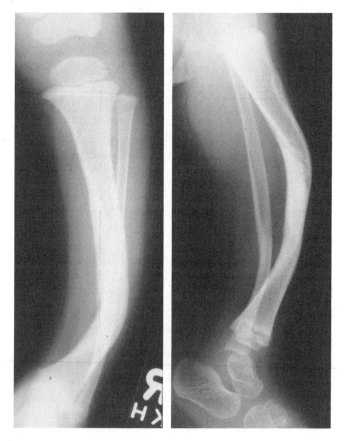

59. State-of-the-art treatment modalities for treatment of tibial pseudarthrosis include:

ANSWERS

54. In type 1, the long arm of chromosome 17; in type 2, the long arm of chromosome 22.

55. Type 1.

56. Scoliosis, pseudarthrosis of the tibia, pseudarthrosis of other long bones (e.g., radius, ulna, fibula), disorders of bone growth (e.g., gigantism), erosive defects from contiguous tumors, multiple fibrous cortical defects, subperiosteal calcifying hematoma.

57. A short, sharply angulated curve, involving only a few vertebral segments (six or fewer); kyphosis and obvious dysplastic vertebrae or ribs may be seen. Treatment is anterior and posterior spinal fusion if progression is recognized. Bracing is ineffective.

58. Osteotomy for angular correction may never heal, and should not be done. Rather, the leg should be protected in an orthosis to prevent fracture and development of frank pseudarthrosis. Some consideration may be given to "prophylactic" grafting in the absence of fracture.

59. Vascularized fibula transfer; prolonged stabilization with ring fixators (such as the Ilizarov); intramedullary fixation with massive onlay grafting.

QUESTIONS

60. Describe the type A (Aitken) proximal femoral focal deficiency (PPFD).

61. Describe the type B (Aitken) PFFD.

62. Describe the type C (Aitken) PFFD.

63. Describe the type D (Aitken) PFFD.

64. Suggest some anomalies associated with PFFD.

65. Management of PFFD prior to walking age should stress:

66. Management of PFFD for the toddler should include:

67. When should definitive management plans be made in cases of PFFD?

68. What is the traditional concept of treatment for most cases of types B, C, and D PFFD?

69. Conversion of PFFD for above-knee (or knee disarticulation) prosthetic fitting usually includes

70. What is a Van Ness rotationplasty?

71. Suggest a surgical conversion to provide stability at the hip level in cases of type D PFFD.

ANSWERS

60. The femoral head is present within an adequate acetabulum. The femur is short. A pseudarthrosis is present in the subtrochanteric region which ossifies by the time of skeletal maturity, resulting in lateral bowing of the proximal femur and relative coxa vara.

ANSWERS

61. The femoral head is present within a dysplastic acetabulum. The femoral shaft is displaced proximally and is short. A defective cartilage bridge between head and shaft does not ossify, resulting in marked subtrochanteric varus.

62. The femoral head never fully ossifies and the acetabulum is severely dysplastic. The femoral shaft tapers to a point which migrates proximally against the pelvis. The shaft moves independently of the hip.

63. The femoral head and acetabulum do not develop. The femoral shaft is represented by the distal condyles and a very small tuft.

64. Longitudinal deficiency of the fibula, short tibia and fibula, absent or dislocated patella, tarsal coalition.

65. Prevention of hip and knee contractures.

66. Fitting of a shoe lift or nonstandard prosthesis.

67. Sufficient ossification must be present to accurately determine the anatomy of the deformity, and sufficient longitudinal growth must have occurred to predict the degree of shortening. Usually this means approximately age 3 to 4 years.

68. Conversion of the limb to a form suitable for above-knee (or knee disarticulation) or below-knee prosthetic fitting.

69. Knee fusion and Syme amputation of the foot.

70. The distal segment, including ankle and foot, is rotated 180 degrees. This permits the ankle to function as a knee joint for prosthetic fitting.

71. Femoral-pelvic arthrodesis, with the stump of the femur "flexed" at a right angle, permits the knee joint to function as a hip.

QUESTIONS

72. What is the basic treatment concept for bilateral PFFD?

73. What is (Renshaw) type I sacral agenesis?

74. What is (Renshaw) type II sacral agenesis?

75. What is (Renshaw) type III sacral agenesis?

76. What is (Renshaw) type IV sacral agenesis?

77. What is the most common type of sacral agenesis?

78. Type II sacral agenesis is frequently associated with:

79. What maternal medical condition may be associated with the etiology of sacral agenesis?

80. What is the neurologic function in patients having sacral agenesis?

81. Suggest treatment concepts for type I sacral agenesis.

82. Suggest treatment concepts for type II sacral agenesis.

83. How successful are lower extremity reconstructive procedures in type IV sacral agenesis?

ANSWERS

72. Observation. These patients usually function much better without prosthetic or surgical interference.

73. Partial, unilateral absence of the sacrum. The vertebral-pelvic junction is usually stable.

ANSWERS

74. Partial, bilaterally symmetric absence of the sacrum. The vertebral-pelvic junction is stable.

75. Total absence of the sacrum, sometimes with partial absence of the lumbar spine. The sides of the lowest vertebra articulate with the pelvis, creating a relatively stable junction.

76. Complete absence of the sacrum and partial to complete absence of the lumbar spine. The lowest vertebra does not form any stable articulation with the pelvis, but rather rests above the posterior ilia, which may be fused.

77. Type II.

78. Myelomeningocele.

79. Diabetes mellitus.

80. Motor paralysis should be within one level of the vertebral deformity. Sensation may be preserved more distally in many cases.

81. The lumbosacral junction is stable and scoliosis usually does not need treatment. The foot deformity should be treated as necessary. These patients should be ambulatory.

82. The lumbosacral junction is stable and many of these patients will be ambulatory. Vertebral anomalies and scoliosis may require treatment. The motor level will determine the deformity seen; treatment closely parallels that for myelomeningocele.

83. They are not successful. The lower extremities are small, flail, with flexion contractures at the hips and knees, and with large popliteal webs. Muscle tissue is completely replaced by loose fat.

QUESTIONS

84. How does one deal with the spinal-pelvic instability in type IV sacral agenesis?

85. Anticipate a lower gastrointestinal problem sometimes seen in cases of type IV sacral agenesis.

86. Suggest another body system which must be evaluated in all cases of sacral agenesis.

87. What is the incidence of idiopathic clubfoot?

88. How often is clubfoot bilateral?

89. Describe the findings at the hindfoot in the physical examination of clubfoot.

90. Describe the findings at the midfoot in the physical examination of clubfoot.

91. Describe the findings at the forefoot in the physical examination of clubfoot.

92. What is the deformity of the talus in clubfoot?

93. Describe the tibiotalar (ankle) joint in clubfoot.

ANSWERS

84. If untreated, the patient "sits" on the distal tip of the spine with the pelvis folded forward beneath the abdomen. A prosthesis can be fashioned with a pelvic-thoracic bucket. Bilateral subtrochanteric amputation can facilitate prosthetic fitting. The lower spine can be fused to the sacrum, using tibias and femora for the graft.

85. The narrowed pelvis causes mechanical obstruction. Pelvic outlet enlargement or colostomy may be needed.

ANSWERS

86. The genitourinary tract. Intravenous pyelogram, renal ultrasound, or similar study is mandatory. Loss of more than one sacral segment is likely to be associated with bladder dysfunction. Unilateral renal agenesis and kidney duplication have been reported.

87. About 1.2/1,000, although the incidence does vary widely with race and sex. The incidence is higher in males. The right foot is affected slightly more often than the left.

88. In about 50% of cases. Bilaterality is even more common in patients having myelodysplasia, arthrogryposis, and diastrophic dwarfism.

89. The hindfoot is positioned in equinus and varus. This causes the heel to appear foreshortened, and often what appears to be the heel is only the fat pad. The tuberosity of the calcaneus is actually more proximal, directly behind the ankle joint. The heel has been described as "keel-shaped."

90. There is no palpable gap between the medial malleolus and tarsal navicular. The head of the talus presents as a prominence on the dorsolateral midfoot.

91. The forefoot is in adduction. Even considering the hindfoot varus deformity, the forefoot is in additional supination. This brings the medial aspect of the first ray into close approximation to the distal medial tibia.

92. The neck of the talus is foreshortened and thickened. The head and neck are deviated medially and plantarward compared to the normal declination. Many believe that this is the primary deformity in clubfoot.

93. Abnormal equinus causes the dome of the talus to extrude anteriorly, i.e., the entire talus is displaced forward in the mortise. There is unresolved controversy as to whether the talus might also rotate medially or laterally in a horizontal plane within the mortise.

QUESTIONS

94. Describe the subtalar joint in clubfoot.

95. What displacement occurs at the talonavicular joint in clubfoot?

96. What deformity may be seen at the calcaneocuboid joint in clubfoot?

97. What is the relative relationship of the medial and lateral columns of the clubfoot?

98. Briefly list several of the theories proposed to explain the cause of clubfoot.

99. What are common findings on the lateral radiograph in clubfoot?

100. What are common findings on the AP radiograph in clubfoot?

101. Discuss the initial management of clubfoot.

102. Forcible dorsiflexion during the conservative treatment of clubfoot may create

103. What is the "nutcracker mechanism"?

104. What are some current concepts regarding surgical correction of the subtalar relationship in clubfoot?

ANSWERS

94. Displacements occur in three planes. Horizontal rotation brings the anterior process of the calcaneus beneath the head and neck of the talus while simultaneously moving the tuberosity laterally toward the fibular malleolus. The calcaneus is also in varus and equinus with respect to the talus.

95. The navicular is displaced medially onto the neck of the talus. The navicular may actually abut the inferior tip of the medial malleolus, forming an abnormal articular facet.

ANSWERS

96. The cuboid is displaced medially and slightly proximally. The articular surface of the anterior calcaneus becomes slanted (angulated) medially.

97. The medial side is shorter, the lateral side longer.

98. Germ plasm defect, arrested fetal development, intrauterine positioning, myofibroblast contraction at the medial foot, neuromuscular defect, circulatory defect, among others.

99. "Parallelism" of the calcaneus and talus is key. This is recognized as a decrease in the lateral talocalcaneal angle (normal, 30–50 degrees), which does not increase on the maximum dorsiflexion lateral view. Talus and calcaneus are together in equinus.

100. Parallelism of the talus and calcaneus is recognized by a decreased AP talocalcaneal (Kite's) angle (normal, 20–40 degrees). A line projected along the lateral border of the calcaneus is not continuous with the cuboid owing to medial displacement. Forefoot adductus is recognized by an increase in the talus–first metatarsal angle (normal, 0––20 degrees, with a positive value indicating forefoot adductus.)

101. Repeated manipulations and the use of some type of holding device. Casts are the most common holding device, although taping and bracing may be effective.

102. An iatrogenic "rocker-bottom foot" or "flat-topped talus."

103. The talus is anteriorly displaced in the ankle mortise, and normal tibiotalar motion is prevented by the contracted capsule and ligaments. With forcible dorsiflexion during manipulation, the talus is compressed between the calcaneus and tibia.

104. McKay and Simons have emphasized the concept of a complete (occasionally sparing portions of the interosseus ligament) subtalar release. This permits correction to include the horizontal rotation, whereas less aggressive posteromedial release addresses only the varus and equinus deformities.

QUESTIONS

105. List the structures of the posterolateral ankle and subtalar joint which must be released to allow correction of the clubfoot.

106. Suggest options for dealing with persistent midfoot adduction after adequate soft tissue release.

107. Parents must be warned about which ipsilateral deformities that are frequently associated with clubfoot?

108. Suggest important concerns prior to initiating treatment of a cavus foot.

109. Suggest a theory of the pathogenesis of cavus foot.

110. Describe pes cavovarus.

111. Describe a test for determination of the flexibility of the hindfoot in pes cavovarus.

ANSWERS

105. Joint capsules, posterior talofibular ligament, calcaneofibular ligament, peroneal tendon sheaths.

106. Lateral column shortening—cuboid decancellation, Evans resection of the calcaneocuboid joint, Lichtblau excision of the anterior calcaneus into the calcaneocuboid joint, Simons vertical wedge resection of the anterior body of the calcaneus.

ANSWERS

107. Calf atrophy, limb length discrepancy, tibial torsion, the affected foot remaining shorter but wider than the contralateral foot despite excellent correction.

108. Cavus foot is almost always a manifestation of neurologic disease. A comprehensive history and physical examination are needed. Radiographs of the spine are basic, and other imaging studies may be indicated. Consultation with a neurologist should be considered.

109. If the anterior tibialis is relatively weak, or the peroneus longus relatively strong, the first ray becomes plantar flexed. The long toe extensors are simultaneously used to substitute for the anterior tibialis, causing clawing of the toes and secondary depression of the distal metatarsals. This is called the "windlass" mechanism. Alternatively, primary paralysis of the intrinsic muscles prevents proper extension of the interphalangeal joints. Again, the clawing of the toes causes secondary depression of the metatarsal heads.

110. The first ray, and sometimes the second, is more plantar flexed than the lateral rays. This relative pronation of the forefoot causes the entire foot to be inverted, with heel varus and elevation of the medial arch.

111. The Coleman block test is performed by placing a block under the affected heel and lateral two rays. The medial rays of the forefoot are allowed to droop toward the floor. The hindfoot position is then assessed visually from behind, or by means of special radiographs (see Figure).

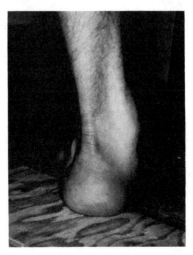

QUESTIONS

112. What is the significance of the block test?

113. Suggest conservative measures for treatment of pes cavus (or cavovarus).

114. Describe surgical concepts for treatment of pes cavus (or cavovarus).

115. Suggest two soft tissue procedures commonly recommended in treatment of pes cavus.

116. Suggest procedures through bone that are commonly recommended for treatment of pes cavus (or cavovarus) in a growing child.

117. Suggest procedures through bone for treatment of pes cavus (or cavovarus) in the mature foot.

118. Describe the difference between a meningocele and a myelomeningocele.

119. Describe rachischisis (myeloschisis).

120. Describe lipomeningocele.

121. Suggest a structural abnormality of the base of the brain that is almost always present in patients having myelomeningocele.

122. What diagnoses should be considered when a myelomeningocele patient shows neurologic deterioration?

ANSWERS

112. If the subtalar joint remains supple and corrects with the block test, then surgical procedures may be directed to correcting forefoot pronation, which is usually due to plantar flexion of the first metatarsal.

113. Cushioning, lateral heel wedges, accommodative orthoses, and stretching exercises may help relieve symptoms. These do not usually reduce the deformity, nor do they usually prevent progression of the deformity.

114. Treatment must be individualized according to the cause, specific deformity, muscle strength, condition and mobility of joints, condition of plantar soft tissues, and patient age.

115. (1) Plantar fascia release, and (2) transfer of long toe extensors to the metatarsal heads.

116. Osteotomy of the first ray to correct plantar flexion; osteotomy of the tuberosity of the calcaneus (Dwyer) to correct the varus and calcaneus position.

117. Various midfoot osteotomies such as dorsal wedge resection or the Japas V-osteotomy; variations of triple arthrodesis.

118. The meningocele sac contains only cerebrospinal fluid (CSF); the myelomeningocele sac includes abnormal neural elements.

119. In rachischisis, there is an absence even of sac; rather, the cord is directly everted and exposed without any covering.

120. The sac contains primarily lipoma which is intermingled with nerve roots, usually at the sacral level.

121. Arnold-Chiari malformation, type II.

122. Hydrocephaly, hydrosyringomyelia, Arnold-Chiari malformation, and tethered cord syndrome.

QUESTIONS

123. Suggest findings or patient complaints that should alert the physician to a possible tethered cord.

124. Suggest tests or procedures that may permit prenatal diagnosis of spina bifida.

125. What is the most common skeletal deformity seen in myelomeningocele?

126. Suggest a role for orthotic management in (paralytic or developmental) myelomeningocele scoliosis.

127. Suggest problems that may be anticipated with spinal orthosis wear.

128. Suggest realistic goals for lower extremity management in thoracic-level myelomeningocele.

129. Describe the expected natural history of the hip in upper lumbar (L1–2) myelomeningocele.

130. Suggest reasonable orthopedic management of the hip in upper lumbar (L1–2) myelomeningocele.

131. Describe the expected natural history of the hip in mid- to low-lumbar (L3–5) myelomeningocele.

132. Suggest reasonable management goals for the hip in mid- to low-lumbar (L3–5) myelomeningocele.

ANSWERS

123. Pain in the low back, buttocks, or posterior thighs; progressive scoliosis; cavus foot deformity; increasing spasticity; loss of muscle strength.

124. Maternal serum alpha-fetoprotein determination (MSAFP); ultrasound; amniocentesis.

125. Scoliosis (in over 50% of patients) related to neurologic levels. The prognosis is worsened by the presence of congenital spinal deformity.

126. Bracing is not definitive management. It may be used as a temporary measure to permit additional growth, or when other medical or social concerns are predominant. A congenital deformity cannot be braced.

127. Insensate skin may break down; growing ribs may deform and further decrease chest capacity; abdominal pressure may interfere with breathing and eating.

128. Prevention of fixed contractures is paramount to facilitate sitting and the use of braces. In the absence of muscle function, this can usually be accomplished by physical therapy, positioning, and orthoses.

129. Muscle imbalance, due to functioning psoas and some adductors, causes progressive contracture and eventual dislocation.

130. First, avoid stiffness. It is usually recommended that the few functioning muscles be released to create a flail situation. Attempts to maintain reduction may be ill advised.

131. Muscle imbalance leads to progressive dislocation.

132. These patients have enough functioning muscle groups and sufficient potential for independent walking that aggressive treatment to maintain reduction of the hip is warranted.

QUESTIONS

133. What operative procedures may be considered for the hip in mid-to low-lumbar (L3–5) myelomeningocele?

134. Suggest a reasonable orthopedic goal for management of the knee in myelomeningocele.

135. Suggest an orthopedic goal for the foot in myelomeningocele.

136. Suggest treatment of the calcaneal deformity in the low-lumbar myelomeningocele patient.

137. Discuss treatment concepts for lower extremity fractures in myelomeningocele.

138. Preoperative planning for spina bifida patients should include consideration of what nonorthopedic systems?

139. About 20 minutes after induction of general anesthesia, prior to skin incision, your spina bifida patient develops a rash, becomes somewhat difficult to ventilate, and experiences a 40-mm Hg fall in systolic blood pressure. What are you seeing?

140. Your T12 spina bifida patient has an erythematous swollen thigh which is slightly warm to the touch. There have been no known accidents. What do you suspect?

141. Your L3 spina bifida patient has a moderately swollen left knee. Radiographs show widening of the physis. This is:

142. What is the factor that differentiates between metatarsus adductus (metatarsus varus) and skewfoot (serpentine foot, Z-foot)?

ANSWERS

133. Open reduction; femoral varus derotation osteotomy; pelvic osteotomy; muscle transfers such as the Sharrard or the external oblique to greater trochanter.

ANSWERS

134. Prevent fixed contractures. Tendon lengthenings are most often employed; tendon transfer is rarely indicated.

135. A plantigrade foot that can be braced. Only with a defect at the sacral level can patients be made brace-free.

136. Section of the dorsiflexors, usually the anterior tibialis and perhaps long toe extensors, may permit successful bracing. Posterior transfer of the anterior tibialis and tenodesis of the Achilles tendon to the tibia or fibula have been described.

137. Osteoporosis is exacerbated by immobilization, leading to postcast fractures. Therefore, minimal immobilization, perhaps only a thick, padded wrap, is indicated.

138. (1) The urologic system: most patients will have a colonized or chronically infected bladder. Preoperative treatment and perioperative antibiotics should be considered. (2) The central nervous system: shunt function must be assured prior to administration of general anesthesia. Formal neurosurgical consultation for preoperative clearance is suggested.

139. The scenario seems to be related to latex allergy. Anaphylactic reactions have been associated with latex allergy in spina bifida patients. The Centers for Disease Control (CDC) has issued a recommendation to avoid latex contact for these patients.

140. Even without known trauma, this is a fracture until proved otherwise. These patients often may even have a slight fever; and frequently call about an "insect bite." Always suspect fracture.

141. Chronic physeolysis (epiphysiolysis). The treatment is immobilization. Subsequent radiographs may show exuberant callus.

142. Heel position. In metatarsus adductus, the heel is in neutral or varus position. In skewfoot, the heel is in valgus position.

QUESTIONS

143. What clinical parameter helps in the decision between observation and active treatment of metatarsus varus?

144. Suggest nonoperative treatment for relatively rigid metatarsus varus in a prewalker.

145. Suggest a criticism of simply reversing shoes, or of the "swung-out" reverse lasted shoe when used to treat metatarsus adductus.

146. There has been a suggestion that metatarsus varus and skewfoot can be further subdivided into simple and complex varieties. What is the discriminator?

147. What pathoanatomy may be related to the relative rigidity of metatarsus adductus?

148. Suggest soft tissue surgery which has been advocated for treatment of resistant metatarsus varus in children younger than 2 years of age.

149. Suggest soft tissue surgery for treatment of resistant metatarsus adductus in the age range of 2 years to about 5 years.

150. A valid criticism of the Heyman, Herndon, and Strong procedure is:

151. Suggest a surgical option for the 10-year-old with persisting metatarsus adductus.

152. When teaching parents to perform stretching exercises for the child's metatarsus adductus, what cautions should be observed concerning heel position?

153. The surgical treatment of a skewfoot may include:

ANSWERS

143. The relative rigidity of the foot. If the foot cannot be easily over-corrected by gentle passive manipulation, some active treatment is indicated.

144. Most authors recommend serial manipulation and casting.

145. These may accentuate heel valgus, creating or exacerbating a skewfoot. Most authors do not feel that shoes will correct the metatarsus adductus deformity.

146. In the complex cases, there is lateral subluxation of the calcaneo-cuboid and talonavicular joints.

147. Some suggest that a true congenital metatarsus varus has medial subluxation of the tarsometatarsal joints. In this analysis, the more flexible varieties may be simple postural variations or may be functionally related to overpull of the abductor hallucis.

148. Release of the abductor hallucis tendon, or release of the first metatarsocuneiform joint.

149. Tarsometatarsal and intermetatarsal release, as described by Heyman, Herndon, and Strong.

150. It frequently leads to midfoot stiffness. Growth arrest of the proximally located physis of the first metatarsal is also a possibility.

151. Multiple metatarsal osteotomy.

152. The heel must be supported in neutral or slight varus. Allowing the heel to move into valgus may create or exacerbate a skewfoot.

153. Grice or similar subtalar stabilization, along with tarsometatarsal release or metatarsal osteotomy in order to address both components of the deformity.

QUESTIONS

154. Contrast childhood discitis with adult vertebral osteomyelitis.

155. Describe the four presentations of childhood discitis.

156. Describe diagnostic tests for childhood discitis.

157. What would an MRI show in a case of childhood discitis?

158. What steps should be taken for isolation of an organism in childhood discitis?

159. Describe treatment concepts for childhood discitis.

160. How long is bed rest continued?

161. How long should immobilization be continued?

162. When should antibiotics be used?

163. Suggest several clinical presentations of tarsal coalition.

ANSWERS

154. Childhood discitis seems to be a much less virulent process, and in many cases is self-limited.

155. (1) Small children may simply refuse to stand or walk; (2) abdominal pain and general malaise is a confusing but frequent presentation; (3) hip syndrome; (4) children of about 5 or 6 years begin to reliably localize symptoms to the lower back. Children are not always febrile with discitis.

ANSWERS

156. The peripheral white blood cell (WBC) count may be unreliable. The erythrocyte sedimentation rate (ESR) is usually elevated, and is probably a better guide than the WBC count. Radiographic findings of disc space narrowing may be delayed up to 3 weeks. Technectium 99m bone scan is usually positive. MRI may be the most sensitive test.

157. Inflammatory swelling of the disc, as well as inflammatory changes in the adjacent vertebral bodies. There will be a relative decrease in signal from the involved disc and surrounding structures on T1-weighted images. The T2-weighted images will show a relative increased signal compared to normal surroundings.

158. Blood cultures are appropriate, and stool cultures are often recommended. If the child responds to the usual treatment, aspiration or biopsy of the disc is not needed.

159. Bed rest or simple immobilization may be sufficient in some cases. Antistaphylococcal antibiotics may be used empirically; if there is good response in the first few days, these may be continued for 3 to 6 weeks with ESR serving as a guide to treatment duration.

160. One to 2 weeks.

161. Some form of activity limitation (immobilization) should be continued until radiographs show reactive bone changes at the adjacent end plates, i.e., until the bony erosion does not show any further progression. This usually takes 4 to 6 weeks.

162. This is controversial. Some authors always use antistaphylococcal antibiotics. Some authors recommend antibiotics whenever there is a suggestion of systemic sepsis such as fever or an elevated peripheral WBC count: otherwise, the patient is given a trial of 2 or 3 days of immobilization, and antibiotics are not used if pain and spasm resolve.

163. Repetitive ankle sprains in an adolescent; peroneal spastic flatfoot; activity-related pain in the subtalar or midtarsal area.

QUESTIONS

164. Where are the most common tarsal coalitions located?

165. Describe findings on a standing lateral radiograph that suggest a diagnosis of tarsal coalition.

166. Request a radiograph for the visualization of calcaneonavicular coalition.

167. Request a radiographic view for the visualization of coalition through the posterior or middle facets of the subtalar joint.

168. Suggest a test which has supplanted many of the specialized radiographic views for diagnosis of tarsal coalition.

169. Describe nonoperative treatment for tarsal coalition.

170. What operation may be recommended for the treatment of calcaneonavicular coalition?

171. What are contraindications to surgical excision of calcaneonavicular coalition?

172. Suggest operative management for symptomatic coalition with degenerative changes of the surrounding joints.

173. What are the major complications associated with treatment of slipped capital femoral epiphysis (SCFE)?

174. What are the treatment goals in SCFE?

ANSWERS

164. Talocalcaneal and calcaneonavicular coalitions are those usually seen. Published series are divided as to which of these two varieties is actually the more frequent.

165. The talus may seem to have a short, broad neck (snub-nosed talus); there may be dorsal beaking of the talus at the talonavicular joint; there may be abnormal elongation of the anterior process of the calcaneus (anteater nose sign).

166. The Sloman oblique, or similar oblique view, in which the beam is generally directed through the sinus tarsi at about 45 degrees.

167. The Harris view ("ski-jump" view) is an axial view of the calcaneus, in which the beam is angled at about 45 degrees. The correct angle of the beam is determined by measuring the angle of the subtalar joint as seen in the standing lateral radiograph.

168. Computed tomography (CT) scan.

169. Oral nonsteroidal anti-inflammatory drugs (NSAIDs); activity modification; various arch supports, pads, and orthoses. In acute or severe cases, a short period (e.g., 3 weeks) of cast immobilization may be tried.

170. Resection of the bar, with interposition of fat or extensor brevis.

171. Radiographic evidence of degenerative changes in the hindfoot or midfoot.

172. Triple arthrodesis. More limited fusion procedures may be tried in selected circumstances.

173. Chondrolysis and avascular necrosis.

174. Prevention of further slipping, and avoidance of complications.

QUESTIONS

175. What is the conventional classification of the time course of SCFE?

176. What is a "pre-slip?"

177. What constitutes a "mild slip?"

178. What constitutes a "moderate slip?"

179. What constitutes a "severe slip?"

180. Which radiographic view is used to classify the severity of a slip?

181. What is the most common hip disorder in adolescents?

182. Is there a racial difference in the incidence of SCFE?

183. Is there a sex difference in the incidence of SCFE?

184. Suggest some factors which tend to stabilize the physis against displacement.

185. Describe the response of the physis to hormonal stimulation.

186. Have any endocrine abnormalities been associated with SCFE, especially "juvenile" SCFE?

ANSWERS

175. Acute: diagnosis within 3 weeks of the onset of symptoms. Chronic: symptoms present for more than 3 weeks. Acute-on-chronic: symptoms present for more than 3 weeks, but with definite exacerbation within 3 weeks.

ANSWERS

176. Radiographs show widening, irregularity, and lucency at the physis but there is no actual displacement of the epiphysis.

177. Various classifications are suggested, but commonly a mild slip is up to one third of the width of the femoral neck.

178. Various classifications are suggested but commonly a moderate slip means femoral head displacement of greater than one third but less than one half of the width of the femoral neck.

179. Various classifications are suggested, but commonly this means femoral head displacement of greater than one half of the width of the femoral neck.

180. Severity is graded according to the view showing the most displacement. Usually, this is a lateral view.

181. Slipped capital femoral epiphysis.

182. Yes, the condition is more common in blacks.

183. Yes, the condition is more common in males.

184. The perichondral ring; transphyseal collagen fibers; mammillary processes at the epiphyseal-metaphyseal interface; the overall contour of the physeal plate, which is convex toward the epiphysis; the physeal inclination angle.

185. Growth hormone (through somatomedin) stimulates cartilage metabolism, and a thick physeal plate is less able to resist shear forces. Sex hormones (estrogens and androgens) cause a decrease in thickness of the physis, and therefore tend to stabilize the plate.

186. SCFE has definitely been associated with hypothyroidism, in which there is a deficiency in the cartilage matrix.

QUESTIONS

187. A 9-year-old girl on dialysis for chronic renal failure continues to have right medial knee pain. Knee radiographs are normal. Which x-ray film would you order next?

188. Describe the body habitus of the typical SCFE patient.

189. Describe the typical presentation of chronic SCFE.

190. How does Kline's line help in the diagnosis of SCFE?

191. Describe the Southwick method of measuring the femoral head–shaft angle.

192. Suggest appropriate steps to take immediately when SCFE is diagnosed.

193. What might be a method of nonoperative treatment?

ANSWERS

187. AP and frog-leg lateral views of the hips. SCFE has been repeatedly associated with renal osteodystrophy and secondary hyperparathyroidism. In fact, these patients tend to slip at many physes (distal tibia, proximal humerus, etc.).

188. The obese, hypogonadal individual would be most typical. One theory suggests that these patients have a subclinical hormonal imbalance, such as relatively low sex hormones. Some patients, by contrast, are tall and thin. Perhaps they have relatively high levels of growth hormones. However, actual hormonal imbalance has not been confirmed in these "typical" patient types.

189. Variable pain in the groin, often radiating to the anteromedial thigh or knee. The affected limb may be shortened 1 to 2 cm. Abduction, internal rotation, and flexion are limited. There may be disuse atrophy of the thigh. The resulting limp is usually a combination of these factors, but the external rotation may be the most obvious change in the gait.

ANSWERS

190. In both the AP and the lateral radiograph, a line projected along the superior margin of the femoral neck should intersect a portion of the femoral head. In SCFE, the line either misses the head entirely, or intersects less of the head when compared with the unaffected side.

191. On a lateral radiograph, a line is drawn connecting the corners of the femoral capital epiphysis, and a line perpendicular to that line is constructed. A third line is projected parallel to the femoral shaft. The angle between the perpendicular and the femoral shaft lines is measured. The normal angle is 0 ± 10 degrees (see Figure).

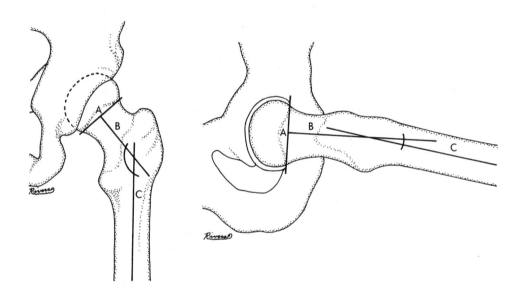

192. The patient must not be allowed to bear weight on the affected extremity. Definitive treatment should be begun urgently in order to prevent further displacement.

193. Spica cast immobilization for 12 weeks has been recommended by at least one author (Steele). However, operative management is currently the standard of care in most areas.

QUESTIONS

194. Suggest criticisms of cast management of SCFE.

195. Describe the usual surgical treatment options for SCFE.

196. What are possible criticisms of pin fixation of SCFE?

197. Suggest criticisms of open bone graft epiphysiodesis.

198. What advantages may there be to open bone graft epiphysiodesis?

199. Discuss the role of reduction in management of SCFE.

200. Discuss the role of traction in reduction of the acute portion of an acute or chronic SCFE.

201. Suggest three categories of osteotomy which may be considered in dealing with displacement of the proximal femur in SCFE.

202. Why are proximal osteotomies (adjacent to the physis) not more popular?

203. What is the criticism of osteotomy at the base of the femoral neck?

ANSWERS

194. Some series show an increased incidence of chondrolysis with casting. Additional displacement can occur if the cast is discontinued too soon.

195. These may consist of internal fixation with pins, or open bone graft epiphysiodesis.

ANSWERS

196. Unrecognized penetration of the pins into the joint has been associated with complications such as chondrolysis. "Nesting" of the tips of several pins may result in avascular necrosis (AVN). Entry holes in the lateral cortex can act as stress risers, especially if located distal to the level of the lesser trochanter. Physeal closure may not be rapid, and overgrowth off the pins can occur. Pin removal is a second operation.

197. The magnitude of the operation is greater than pinning, and the technique may be unfamiliar to many. Curettage of the physis may actually destabilize the slip further, risking additional displacement. Postoperative casting may be indicated, especially in acute cases.

198. Most series show extremely low rates of chondrolysis or AVN— much lower than most series of pinning. Physeal closure after operation may be more rapid. There is no second operation for hardware removal.

199. Reduction of chronic slips is contraindicated because of high AVN rates. Reduction of acute slips is controversial for that same reason. Some slips present so acutely that they may more properly fit into a category of type I physeal fractures; reduction is probably indicated in this small subset.

200. Some series suggest that traction including internal rotation may effect a "gentle" reduction of the acute portion of the slip. Traction is also sometimes used to decrease symptoms of synovitis prior to surgical intervention.

201. Osteotomy may be performed in the proximal femoral neck adjacent to the physis, at the base of the femoral neck, or more distal in the intertrochanteric or subtrochanteric region.

202. Although osteotomy at this level (Dunn, Fish) more directly restores the anatomy, the AVN rates have been prohibitive in most series.

203. Once again, osteotomy at this level (Kramer) places the vascular supply of the femoral head at risk.

QUESTIONS

204. Suggest a criticism of inter- or subtrochanteric osteotomy.

205. What happens to hip motion when SCFE is successfully stabilized in situ?

206. What happens to bony deformity when SCFE is successfully stabilized in situ?

207. Suggest the late outcome of SCFE.

208. What descriptive label is given to the late deformity of SCFE?

209. Describe the clinical presentation of chondrolysis.

210. Suggest radiographic findings in chondrolysis.

211. What other study may be helpful in the diagnosis of chondrolysis?

212. Suggest factors which may be associated with the development of chondrolysis.

213. Suggest nonoperative treatment which may be offered for chondrolysis.

214. What operative treatment may be offered for chondrolysis?

ANSWERS

204. These compensatory operations (Southwick) improve the femoral head-to-acetabulum relationship by actually creating another deformity at the level of the trochanters. This may complicate later reconstructive surgery such as total hip arthroplasty.

ANSWERS

205. Motion may never return to normal, but there is significant improvement and restoration of motion within the first 6 months.

206. There is a documented tendency toward improvement. The anterolateral "hump" of femoral neck is resorbed as some reactive new bone is laid down at the inferomedial neck. Trochanteric overgrowth may increase, as may limb length discrepancy, depending on the growth remaining.

207. The worst results are in those cases having complications of AVN or chondrolysis. In uncomplicated cases, the occurrence of osteoarthritis depends on the amount of residual deformity.

208. "Pistol grip" deformity of the proximal femur.

209. Increasing stiffness of the hip, with loss of motion in all planes. Muscle spasm and pain are variable.

210. Joint space narrowing ($<50\%$ of the contralateral side, or $<2mm$), periarticular osteoporosis, premature closure of the greater trochanteric apophysis.

211. Technectium 99m bone scan may show increased uptake on both sides of the joint. In uncomplicated SCFE, acetabular uptake is not expected.

212. Pins left protruding into the joint, prolonged immobilization, residual deformity with joint incongruity, black or Hawaiian race, female sex.

213. The treatment goal is to restore motion to the joint. This may include a period of traction and institution of continuous passive motion (CPM). NSAIDs may be prescribed. As motion improves, restricted ambulation with crutches can be allowed.

214. If motion cannot be restored by conservative means, some authors suggest soft tissue releases including adductors, iliopsoas, and subtotal capsulectomy. Postoperatively, CPM is resumed.

QUESTIONS

215.   Suggest operative treatment for AVN with segmental collapse.

216.   Suggest operative treatment for severe chondrolysis or whole-head AVN.

217.   Suggest probable organisms which cause osteomyelitis or septic arthritis in the neonate.

218.   Suggest probable organisms which cause osteomyelitis or septic arthritis in young children, ages about 6 months to about 4 years.

219.   Suggest probable organisms which cause osteomyelitis or septic arthritis in children older than age 5 years.

220.   Suppose a neonate presents with signs of bilateral femoral osteo-myelitis, as well as bilateral forearm swelling (see Figure). What specific infectious process should be considered?

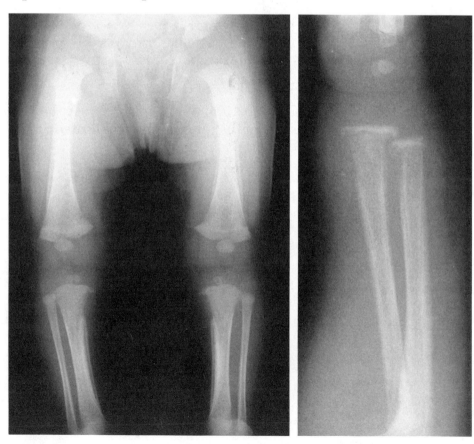

ANSWERS

215. The Sugioka intertrochanteric osteotomy is designed to rotate an uninvolved section of the femoral head into the weightbearing position.

216. Hip arthrodesis is a realistic option in this age group. Total hip arthroplasty is usually not recommended for these young patients.

217. Group B streptococci, *Staphylococcus aureus*, gram-negative coliforms.

218. *S. aureus, Haemophilus influenzae*, group B streptococci, group A streptococci.

219. *S. aureus* is the predominant organism.

220. Congenital syphilis classically shows bilateral, symmetric involvement.

QUESTIONS

221. Suppose a black child presents with osteomyelitis and a very low hematocrit. What particular conditions should be considered?

222. Suggest a common dilemma in the diagnosis of osteomyelitis in a sickle cell patient.

223. Can nuclear medicine studies help with the sickle infarct vs. osteomyelitis dilemma?

224. Needle aspiration of metaphyseal bone may be performed as part of the diagnostic evaluation for osteomyelitis. Should this step be delayed until after a ^{99m} Tc bone scan?

225. Aspiration of a swollen, tender, joint yields fluid with a WBC count of 20,000. The Gram stain shows many polymorphonuclear neutrophils (PMNs), but no organisms. Still, you strongly suspect infection on the basis of other systemic signs. How do you proceed?

226. Other than direct aspiration of the infected bone or joint, suggest methods of isolating the infectious organism.

227. Suggest special etiologic considerations for an apparent septic knee in an adolescent who does not look "sick."

228. How do weight training and weightlifting differ?

229. Discuss some effects of weight training on prepubescent children.

ANSWERS

221. Sickle cell screening should be part of the evaluation. Sickle cell disease predisposes to salmonella infection of the bone. Salmonella osteomyelitis is also associated with related hemoglobinopathies, such as Hb SC and Hb SB thalassemia.

ANSWERS

222. Bone infarct is common, and the symptoms are nearly identical to osteomyelitis. Differentiation is sometimes made directly, by needle aspiration of the bone. High spiking fever suggests infection rather than infarct.

223. Some series suggest that increased uptake on ^{99m}Tc bone scan and increased uptake on gallium scan indicate infection. By contrast, the infarction of sickle crisis may show increased activity on ^{99m}Tc but a decrease on Ga scan.

224. Not necessarily. It has been experimentally established that needle aspiration does not cause a false-positive bone scan. Of course, that presumes that a suspicious area can be identified by physical examination or routine radiography. With uncooperative children, sometimes the bone scan is the only modality which can localize the site of infection.

225. This scenario suggest metaphyseal osteomyelitis with formation of a "sympathetic effusion." Proceed with aspiration of the adjacent metaphysis.

226. Since most childhood bone and joint sepsis seems to be hematogenous, blood cultures are positive in approximately 50% of cases. Other sites of infection must be sought, especially upper respiratory.

227. Do not neglect the possibility of sexually transmitted disease. Gonorrhea and Reiter's syndrome are examples.

228. The different terms are meant to distinguish the training technique from the competitive sport. Weight training implies that progressive resistance exercise techniques, whether with free weights or machines, are used in a controlled program designed to enhance one's strength, size, and power. Power lifting or Olympic weightlifting refers to competition, usually on the basis of single repetition for maximal load.

229. These children can increase strength, but this increase is thought to be due to recruitment and synchronization of muscle fibers. Actual hypertrophy of motor units does not occur, probably owing to the lack of circulating androgens in this age group.

QUESTIONS

230. What about the safety of strength training for prepubescent children?

231. Describe "Little Leaguer's shoulder."

232. Describe "Little Leaguer's elbow."

233. What is "swimmer's shoulder"?

234. A 12-year-old female gymnast complains of pain at the distal radius. What might be seen on a radiograph?

235. Suggest the repetitive stress mechanism which causes popliteus tendinitis.

236. How does femoral version differ from femoral torsion?

237. What is the mean femoral anteversion at birth and at skeletal maturation?

238. What is the normal tibial lateral rotation noted at birth and at maturity?

239. What physiologic contractures are noted in the newborn?

ANSWERS

230. Policy statements from the major concerned medical groups, such as the American Academy of Pediatrics, all stress the use of submaximal resistance in a controlled, supervised setting. In this type of setting, physeal fractures and stress fractures may occur, but are uncommon. The common injuries are muscle pulls and tendinitis. There does not seem to be any direct harm to the physeal plate from the controlled use of submaximal loads.

231. This typically presents as an insidious, progressive, deep pain in the dominant shoulder of a Little League pitcher. Repetitive stress can cause an epiphysiolysis of the proximal humerus. The physical

ANSWERS

examination may be very nondescriptive, but the radiograph shows widening and irregularity of the proximal humeral physis. The treatment is rest, followed by stretching to reestablish full range of motion, and strengthening to assure muscle balance. Attention must be directed to correcting the mechanics of pitching. If recognized and treated, there are no known sequelae.

232. Elbow problems in Little League pitchers are almost always repetitive stress injuries due to valgus forces. This particular condition is due to tension stress at the medial epicondylar apophysis. The symptom is pain at the medial side of the elbow. The physical findings are local swelling, sometimes with ulnar nerve dysfunction. Radiographically, the epicondyle may be enlarged, sclerotic, or even fragmented, with widening of the physeal plate.

233. This repetitive stress injury is an impingement syndrome of the shoulder which occurs in many overhead sports, most typically freestyle swimming.

234. The repetitive stress syndrome which occurs in this situation is an epiphysiolysis at the distal radius. The physeal plate may be widened and irregular, with lucent defects in the adjacent metaphysis. The process responds to rest.

235. This is caused by excessive internal rotation of the tibia during running or similar activity. Excessive pronation of the forefoot, running on banked surfaces, and running on hills have all been implicated.

236. Version describes rotation within normal ranges. Torsion describes abnormal rotation deviating from the mean by 2 SD or more.

237. At birth femoral anteversion averages 40 degrees and decreases to 15 degrees at skeletal maturation.

238. Lateral rotation at birth is approximately 5 degrees and at maturity averages 15 degrees.

239. Mild hip flexion and lateral rotation contracture maintain the infant's lower extremities in a position of lateral rotation throughout the first year of life.

QUESTIONS

240. Using the foot progression angle (FPA) as an index for intoeing, define mild, moderate, and severe intoeing.

241. What torsional abnormality is associated with the "eggbeater" running pattern?

242. True or false? In the management of lower extremity rotational deformities, the following treatment methods have been proved effective: (1) twister cables; (2) shoe modifications; (3) Dennis-Browne bar.

243. The most common cause for intoeing in the second year of life is:

244. The most common cause for intoeing after the age of 3 years is:

245. True or false? The natural history of flexible pes planus is favorably altered by the use of arch supports and UCB heel cups.

246. True or false? Rotational osteotomies can be considered as a definitive form of treatment in children after the age of 8 if a persistent deformity, exceeding 3 SD, is causing cosmetic or functional problems.

247. True or false? Untreated femoral antetorsion results in degenerative arthritis.

248. Describe the two types of physiologic bowing.

249. When is resolution of physiologic bowing usually noted?

250. True or false? Bracing will hasten the resolution of physiologic bowing.

251. At what age is physiologic knockknee most commonly encountered?

ANSWERS

240. Mild intoeing: -5 to -10 degree FPA; moderate intoeing: -10 to -15 degree FPA; severe intoeing: -15 degree or greater FPA.

241. Femoral antetorsion.

242. False.

243. Medial tibial torsion.

244. Femoral anteversion.

245. False. The natural history of treated and untreated children is identical.

246. True.

247. False.

248. (1) Lateral tibial bowing is noted in the first year of life, with complete resolution the rule. (2) Physiologic bowing involving the distal femur and proximal tibia occurs during the second year, is associated with medial tibial torsion, and is more common in blacks.

249. Between age 2 and 3 years.

250. False. Bracing does not affect the natural history of physiologic bowing.

251. Between the ages of 3 and 4 years.

QUESTIONS

252. Describe the best age and method of treatment for persistent valgus deformities secondary to unresolved genu valgum with femorotibial angles exceeding 15 degrees valgus.

253. In a standing AP radiograph of a 3-year-old child's lower extremity, a proximal metaphyseal tibial bowing is noted. The metaphyseal-diaphyseal angle approximates 15 degrees. The medial tibial physis and *metaphysis* suggest a disorganized growth pattern. The most likely diagnosis of the described deformity is:

254. Describe the presently accepted thinking on the etiology of Blount's disease.

255. The most effective management of bilateral Langenskiöld type III tibia vara deformities in a 4-year-old child should consist of:

256. The risk of recurrence of Blount's deformity following osteotomy is directly correlated with:

257. True or false? Adolescent tibia vara is commonly a bilateral deformity.

258. Posttraumatic genu valgum is most commonly seen secondary to what injury?

259. True or false? The development of posttraumatic valgus deformities after proximal tibial fracture is secondary to poor reduction of these fractures.

260. A 4-year-old child presents with bilateral lower extremity varus deformities, falls below the 5th percentile in height, is noted to have low calcium and phosphorus and a high alkaline phosphatase activity. The most likely diagnosis for this patient is:

261. True or false? The most common cause of bilateral pathologic valgus deformities in childhood is secondary to renal disease.

ANSWERS

252. Hemiepiphysiodesis or medial distal femoral physeal stapling at or about the age of puberty. Osteotomy may be indicated in severe cases.

253. Blount's disease.

254. Blount's disease is thought to be an osteochondrosis secondary to excessive mechanical stress, which converts a physiologic bowing into tibia vara in a susceptible individual.

255. Bilateral proximal tibial and fibular valgus and derotation osteotomies, with prophylactic fasciotomies.

256. Age at surgery over 5 years, and physeal bar formation.

257. False. Adolescent tibia vara is most often seen as a unilateral deformity in obese black males.

258. Proximal tibial metaphyseal fractures (Cozen's fracture).

259. False. The development of posttraumatic genu valgum may be due to trauma-induced differential growth of the medial aspect of the proximal tibial physis. Meyers reported interposed periosteum. Lonon reported interposed pes anserine.

260. Rickets-induced lower extremity bowing.

261. True.

QUESTIONS

262. True or false? Posteromedial bowing of the tibia is characterized by spontaneous improvement with subsequent growth.

263. The most likely surgical procedure that a child with posterior medial bowing of the tibia will undergo is:

264. True or false? Congenital dislocation of the knee is often associated with arthrogryposis, myelodysplasia, and Larsen's syndrome.

265. True or false? Congenital dislocation of the knee is occasionally associated with hyperextension intrauterine position and responds well to manipulation and casting into flexion.

266. True or false? Congenital dislocation of the hip and knee are frequently associated.

267. True or false? Open reduction and quadricepsplasty of a congenital knee dislocation is indicated if less than 30 degrees of flexion can be achieved by 3 months of age.

268. True or false? Anterolateral bowing of the tibia can progress to tibial pseudarthrosis.

269. Lateral patellar dislocation is associated with what lower extremity deformities?

270. Recurrent patellar subluxation in adolescents frequently has a number of predisposing factors. List them.

271. The "miserable malalignment syndrome" is a common cause of persisting lateral patellar subluxation. Describe the rotational profile of these children.

272. Describe the pathologic changes associated with osteochondritis dissecans in the adolescent.

ANSWERS

262. True.

263. Epiphysiodesis of the contralateral limb for persistent limb length discrepancy.

264. True.

265. True.

266. True.

267. True.

268. True.

269. External tibial rotation, genu valgum, and knee flexion contracture.

270. Generalized joint laxity, genu valgum, increased Q-angle, patella alta, incongruence of the patellofemoral joint, hypoplasia of the vastus medialis, lateral retinacular contracture, lateral condylar hypoplasia.

271. Femoral antetorsion with external tibial torsion.

272. Periarticular osseous necrosis with overlying cartilage softening, occasionally associated with fragment displacement.

QUESTIONS

273. Describe the most common location of osteochondritis dissecans in the knee.

274. Which radiographic view most often identifies osteochondritis dissecans?

275. What is the best management for the nondisplaced osteochondritis dissecans of the medial femoral condyle identified in a skeletally immature male?

276. What is the appropriate management of loose fragments of osteochondritis dissecans in the skeletally mature adolescent?

277. Describe the pathologic changes in Osgood-Schlatter disease.

278. At what age is Osgood-Schlatter disease most common?

279. What is the natural history of Osgood-Schlatter disease?

280. In the presentation of Osgood-Schlatter disease, what study is mandatory to rule out other possible abnormalities such as tumors?

281. Which of the following treatment modalities are contraindicated in Osgood-Schlatter disease? (1) Rest and immobilization; (2) isometric knee exercises; (3) knee pads; (4) steroid injections.

282. Sinding-Larsen-Johansson syndrome, also known as juvenile jumper's knee, is associated with what abnormality?

283. Describe the most common cause and location of Baker's cyst in childhood.

284. Describe the natural history of Baker's cyst in childhood.

ANSWERS

273. The lateral aspect of the medial femoral condyle.

274. Tunnel view of the knee.

275. Activity modification and a short period of immobilization supplemented with isometric strengthening exercises of the knee.

276. If the fragment is less than 5 mm, simple excision. If the fragment is larger, placement into the recipient bed and internal fixation is suggested.

277. Apophysitis secondary to repetitive microtrauma results in inflammation and new bone formation at the tendon-bone junction.

278. In boys, age 13 to 14 years. In girls, age 10 to 11 years.

279. In the majority of cases, complete resolution in 1 to 2 years of onset.

280. AP and lateral radiographs of the knee.

281. Steroid injections, because they can induce weakening of the patellar tendon and subcutaneous fat necrosis.

282. Traction apophysitis of the distal pole of the patella secondary to repetitive stress.

283. Synovial popliteal cysts which arise between the semimembranosus and gastrocnemius tendons.

284. Spontaneous resolution with 2 to 5 years.

QUESTIONS

285. Describe the most common type and location of discoid meniscus.

286. The Wrisberg discoid meniscus may become symptomatic due to increased meniscal mobility causing symptoms of snapping, locking, and pain. At what age are symptoms most likely to present in children with this disorder?

287. The optimal treatment of symptomatic discoid meniscus consists of:

288. Describe the percent growth contributions provided by the distal femoral and proximal tibial physes.

289. What is the relationship of the length of the femur to that of the tibia?

290. The most common cause for discrepancies between apparent leg length as measured from the umbilicus to the medial malleolus and true leg length as measured from the anterior superior iliac spine to the medial malleolus is:

291. Leg length discrepancies present as either static or dynamic processes during the growth of a child. In a child who sustains a midshaft femur fracture and is allowed to heal with 4 cm of overlap, the pattern of leg length discrepancy that is most likely to occur is:

292. In a larger child, scanograms appear to be more accurate than teleroentgenograms. The reason for this is:

293. True or false? The most accurate and predictable method for determining future growth is the radiographic assessment of past growth.

294. True or false? The straight-line graph method is based on the data of Green and Anderson.

295. Describe the best treatment for the following leg length discrepancies: (a) 0–2 cm; (b) 2–6 cm; (c) 6–15 cm; (d) >15 cm.

ANSWERS

285. Complete discoid meniscus involving the lateral compartment.

286. Between the ages of 12 and 13 years.

287. Meniscal stabilization and meniscoplasty, with complete excision serving as a last resort.

288. The distal femoral physis provides 37% and the proximal tibial physis 28% of the growth of the lower extremities. Combined, these two physes contribute 65% of the growth of the lower extremities.

289. The femur constitutes 54% of the total length of the lower extremity with the tibia making up the additional 46%.

290. Pelvic obliquity (which may be secondary to supra- or intrapelvic causes).

291. Static deformity.

292. Scanogram technique avoids the risk of magnification by providing an exposure perpendicular to each joint.

293. True.

294. True.

295. (a) No treatment is necessary; (b) epiphysiodesis or contralateral limb shortening; (c) consideration of lengthening of the shortened limb; (d) consideration of prosthetic fitting.

QUESTIONS

296. What is the maximum degree of shortening that can be achieved in the tibia and femur before complications of excessive shortening (muscle weakness) become evident?

297. What potentially fatal complication has been associated with the closed femoral shortening technique with IM rod insertion?

298. True or false? The complications of lengthening can be minimized by careful attention to the biologic considerations such as lengthening in the metaphyseal region, avoidance of power equipment during osteotomy, delay in onset of distraction to allow the regenerate callus to form, and distraction at a rate of 1 mm/day or less in numerous small increments.

299. What four disease processes can frequently be associated with elevated creatine phosphokinase (CPK) levels?

300. Which electrodiagnostic study can be used to differentiate a myopathic from a neuropathic process?

301. Which hereditary muscle disorder is characterized by difficulty in postcontraction relaxation and has a characteristic EMG finding suggestive of rapid repetitive discharges?

302. True or false? Nerve conduction velocities will remain normal in patients with anterior horn cell disease, spinal nerve root injury, and in myopathy.

303. True or false? Type II muscle fibers are characterized by fast-twitch potential, high glycolytic and adenosine triphosphatase (ATPase) activity, and low oxidative metabolism activity.

304. What is the normal ratio of type I to type II muscle fibers in skeletal muscle?

305. Describe the typical histologic changes of muscle tissue in myopathy.

ANSWERS

296. In general the tibia can be shortened by 3 cm and the femur by up to 5 cm.

297. Fat embolism syndromes.

298. True.

299. (1) Duchenne's muscular dystrophy; (2) type IV spinal muscular atrophy; (3) dermatomyositis; (4) limb girdle dystrophy.

300. Electromyogram (EMG). Neuropathic changes are seen as fibrillation potentials, which are characterized by prolonged polyphasic high-voltage action potentials. Myopathic disorders show low-voltage polyphasic action potentials.

301. Myotonia dystrophica.

302. True. Nerve conduction velocities should not be affected by spinal cord, nerve root, or muscle disorders.

303. True. Type I fibers are characterized by slow-twitch, high oxidative capacity, and a low ATPase level. Type III fibers appear to have characteristics intermediate between types I and II.

304. 1:2.

305. Type I fiber predominance, muscle cell phagocytosis, low-grade inflammatory reaction, replacement fibrosis.

QUESTIONS

306. Name three neuromuscular disorders in which electrocardiogram abnormalities have been identified.

307. Name three neuromuscular conditions that have been associated with an increased risk of malignant hyperthermia.

308. Duchenne's muscular dystrophy is an X-linked recessive disorder. What is the name and the function of the protein that is not synthesized if this defect is present?

309. What is the incidence of Duchenne's muscular dystrophy and the rate of a positive family history in index cases?

310. What is the key factor in deterioration of gait in a child with Duchenne's muscular dystrophy?

311. What is the significance of a positive Gower maneuver?

312. What is the clinical significance of Maryon's sign?

313. True or false? Calf muscle enlargement of Duchenne's muscular dystrophy occurs in an attempt to compensate for weak proximal musculature.

314. The development of scoliosis occurs in nearly all children with muscular dystrophy. Rapid progression is frequently noted once the child becomes confined to the wheelchair, usually at age 10 to 12. These curves do not respond to bracing. Should surgery be considered, which technique provides the most consistent results?

315. In a child who develops a pattern of muscular weakness similar to Duchenne's muscular dystrophy, but whose symptoms started after the age of 8 years, and who continues to ambulate beyond the age of 20 years, the most likely diagnosis is:

ANSWERS

306. (1) Duchenne's muscular dystrophy; (2) Friedreich's ataxia; (3) myotonia dystrophica.

307. (1) Myelodysplasia; (2) Duchenne's muscular dystrophy; (3) congenital myopathies associated with increased CPK enzyme levels.

308. Dystrophin. This protein functions in calcium hemostasis at the level of the sarcoplasmic reticulum.

309. Duchenne's muscular dystrophy is noted in 1 in 3,000 live male births and a positive family history can be obtained in 60% of cases.

310. Development of quadriceps weakness with loss of muscle power below 3/5.

311. In this maneuver, a child lying prone on the floor needs to climb up on his legs using his arms to obtain the upright position. This is strongly suggestive of pelvic muscle and quadriceps weakness.

312. This sign, which represents a tendency for a child to slip through the examiner's arms with both arms going into full abduction, suggests shoulder girdle weakness.

313. False. Calf pseudohypertrophy is associated with progressive clinical weakness of the ankle plantar flexors and development of heel cord contracture.

314. In general, children with curves over 40 degrees are best managed by stabilization using Luque rods and sublaminar wires and the Galveston technique. The goal should be to operate on these children while their curve is flexible and their forced vital capacity remains over 30%.

315. Becker's muscular dystrophy.

QUESTIONS

316. Polymyositis presents as an inflammatory myopathy of childhood. What is one important differentiating feature between this disorder and muscular dystrophy?

317. Poliomyelitis is an acute viral infection which attacks a specific location of the spinal cord. At what level does this damage occur?

318. In a child with residual polio, a mild lumbar scoliosis and pelvic obliquity are identified. What test is most important in evaluating the cause of the pelvic obliquity as supra- or infrapelvic?

319. The postpolio syndrome has been described as development of progressive fatigue, muscle weakness, and muscle atrophy, occurring 30 years or more after acute polio syndrome. There are presently two theories to explain this phenomenon. Describe them.

320. List the risk factors associated with developmental hip dislocation.

321. What percentage of patients presenting with developmental dislocation of the hip will demonstrate a congenital muscular torticollis?

322. What pathologic abnormality is most often responsible for an irreducible congenital dislocated hip?

323. What is the incidence of established congenital dislocated hip?

324. Are there racial influences on the incidence of dislocation?

325. In an established complete hip dislocation, a false acetabulum occasionally develops. What is the genesis and character of the tissue forming the false acetabulum?

326. The natural history of developmental subluxation and developmental dislocation have been studied and categorized. Which has the worst prognosis as far as early onset of severe arthritis?

ANSWERS

316. These children appear mildly systemically ill and their muscles are tender in contradistinction to patients with muscular dystrophy.

317. The anterior horn cell of the spinal cord and motor nuclei of the brainstem.

318. The Ober test indicates a hip abduction contracture secondary to iliotibial band or gluteus medius contractures, suggesting an infra-pelvic pelvic obliquity.

319. (1) The possibility of a continued reactivitation of the poliovirus in the anterior horn cell. (2) A partial permanent injury to the anterior horn cells, which were not completely destroyed during the acute phase, which years later may show premature degeneration and death.

320. Female sex, familial ligamentous laxity, breech position, first-time mothers with large infant birth weight, genetic factors, postnatal positioning.

321. 20%.

322. Hourglass deformity of the hip capsule.

323. The overall incidence is 0.65/1,000 live births. The rate in males is 0.12/1,000 and in females 1.1/1,000.

324. Yes. Black infants have a much lower incidence with a rate of 0.46/1,000.

325. The false acetabulum is lined with fibrocartilage which originates from metaplasia of the hip joint capsule between the femoral head and the ilium.

326. Subluxation. Also, patients with complete dislocations who demonstrate a well-developed false acetabulum frequently have more severe symptoms.

QUESTIONS

327. In the treatment of congenital dislocated hip, which complication substantially worsens the prognosis of the hip beyond that of the natural history of the untreated hip?

328. Beyond careful serial physical examinations in the first days and weeks of life, which diagnostic study offers the best assurance of a stable concentric reduced hip?

329. In arthrography of a normal hip joint the "thorn sign" represents

330. While the acetabular index is noted to be highly variable and dependent on pelvic position, what acetabular angle should be considered highly suspect of a hip abnormality?

331. A 4-day-old infant presents with left hip dysplasia characterized by positive Ortolani and positive Barlow signs. The right hip appears stable. A Pavlik harness is chosen as a means of obtaining initial reduction. Describe the accepted optimal hip position to achieve reduction.

332. This infant has now been treated with the harness for 4 weeks but the left hip remains unstable on examination with positive Ortolani and positive Barlow signs. What should the next course of action be?

333. Following a 2-month period of hip spica casting, the left hip stabilizes. The spica cast is removed and an abduction splint is used at night and naptimes. At 1 year of age concentric reduction with an acetabular index equal to the uninvolved side is noted. Physical examination is perfectly normal. At this point you recommend

334. A 12-month-old infant presents with a complete dislocation of the left hip identified secondary to a limp. There are significant changes of adaptive shortening, a significant limitation in abduction, and examination reveals this hip to be negative for Ortolani's sign. What is the appropriate treatment plan for this hip?

ANSWERS

327. Avascular necrosis.

328. Dynamic ultrasonography of the hip performed by an experienced ultrasonographer.

329. The free border of the labrum extending up from the acetabulum right over the superior aspect of the femoral head.

330. Acetabular indices greater than 35 degrees warrant careful radiographic follow-up.

331. Ninety to 100 degrees of forward flexion achieved by tightening the anterior straps, and 45 to 50 degrees of hip abduction maintained by placement of the anterior straps along the anterior axillary line. The posterior straps serve as tethers to prevent adduction beyond 20 degrees. Rotation of the limbs should be essentially neutral and the anterior straps should pass across the axis of the knee.

332. Abandon the Pavlik harness treatment and proceed with alternatives such as spica cast application.

333. Continued follow-up through maturity. Approximately 20% of children with apparently normal hips at 1 or 2 years of age develop late and significant acetabular dysplasia.

334. A home skin traction program carried out in a modified Bryant's position until simple positional reduction can be achieved without force; adductor tenotomy to improve the safe zone of Ramsey; and spica casting in the human position, with the hips flexed 90 degrees, in neutral rotation, and with 45 to 50 degrees of abduction. This is followed by a CT scan to document concentric reduction.

QUESTIONS

335. A 3-year-old child is diagnosed with a missed dislocation of the left hip. At this point the treatment plan would include

336. Following this procedure, excellent concentric reduction is obtained and maintained. In spite of a concentric reduction, 3 years later an acetabular dysplasia persists with the acetabular index approximately 35 degrees. Recommendations at this point in time should include

ANSWERS

335. Formal open reduction of the left hip followed by varus and short-ening derotation osteotomy.

336. The innominate osteotomy of Salter.

CHAPTER 3

Pediatric Trauma

Timothy S. Loth, M.D.

QUESTIONS

1. What are the indications for surgery in fractures of the proximal humeral physis?

2. How are closed fractures of the distal end of the clavicle treated in children?

3. What are the key elements of acromioclavicular (AC) dislocations in children? How should they be treated?

4. How should fractures of the base of the coracoid be treated in children?

5. How should voluntary dislocation of the shoulder be treated in children?

6. What is the ossiculum terminale? When does it appear and fuse?

7. At what age does pseudosubluxation of C2–3 and C3–4 become less frequent?

8. At which level do most children's cervical spine injuries occur?

ANSWERS

1. Surgery is rarely indicated. In a child 12 years or older with non-reducible fracture secondary to biceps tendon entrapment, perform open reduction. Salter-Harris grades III and IV are treated with open reduction with smooth Steinmann pin fixation. Teenagers take 6 to 7 weeks to achieve solid union.

2. Excellent results can be expected with closed treatment regardless of displacement. A figure-8 bandage, sling, or collar and cuff are applied. Anticipate remodeling up to the age of 16.

3. These are physeal separations or fractures of the distal clavicle, whereby the clavicle is displaced upward through a dorsal longitudinal split in the periosteal tube. The periosteal tube remains intact inferiorly, and the AC ligaments and the coracoacromial (CA) ligament remain attached to the periosteal tube. Spontaneous healing will occur without need for surgery. Severe displacement (Rockwood type IV, V, and VI) with entrapment of the clavicle in the trapezius and deltoid or beneath the corocoid usually requires open reduction and internal fixation is carried out.

4. Nonoperatively.

5. If emotionally unstable, no surgery. If instability continues to be a problem after a 6- to 12-month period of active rehabilitation and if the patient is cleared as being emotionally stable, reconstruction may be considered.

6. The ossiculum terminale is an ossification center of the tip of the odontoid. It appears at about age 3 to 6 years of age and fuses to the odontoid by age 12.

7. Over age 8. Between 19% and 40% of children less than 8 years old have C2–3 pseudosubluxation. With neck flexion, translation can measure up to 4 mm.

8. Most occur between the occiput and C3 or C4; this is the reverse of adult cervical-spine injuries, most of which occur at C4 or below.

QUESTIONS

9. Which four lesions occur at the atlantoaxial segment in children?

10. In children, what is an acceptable atlantodens interval (ADI)?

11. How is posttraumatic C1–2 instability treated in children?

12. How should type I (Fielding and Hawkins) atlantoaxial displacement secondary to inflammation be treated?

13. How should atlantoaxial rotary displacement be approached in a child?

14. Describe the treatment of odontoid fractures in children.

15. What is the incidence of progressive spinal deformity in immature children (girls less than 12 years old, boys less than 14) with para- or quadriplegia?

16. In a child age 2 to 6 years, the spontaneous collapse of a single vertebra suggests what diagnosis?

17. In which childhood conditions does one see multiple vertebral collapse?

18. When does spondylolysis occur in children?

ANSWERS

9. (1) Traumatic ligament tear; (2) rotary subluxation deformity, (3) odontoid "epiphyseal" separation, and (4) ligament laxity secondary to inflammation.

ANSWERS

10. Less than 4.5 mm. Over 5 mm is indicative of ligament incompetence in association with a history of trauma.

11. Extension reduction and surgical stabilization followed by 8 to 12 weeks in a halo or Minerva jacket.

12. Type I rotary displacement has no associated anterior shift of C1 and can be treated with soft collar and analgesics. If still present after 1 week, bed rest, halter traction, and analgesics usually are effective.

13. Most cases are mild, presenting with stiff necks for which a soft collar, analgesics, and possibly halter traction for several days may be necessary. If anterior displacement of C1 is demonstrated, halter traction for correction is followed by Minerva jacket or halo vest immobilization in the corrected position for 6 weeks. C1–2 fusion is indicated for neurologic involvement, persistent anterior displacement, failure to maintain or achieve correction if the deformity has been present for more than 3 months, or recurrence of deformity following 6 weeks of immobilization.

14. These are epiphyseal fractures through the synchondrosis. They are treated with reduction in recumbency and hyperextension followed by use of a Minerva jacket for 6 weeks. Lateral flexion-extension films are obtained after removal of the jacket to assess healing.

15. Eighty-six percent to 100%.

16. Eosinophilic granuloma (vertebral plana).

17. Gaucher's disease, mucopolysaccharidosis, lymphoma, metastatic disease, osteogenesis imperfecta.

18. After walking age—most commonly by 7 to 8 years of age.

QUESTIONS

19. What problems are encountered in pelvic fractures in children? What problems are associated with hip fractures in this age group?

20. When does the triradiate cartilage fuse?

21. What are the current recommendations for treatment of anterior-superior iliac spine, anterior-inferior iliac spine, and ischial tuberosity avulsion fractures in children?

22. How should pelvic straddle fractures in children be treated?

23. How should Malgaigne (vertical sheer) fractures in children be treated?

24. Describe the treatment of children's central acetabular fracture-dislocations.

25. What are the two types of transepiphyseal femoral neck fractures in children? Describe their treatment.

26. What problems are common with transepiphyseal fractures?

27. What is the major problem with transcervical fractures in children?

ANSWERS

19. Pelvic fractures are associated with severe trauma with short-term risks to life and limb. In the long term, however, most do well. Hip fractures, on the other hand, are associated with many complications (nonunion, coxa vara, avascular necrosis) and necessitate early agressive treatment.

ANSWERS

20. At age 16 to 18 years in males, 12 to 14 in females.

21. Bed rest for several days, then crutches for 4 to 5 weeks; return to athletics in 10 to 16 weeks. Marked displacement (1–2 cm) of ischial tuberosity avulsions in athletes may benefit from open reduction and internal fixation.

22. Bed rest for 4 to 6 weeks with hip flexion to relieve pull on the abdominal muscles. Traction is not necessary since the limbs are not affected. A pelvic sling is not necessary.

23. These are chondro-osseous separations in contrast to adult ligamentous injuries, and reduction is achieved with skeletal traction and a pelvic sling for 3 to 6 weeks. Rarely, external fixation, open reduction and internal fixation, and a spica cast may be necessary. These fractures will heal in 6 weeks if reduced.

24. Distal femoral pin traction. If not satisfactory, add lateral traction. Open reduction and internal fixation has not improved the essentially poor results associated with this injury.

25. (1) Transepiphyseal fracture without dislocation: treatment is closed reduction with longitudinal traction, abduction, and internal rotation, then fixation with smooth pins, and a spica cast for 6 weeks. (2) Fracture associated with hip dislocation: one attempt at closed reduction is made; if unsuccessful, open reduction through Watson-Jones or Smith-Peterson exposures is carried out with smooth pin fixation and a spica cast for 6 weeks.

26. Avascular necrosis (AVN) of the femoral head, premature closure of the proximal femoral physis, and nonunion.

27. The rate of AVN is 40%, with higher rates in displaced neck fractures.

QUESTIONS

28. How should transcervical femoral fractures in children be treated?

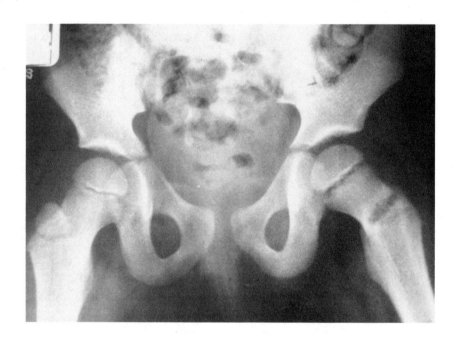

29. What are the major problems associated with displaced cervicotro-chanteric fractures in children?

30. Describe the treatment of cervicotrochanteric fractures in children.

31. Describe the treatment of intertrochanteric fractures in children.

32. After a hip fracture malunion in a child, what degree of coxa vara will produce an unacceptable result, possibly requiring a valgus intertrochanteric osteotomy?

33. Describe the treatment of femoral neck stress fractures in children.

ANSWERS

28. Nondisplaced fractures are treated by pin fixation and a spica cast for 6 weeks. Displaced fractures are treated by closed reduction (like adult neck fractures: traction, ABD, internal rotation), with pins, and a spica cast for 6 weeks. This can prevent coxa vara and nonunion. Aggressive treatment probably does not affect the incidence of AVN or growth arrest.

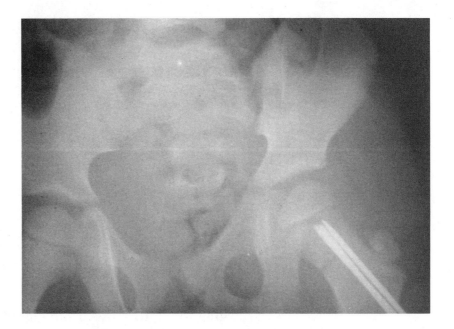

29. AVN (the rate is 25%) and coxa vara, if not reduced and pinned.

30. Nondisplaced fractures are treated by abduction hip spica cast for 6 weeks with close follow-up with good radiographs to be sure coxa vara does not develop. Displaced fractures are treated by closed reduction and pinning without crossing the physis.

31. Skin or skeletal traction followed by a spica cast; internal fixation for fractures in which reduction cannot be achieved or maintained.

32. While this depends on the age of the child, malunion with neck-shaft angles of less than 110 degrees may require corrective osteotomy.

33. The treatment is the same as in adults: the transverse type occurring in the superior neck should be pinned; the compression type in the inferior neck is treated by nonweightbearing for 6 weeks, then partial weightbearing for 6 weeks.

QUESTIONS

34. Describe the treatment of a traumatic dislocation of the hip in a child.

35. How should birth femoral fractures be treated?

36. How should ipsilateral femur and tibia fractures be treated in children?

37. Describe the treatment of bilateral femoral shaft fractures in a child.

38. Describe the treatment of femoral shaft fractures in infants, 2 to 10-year-olds, 10- to 15-year-olds, and children older than 15 years.

39. What is acceptable shortening and angulation in children 2 to 10 years old with femur fractures treated with immediate spica casts?

40. In managing the 2- to 10-year-old child with a femur fracture in traction, what is the desired amount of shortening?

41. Describe the treatment of femur fractures in children 10 to 15 years of age.

ANSWERS

34. Emergent closed reduction, then skin traction for 1 week followed by nonweightbearing crutch ambulation for 3 weeks.

35. With an immediate spica cast in 45 degrees of hip abduction, 90 degrees of flexion, and 15 degrees of external rotation, or modified Bryant's traction.

36. Treatment is 90/90 distal femur traction and a short leg cast. In polytraumatized or head-injured children, internal or external fixation may be considered.

37. Bilateral split Russell or 90/90 traction. Children older than 14 to 15 years may be treated with IM nailing.

38. Infants are treated in an immediate spica cast. In children 2 to 10 years old, if on resting radiograph there is less than 2 cm shortening, then a spica cast is applied; If there is more than 2 cm shortening, treatment is split Russell traction. In children aged 10 to 15 years treatment is 90/90 traction and a spica cast when sticky. Children 15 years or older are treated like adults (internal fixation or distal tibial traction followed by a femoral cast brace).

39. Up to 2 cm shortening, up to 20 to 30 degrees of angulation in the anteroposterior (AP) plane, and up to 10 to 15 degrees of varus or valgus angulation. Increased angulation is acceptable in the younger child in this group. Follow the patient weekly for 3 weeks with radiographs. Then return at 6 to 8 weeks after injury for radiograph out of plaster.

40. One to 1.5 cm. After 2 to 3 weeks in traction, apply a spica cast.

41. Treatment is 90/90 traction with a hip spica cast when the fracture is not tender (3–6 weeks). Total treatment time is 8 to 12 weeks. There is a greater tendency to shortening in these patients. Half-pin external fixation or unreamed IM nail are alternative methods.

QUESTIONS

42. Describe the treatment of distal femoral epiphyseal separations.

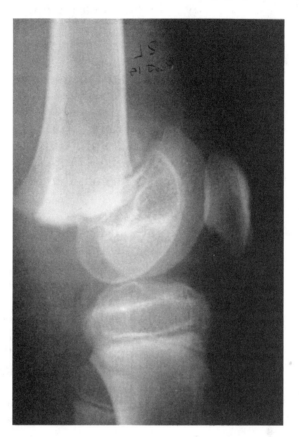

43. Describe the treatment of talus neck fractures in children.

44. What is the management of children with posttraumatic AVN of the body of the talus after union of a talar neck fracture?

45. What are the mechanisms of injury in medial and lateral transchondral dome fractures of the talus?

46. Describe the treatment of transchondral dome fractures of the talus in a child.

ANSWERS

42. Salter-Harris grades I and II are treated with closed reduction with traction, tilt, and reduction. Anterior displacement is treated with a cast in slight to moderate knee flexion for 6 weeks. Posterior displacement is treated with a cast in extension. Medial or lateral displacement is treated with a cast molded to hold reduction. If displaced, Salter-Harris grades III and IV are treated by skewering the fragment with a Steinmann pin percutaneously. Under fluoroscopy, the fracture is reduced and pinned. Open reduction and internal fixation is reserved for cases that cannot be treated as above.

43. The treatment is similar to treatment in adults. Patients with non-displaced fractures are treated in nonweightbearing cast until the fracture is united, then 2 weeks in a short leg weightbearing cast. Displaced fractures are treated by closed reduction (acceptable limits in closed reduction are 5 mm of displacement, 5 degrees of malalignment). If acceptable, a long leg nonweightbearing cast is applied for 4 to 6 weeks (until united, then a short leg weightbearing cast for 2 weeks). Occasionally, it may be necessary to put the foot in plantar flexion and eversion to maintain reduction, but the fracture usually is stable enough to achieve a neutral ankle position. If unacceptable, open reduction and internal fixation is done through a dorsomedial approach over the neck of the talus, keeping medial to the extensor hallucis longus to avoid damage to the anterior tibial vessels. With minimal exposure to allow reduction, internal fixation is done with Kirschner wires or cancellous screws. The patient is followed monthly for the first 6 months since AVN usually shows up within the first 6 months.

44. No conclusive series have documented the advantages of weightbearing or nonweightbearing. Nonweightbearing until revascularization is evident is a worthy goal, although not easily achieved in a child.

45. In medial fractures, plantar flexion inversion produces a posteromedial lesion. In lateral fractures; dorsiflexion and inversion produce an anterolateral lesion.

46. One may try cast immobilization for 1 to 2 months for stage I and II lesions (Anderson modification of Berndt/Hartz classification. Stages II, IIA, III, and IV can be treated with arthroscopic drilling, curettage, and sometimes excision.

QUESTIONS

47. Describe the treatment of calcaneal fractures in children.

48. What is the most common location for stress fractures in children?

49. How do you treat children with tibial stress fractures?

50. What is the recommended treatment for tibial fractures in meningomyelocele or cerebral palsy patients?

51. What are the four prevalent theories regarding valgus angular deformity after proximal tibial greenstick fractures?

52. Describe the treatment of proximal tibial metaphyseal fractures.

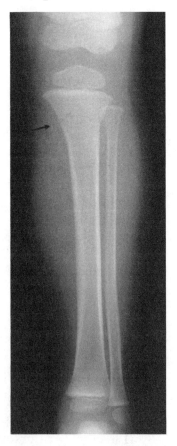

53. Describe the treatment of children's ankle fractures.

ANSWERS

47. A nonweightbearing cast is applied for 4 to 6 weeks. Then, activities are allowed, as tolerated. The fractures remodel up to about 15 years of age.

48. The tibia.

49. Rest. For an active noncompliant child; a long leg cast for 4 to 6 weeks.

50. Immobilization for 1 to 2 weeks in a bulky dressing or posterior molded padded splint. After splint removal, fit the child in an orthosis for early standing and walking. Physeal injuries are usually nondisplaced and need only immobilization for brief periods.

51. (1) Medial tibial overgrowth, (2) inadequate reduction with interposed periosteum, (3) lateral fibular tether, or (4) growth inhibition. Medial tibial growth stimulation appears to be the most likely explanation.

52. Obtain AP films with the leg extended. Any valgus angulation must be corrected by closed manipulation under anesthesia and a long leg cast with the knee in extension for 6 weeks. If the valgus deformity recurs, the fracture should be remanipulated. If reduction is not successful and a residual valgus deformity or medial fracture gap remains, open the fracture and remove soft tissue, reduce, and then apply the cast.

53. Salter-Harris grades I and II are treated by closed reduction and a long leg cast for 3 weeks, then a short leg cast for 3 weeks. Salter-Harris grades III and IV are treated by closed reduction under general anesthesia. If any displacement is present, treat with open reduction and internal fixation (ORIF), 3 weeks in a long leg cast, and 3 weeks in a short leg weightbearing cast. Juvenile Tillaux and triplane fractures are treated by closed reduction through foot internal rotation. If any displacement is noted after reduction on CT or tomos, ORIF is carried out. For two-fragment triplane fractures, an anterolateral approach is used to reduce anterolateral fragment. For three-fragment triplane fractures, the medial fragment is reduced first, then the anterolateral fragment.

QUESTIONS

54. How should patellar fractures in children be treated?

55. How should you treat ankle ligament tears in children?

56. What is a Sinding-Larsen-Johansson lesion?

57. Describe the treatment of symptomatic Osgood-Schlatter disease.

58. Give some general guidelines as to how much shortening in displaced tibiofibular fractures is acceptable in children?

59. What are some average healing times for closed and open displaced tibiofibular fractures in children?

60. How much angular deformity is acceptable in children's tibiofibular fractures?

61. What is the recommended treatment for bicycle spoke injuries to a child's foot?

62. What is a good test for injury to Lisfranc's joints?

63. What can prevent closed reduction of a Lisfranc joint dislocation?

ANSWERS

54. Nondisplaced with less than 4 mm of diastasis, and less than 3 mm of articular step-off, treat with a cast in extension. Displaced transverse fractures are treated with open reduction and internal fixation with tension band wire and repair of the retinaculum. Medial or lateral marginal fractures are excised.

55. Complete tears of the entire medial or lateral ligamentous complex warrant repair. In partial tears, apply cast or cast brace with early weightbearing.

ANSWERS

56. New bone formation adjacent to the anterior aspect of the distal pole of the patella following the onset of knee pain with associated limp. Radiographs demonstrate healing phase of an avulsion of the ligament from the distal pole of the patella. These usually occur in preadolescents. The acute phase is treated with a cylinder cast for 3 to 4 weeks.

57. Quadriceps strengthening, with hamstring stretching and activity modification. If symptoms persist, a cylinder cast is applied with the knee in extension for 3 to 4 weeks. Rarely, excision of ossicles after closure of the growth plate may be necessary.

58. In children aged 1 to 5 years, shortening of 5 to 10 mm is acceptable; in children aged 5 to 10, up to 5 mm is acceptable, in children over 10 years old, no shortening is acceptable.

59. Closed fractures heal in 5 to 13 weeks, open fractures in 3 to 5 months.

60. Five degrees of varus or valgus deformity is acceptable. Ten degrees of recurvatum deformity is acceptable. The tibia remodels surprisingly little (on average, only 10%).

61. Obtain a radiograph. Admit the child and elevate the foot in a bulky dressing. Necrosis of soft tissue and skin requires debridement and a split-thickness skin graft.

62. Gentle passive supination and pronation of the forefoot, with the hindfoot held fixed with the other hand, will elicit tarsometatarsal pain in Lisfranc joint injuries.

63. An anterior tibial tendon entrapped between fracture fragments at the base of the second metatarsal, and unreduced small fracture fragments. The key to obtaining reduction is reducing the second metatarsal base, after which the others tend to fall into place. They are then pinned with 0.062 Kirschner wires.

QUESTIONS

64. How are birth clavicle fractures treated?

65. How are birth humerus fractures treated?

66. How are birth femur fractures treated?

67. How are stress fractures of the femoral neck treated in children? What are the two types?

68. What are the features of active and latent unicameral bone cysts?

69. How should flexion-type supracondylar humerus fractures in children be treated?

70. What is the major complication of the flexion supracondylar fracture of the humerus?

71. How are nondisplaced lateral condyle fractures of the humerus treated?

72. How are moderately displaced lateral humerus condyle fractures treated?

ANSWERS

64. Most are not treated. Large babies (>9 lb) are immobilized with a Velpeau bandage.

ANSWERS

65. Velpeau bandage with an abduction pad to facilitate humerus abduction for 10 to 14 days. The humerus will remodel up to 50 degrees of angulation. Associated radial nerve palsy usually resolves in 6 to 8 weeks.

66. A one-and-one-half hip spica with the knee in slight flexion is applied. The knee is flexed more when the fracture is in the proximal femur.

67. Treatment is protected ambulation and possibly bed rest. The two types are (1) the transverse type, demonstrated radiographically by a lucency at the superior part of the femoral neck. These can become displaced and should be internally fixed with cancellous screws. (2) The compression type has a haze of callus on the inferior aspect of the neck. Displacement rarely occurs.

68. If active cysts abut on the epiphyseal plate, they still possess growth potential, whereas latent cysts are some distance from the growth plate and have less potential for growth. Ten percent of cysts that present with pathologic fracture will heal completely.

69. Closed reduction in extension with percutaneous pinning or open reduction and internal fixation.

70. Ulnar nerve injury. Elbow stiffness is frequent. Unsatisfactory results in displaced fractures are common. Parents should be told immediately that this is a difficult and problematic fracture with a high frequency of poor outcome.

71. With less than 2 mm of displacement, the articular surface is intact and the condylar fragment is hinged open laterally. There is no lateral shift of the olecranon. Treatment is posterior splint with the elbow flexed more than 90 degrees for 3 to 5 days. If there is no displacement on follow-up radiographs, then a long arm cast is applied for 3 weeks.

72. With moderate displacement, the fracture extends completely through the articular surface allowing additional displacement and olecranon shift. Hyperflexing and pronating the forearm can often effect reduction. This is followed by percutaneous pin fixation.

QUESTIONS

73. How are displaced and rotated lateral condyle fractures treated?

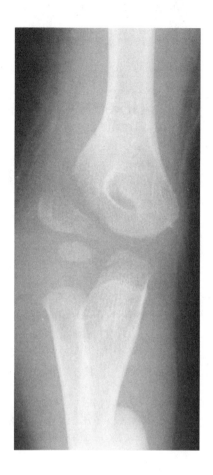

74. What complications occur in humerus lateral condyle fractures?

75. What problems occur in children with displaced medial condyle fractures of the humerus?

76. How should medial humeral condyle fractures in children be treated?

77. What is the most important stabilizer of the distal radioulnar joint?

78. How are Galeazzi fracture-dislocations in children treated?

79. What is Baumann's angle?

ANSWERS

73. By closed reduction and percutaneous pinning if needed. The best way is open reduction and internal fixation through Kocher's approach.

74. Malunion resulting in cubitus valgus and varus; nonunion or delayed union resulting in lateral condyle overgrowth and spur formation; ulnar nerve palsy secondary to cubitus valgus.

75. Nonunion and growth disturbance (cubitus valgus and varus).

76. Open reduction and internal fixation.

77. Triangular fibrocartilage complex.

78. Treatment is closed reduction in longitudinal traction, with correction of radius angulation. With the radius out to length, the distal radioulnar joint is reduced and held in full supination in a long arm cast for 6 weeks. In a child over 12, if satisfactory reduction is not obtained, treatment is open reduction and internal fixation of the radius with a four-hole plate and closed reduction of the distal radioulnar joint.

79. On the AP view of the humerus, Baumann's angle is formed by the physeal line of the lateral condyle and a line perpendicular to the long axis of the humerus; it is most useful when compared with the normal side. Normal is about 11 degrees.

QUESTIONS

80. Which fat pad can be normally seen in an elbow?

81. What is the mechanism of injury for most supracondylar fractures of the humerus in children?

82. What is the most common nerve injury in children with supracondylar fractures?

83. How should a pulseless hand associated with a supracondylar humerus fracture be treated?

84. What injuries are associated with fractures of the radial head?

85. What are the indications for surgery of a child's medial epicondyle fracture?

86. How should proximal humerus fractures in infants to age 1 year be treated?

87. How should proximal humerus fractures in children 1 to 5 years old be treated?

88. Describe the treatment of proximal humerus fractures in the 5 to 12-year-old age group.

ANSWERS

80. The anterior fat pad. The posterior fat pad is not seen unless displaced from the olecranon fossa by an elbow effusion.

81. Elbow hyperextension which allows the olecranon to impact posteriorly producing an extension-type supracondylar fracture.

82. Radial nerve injury.

83. If after closed reduction signs of vascular compromise persist (i.e., loss of pulses, loss of active function of the forearm muscles), consider immediate exploration or application of traction followed by brief observation. Operate if marked improvement has not occurred after 1 hour of traction.

84. Rupture of the triceps, elbow dislocation, Essex-Lopresti injury.

85. Fracture fragments in the joint that cannot be manipulated out; ulnar nerve dysfunction; large fragments displaced to the joint level; an elbow that is unstable to valgus stress.

86. These fractures are usually Salter-Harris I. Reduction is by gentle traction in a position of 90 degrees of flexion and 90 degrees of abduction. Reduce the fracture by pushing the metaphysis through the periosteum back (posteriorly and medially) into the periosteal tube. If stable after reduction, immobilize the arm against the trunk. If unstable, maintain the arm in the abducted position with some external rotation. The fracture gets sticky in 3 to 4 days. Protect from hyperextension and adduction for 2 weeks.

87. Any apposition of fracture fragments with less than 70 degrees of angulation can be accepted. If a satisfactory position cannot be obtained, an abduction splint or traction may be necessary.

88. Angulated fractures that are displaced greater than 50% of the shaft diameter should be reduced. It may be necessary to hold the reduction in a shoulder spica in flexion, abduction, slight external rotation, or overhead traction for 2 weeks.

QUESTIONS

89. Describe the treatment of proximal humerus fractures in the group aged from 12 years to maturity.

90. In a child with 1 year of growth remaining, how much angulation and displacement can be accepted in fracture of the proximal humeral physis?

91. In a child, what differentiates separation of the distal humeral physis from a dislocated elbow?

92. How are fractures of the distal humeral physis treated?

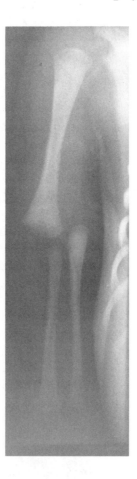

93. What should always be considered regarding the cause of fractures of the distal humeral physis?

94. What is Little Leaguer's elbow?

ANSWERS

89. There is less remodeling potential than in younger children and less potential as maturity is approached. These fractures may be difficult to reduce and hold. Muscular pull on the proximal physeal fragment causes it to flex, abduct, and rotate slightly externally. The best position to maintain reduction is the "salute position" with the arm in 90 degrees of abduction, the humerus brought forward 45 degrees, and the extremity rotated to place the hand in front of the face. The arm can also be held in traction; in prefabricated and custom splints; and with percutaneous pinning or open reduction and internal fixation. Open reduction is, however, seldom, if ever, indicated. Reduction in this age group can often be done using a bupivacaine hydrochloride (Marcaine) block from a posterolateral approach with application of the salute cast or splint.

90. Forty-five degrees of angulation and 50% displacement.

91. In an elbow dislocation, the proximal radius and ulna usually are displaced posterolaterally and the relationship between the proximal radius and lateral condyle epiphysis is disrupted. In the physeal separation, the displacement is usually posterior and medial. An arthrogram is helpful in cases in which ossification centers are not present.

92. By closed reduction with the elbow flexed and pronated; pin fixation is helpful in maintaining reduction in older children.

93. Child abuse.

94. Medial epicondyle stress fracture.

QUESTIONS

95. How should fractures of the medial epicondyle in children be treated? What are the indications for surgery?

96. How should avulsions of the lateral epicondylar epiphysis be treated?

97. How should distal humeral T-condyle fractures in children be treated?

98. Describe the Wilkins classification of children's proximal radius fractures.

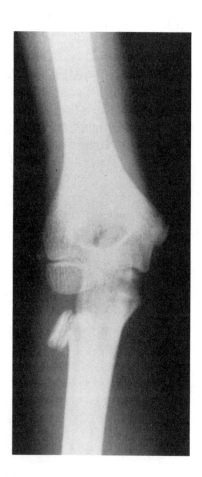

ANSWERS

95. Minimally or nondisplaced fractures are treated with a posterior splint for 1 to 2 weeks, followed by active range-of-motion exercises. Moderately (>5–10 mm) displaced fractures, in an athlete who needs a stable elbow (e.g., gymnast, baseball pitcher, wrestler) or in the presence of valgus instability, are treated with open reduction and internal fixation (ORIF). If the patient is not an athlete or if there is no instability, immobilize the elbow in hyperflexion for 2 weeks. Then begin active range-of-motion exercises. Fragments in a dislocated joint can be removed with closed manipulation; if unsuccessful, perform open extraction with ORIF or resection of the medial epicondyle. If ulnar nerve dysfunction is present, consider ORIF concomitant with exploration of the ulnar nerve. Anterior transposition of the ulnar nerve is not necessary. For Little Leaguer's elbow, modify the throwing activities to prevent permanent dysfunction.

96. Immobilize the joint for comfort, then begin active range-of-motion exercises. Unless the fragment is entrapped in the joint, nonoperative treatment is indicated.

97. By closed reduction, traction, then casting, and sometimes open reduction and internal fixation if closed reduction is inadequate. Most patients lose motion regardless of the type of treatment.

98. The Wilkins classification of children's proximal radius fractures comprises three groups, based upon the mechanism of injury and the direction of displacement of the radial head. Type II are neck-displaced fractures consisting of subtype A: angular, and subtype B: torsional injuries. Type III consists of stress injuries and includes osteochondritis of the radial head (subtype A) and neck physeal injuries with angulation (subtype B). Type I valgus fractures are divided into subtype A, Salter-Harris I and II fractures of the proximal radial physis; subtype B, Salter-Harris IV fractures of the proximal radial physis; and subtype C, fractures of the proximal radial metaphysis only. Type I fractures associated with dislocation of the elbow are subtype D, which are reduction injuries, and subtype E, which are dislocation injuries.

QUESTIONS

99. How are children's radial head and neck fractures treated?

100. How should children's flexion olecranon fractures be treated?

101. How are children's extension olecranon fractures treated?

102. How are children's shear olecranon fractures treated?

103. How should posterior elbow dislocations in children be treated?

104. What pathologic events lead to recurrent elbow dislocations?

105. What are the radiographic features seen in congenital dislocation of the radial head?

106. You return home after the Orthopedic Department's Christmas party to find that your 4-year-old son is crying and lying in bed watching TV. He complains of pain in the right elbow. The baby sitter admits to no history of trauma. The child developed elbow pain after being swung around by the arms, while playing. Physical examination reveals no bony deformity. The elbow is held in a slightly flexed position. The olecranon is in normal relationship to the lateral and medial epicondyles. Most of the tenderness is localized to the radial aspect of the joint. Range of motion is limited by pain. What is the most likely diagnosis?

ANSWERS

99. As conservatively as possible. They usually lose pronation and supination regardless of whether anatomic reduction is obtained. Fortunately, they usually do not have pain from injury residua. With 0 to 30 degrees of angulation, no reduction is needed; treatment is 7 to 10 days of immobilization, then range-of-motion exercises. With greater than 30 degrees of angulation, treatment is closed reduction; 45 degrees of angulation is acceptable. If the passive range of supination and pronation is 60 to 70 degrees in both directions, one should consider accepting the reduction. If residual angulation is greater than 45 degrees, consider open reduction with internal fixation (ORIF). If the fragment is com-

ANSWERS

pletely displaced and cannot be reduced, treatment is open reduction and internal fixation with oblique pins. After closed reduction, immobilize in 90 degrees of elbow flexion and slight pronation. Begin active range-of-motion exercises in 7 to 10 days.

100. Nondisplaced fractures are immobilized in 40 to 60 degrees of flexion for several weeks. Displaced fractures are treated by open reduction and internal fixation with tension band wiring, absorbable suture, and axial screws.

101. The elbow is placed in extension and manipulated; with this correction, the radial head will reduce spontaneously. Follow closely for 1 to 2 weeks. Remanipulation may be necessary. ORIF may be needed in displaced fractures.

102. The distal fragment is displaced anteriorly. The posterior periosteum remains intact. Use the posterior periosteum as a hinge for closed reduction. Immobilize in elbow flexion to keep the fracture reduced. If reduction cannot be achieved or held, perform open reduction with screw fixation.

103. By closed reduction. Supinate or hypersupinate the forearm to unlock the radius and ulna from the humerus; then reduce. The elbow is placed in a cast in 90 degrees of flexion, in midpronation for 5 to 7 days, then the cast is removed and active range-of-motion exercises are begun.

104. The posterior lateral (radial) ligamentous and capsular structures heal in a lax position after reduction of the first dislocation. The medial collateral ligament also becomes attenuated.

105. A short ulna or long radius, a hypoplastic or absent capitellum, a partially defective trochlea, a prominent medial epicondyle, a dome-shaped radial head with a long neck, and grooving of the distal humerus. These defects can also be seen in longstanding posttraumatic dislocations.

106. Nursemaid's elbow, also known as subluxation of the radial head.

QUESTIONS

107. How are subluxations of the radial head reduced?

108. How should plastic deformation of the forearm bones in children be treated?

109. In what direction does the radial head dislocate in Monteggia fractures?

110. Describe the Bado classification of Monteggia fractures.

111. Describe the treatment for each Bado classification of Monteggia fracture.

112. What prevents achieving or maintaining reduction in a child's Bado I Monteggia fracture?

113. What should be done if the radial head cannot be reduced or maintained?

114. What constitutes a nondisplaced olecranon fracture?

115. How should sternoclavicular injuries in children be treated?

ANSWERS

107. By full supination. If the radial head is not reduced, proceed to full flexion of the elbow. If recurrent, i.e., three episodes or more, then apply a cast for 3 weeks. Usually no immobilization is needed.

108. The forearm is manipulated to correct the deformity, and then placed in a long arm cast for 6 weeks. Loss of motion (supination and pronation) will result if left uncorrected. In children less than 10 years of age, some remodeling can help correct the bowing.

109. In the same direction as the apex of the ulnar fracture in all cases.

ANSWERS

110. *Type I* (most common, in 60%–80%) is an anterior dislocation of the radial head with an apex anterior angulated ulna fracture. *Type II* is posterior dislocation of the radial head, with an apex posterior ulna fracture. *Type III* is lateral or anterolateral dislocation of the radial head, with fracture of the ulnar metaphysis. *Type IV* (5% or less) is anterior dislocation of the radial head with fracture of the proximal one third of the radius and fracture of the ulna at the same level.

111. Most authors agree that treatment should include closed manipulation in children. In type I, the elbow is flexed with longitudinal traction and the forearm is supinated fully to effect reduction of the ulna. The radial head will then slip back into the reduced position with gentle pressure from the thumb on the radial head. The arm is immobilized in a long arm cast 4 for 6 weeks in 100-degree elbow flexion and full forearm supination. In type II, longitudinal traction with the elbow extended allows the head to reduce. A long arm cast is applied with the elbow extended for 4 weeks until the ulna fracture is healed. In type III, the elbow is extended, and pressure is applied over the radial border of the ulna. Usually this will reduce the lateral dislocation of the radial head as well. The patient is then placed in a long arm cast with the elbow in 90 degrees of flexion, and the forearm supinated for 4 weeks. Type IV fractures are treated by closed reduction with supination. If closed reduction fails, open reduction and internal fixation is performed.

112. Improper position of the elbow, i.e., less than 110 degrees of flexion; an infolded annular ligament; the radial head buttonholed through the capsule.

113. Open reduction with internal fixation of the ulnar fracture using a smooth IM pin usually allows radial head reduction.

114. Displacement of less than 2 mm with the elbow at 90 degrees and the patient able to actively extend the elbow (triceps still attached).

115. Since the sternal end of the clavicle growth plate does not close until age 23 to 25 years, most of these injuries are Salter-Harris I or II epiphyseal separations. Treatment is nonoperative.

QUESTIONS

116. True or false? Injuries in children that are suspicious for child abuse need to be reported to the appropriate state authority.

117. True or false? The incidence of child abuse is estimated to approach 1.0% to 1.5% of all children yearly.

118. True or false? Child abuse is most common in children under the age of 3 years.

119. True or false? The most likely perpetrator of child abuse is a parent.

120. Describe the hallmark findings of the skin lesions typical of child abuse.

121. True or false? Closed head injury is a frequent cause of disability and death in victims of child abuse.

122. Describe the fractures suspicious for child abuse commonly seen in orthopedic practice.

123. Evaluation of a child with a musculoskeletal injury secondary to suspected child abuse should include

124. What percentage of femoral fractures in children under the age of 4 years are secondary to child abuse?

125. What percentage of children presenting with femur fractures under the age of 2 years related to abuse?

ANSWERS

116. True. State and federal laws on child abuse make reporting mandatory and place the onus of reporting on the treating physician.

117. True.

118. True. Approximately 78% of abused children are under the age of 3; 50% are under the age of 1.

119. True. In approximately 95% of cases the child is abused by the parent(s).

120. Bruising in a linear pattern, and lacerations and burns over the perineum, trunk, back, and buttock are typical.

121. True. A careful neurologic assessment and visual inspection of the head and scalp along with AP and lateral skull films are indicated.

122. Epiphyseal and metaphyseal fractures (corner fractures), usually secondary to a torsion or pulling mechanism; multiple fractures in different phases of healing; diaphyseal fractures of the femur and humerus, not associated with a documented history of significant trauma; posterior rib fractures; spinal compression fractures.

123. Admission to the hospital; social service consult to evaluate the family situation and facilitate mandated reporting; a skeletal survey and, if necessary, bone scan to identify other areas of injury; clinical photographs if significant skin lesions are noted; definitive management of the orthopedic problem. Discharge can be considered only after resolution of the circumstances surrounding the child's injury have been answered and the child can be discharged into a safe environment.

124. 30%.

125. 80%.

QUESTIONS

126. What specific type of diaphyseal fracture pattern appears to be associated with abuse?

127. True or false? An isolated clavicle fracture is frequently encountered in child abuse cases.

128. An important differentiating feature between birth trauma fractures usually involving the humerus, clavicle, and femur, and those of child abuse is

129. True of false? Infants frequently sustain long-bone fractures of the humerus and femur in falls from the bed in the first year of life.

130. What percentage of Salter-Harris I and II fractures of the proximal tibia epiphysis are nondisplaced?

131. How can one make the diagnosis of a nondisplaced proximal tibia Salter-Harris I or II fracture?

132. Describe the treatment of proximal tibia epiphyseal fractures.

133. What complications can occur after separation of the proximal tibial epiphysis?

ANSWERS

126. Spiral and oblique fractures associated with significant rotational force.

127. False. Clavicle fractures make up less than 6% of child abuse fractures.

128. In birth trauma–related fractures, radiographic callus should be present by the 11th day of life. Fractures presenting after the 11th day of life without callus formation may be secondary to abuse.

129. False. While 30% of infants reportedly have a falling incident in the first year of life, long-bone fractures are exceedingly rare from this mechanism of injury. A history of a fall-induced fracture of the femur or humerus is suspicious for child abuse.

130. Fifty percent of type I fractures and 30% of type II fractures.

131. Stress radiographs. Sometimes tomograms and a CT scan can aid in quantitating the amount of displacement.

132. Nondisplaced Salter-Harris I–III fractures are treated in long leg cast immobilization. Monitor closely for displacement on follow-up. Displaced Salter-Harris grade I–IV fractures are treated by closed reduction in the operating room with application of a long leg cast. If unstable or not adequately reduced, use percutaneous pin or screw fixation, or open reduction with internal fixation.

133. (1) Recurrent deformity from loss of reduction. This may require remanipulation if displacement occurs at 1 week, or if unstable initially, one should proceed to percutaneous pin fixation or open reduction and internal fixation. (2) Vascular impairment. (3) Compartment syndrome. (4) Premature growth arrest with angular deformity or limb length discrepancy. (5) Nerve palsy.

QUESTIONS

134. What are the differences between Osgood-Schlatter disease and tibial tubercle avulsion fractures?

135. Describe the Watson-Jones classification of tibial tubercle avulsions.

136. How are tibial tubercle avulsion fractures treated?

137. What factors predispose to chronic subluxation of the patella?

138. Describe the treatment of osteochondral fragments secondary to a dislocated patella in children.

ANSWERS

134. Osgood-Schlatter disease is an avulsion of the anterior surface of the apophysis. It is characterized by insidious onset and intermittent mild symptoms. It usually responds to symptomatic treatment; the prognosis is good (occasionally an ununited ossicle may be symptomatic). Acute traumatic tubercle avulsion is a separation through the physis of the tubercle characterized by acute pain, swelling, and often an inability to stand or ambulate. Often open reduction and internal fixation is needed. The prognosis for rapid recovery is excellent.

135. Type I avulsions are fractures across the secondary ossification center at the level of the posterior border of the insertion of the patellar ligament (*A*). Type II occur at the junction of the primary and secondary ossification centers of the tibia (*B*). In type III, the fracture propagates upward across the epiphyseal plate and into the knee joint (Salter-Harris III) (*C*).

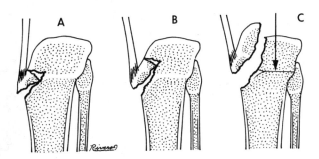

136. Most grade I fractures can be reduced and treated in a cast with the knee in extension. If, after reduction, more than 5 mm of displacement persists, open reduction and internal fixation (ORIF) should be performed. Displaced grade II and III fractures usually require ORIF.

137. Hypoplasia of the lateral femoral condyle, genu valgus, lateral tibial torsion, hypoplastic patella, patella alta, quadriceps insufficiency, and an increased Q angle.

138. Replace large fragments from the weightbearing surfaces as soon as possible using small threaded Steinmann pins or screws. Small fragments should be removed arthroscopically or through an arthrotomy.

QUESTIONS

139. Describe the Meyers-McKeever classification of tibial intercondylar eminence fractures.

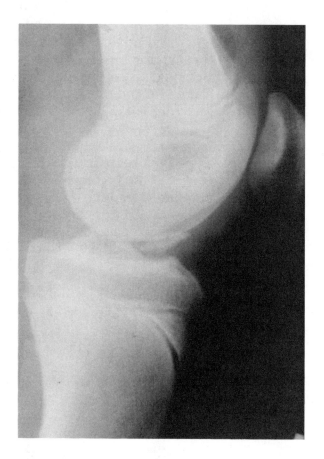

140. Why is the AP radiograph valuable in the evaluation of intercondylar eminence fractures?

141. Describe the treatment for intercondylar eminence avulsions.

142. What are the three types of partial physeal arrests?

143. What is the most common complication of surgical management of partial growth arrest?

ANSWERS

139. *Type I* is nondisplaced. *Type II* is a hinged fracture elevated anteriorly with the posterior rim of the avulsed fragment maintaining contact with the fracture bed. *Type III* is a completely displaced fracture.

140. The dimension of the fragment in the coronal plane is a significant factor in the choice of treatment. If the fragment is displaced and extends beneath the articular surfaces of the adjacent tibial condyles, there may be interposition of the anterior portions of the menisci between the displaced fragment and its bed, which could impede closed reduction.

141. Closed reduction. Knee aspiration, general anesthesia, and full knee extension to 20 degrees of flexion usually produce reduction. If full extension is not obtained, the reduction is probably not complete. This is because the avulsed fragment is prevented from reduction by the interposed lateral meniscus. Treatment is arthrotomy, reduction, possibly suture fixation, and a cast with the knee in extension. The fragment could also be manipulated and fixed arthroscopically. Type III avulsions usually cannot be reduced through closed techniques, and ORIF should be anticipated.

142. Type I is peripheral; type II is central; and type III is combined (sequelae of Salter-Harris grades III and IV).

143. Rebridging.

QUESTIONS

144. A 5-year-old right hand–dominant girl fell while riding her bicycle, sustaining a closed supracondylar humerus fracture seen on radiograph. The radial and ulnar pulses are not palpable. How should this patient be treated?

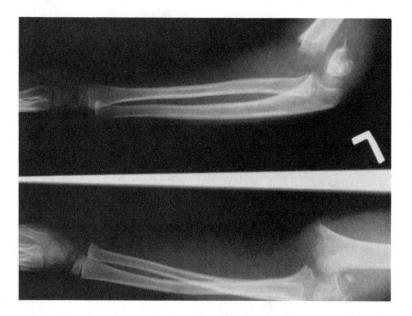

145. Before reaching the operating room, it is noted that the patient has lost her ability to flex the thumb interphalangeal (IP) joint as well as the index finger distal interphalangeal (DIP) joint. No sensory changes are noted. Passive flexion and extension of the digits does not produce excessive pain. What is causing this problem?

146. What is the treatment of choice for anterior interosseous nerve palsy associated with a displaced supracondylar fracture?

ANSWERS

144. A supracondylar fracture with a pulseless hand should be expeditiously reduced. The loss of pulse may be indicative of either arterial spasm secondary to stretch, direct trauma, arterial thrombosis, or arterial severance. If after reduction of the fracture the extremity remains pulseless, surgical exploration of the brachial artery should be performed. Waiting an hour after the reduction for resolution of the spasm is reasonable. However, because the patient has usually been taken to the operating room for closed reduction with percutaneous pinning or open reduction and internal fixation of this type of supracondylar fracture, most surgeons would immediately explore and repair any damage to the artery if the pulse did not rapidly return after reduction. Traction and reduction of the displaced supracondylar fracture has also been advocated with close monitoring for return of pulse. If the pulse has not been restored within an hour of the institution of traction, then exploration of the artery is advised.

145. The patient most likely has a neuropraxia of the anterior interosseous nerve.

146. In this particular case, while exploring the brachial artery one should also evaluate the median nerve and the anterior interosseous branch for damage. In most cases of closed supracondylar fracture without vascular impairment, following open or closed reduction the patient should be followed clinically. The vast majority should resolve spontaneously over the course of several months.

QUESTIONS

147. Describe the initial treatment approach to the fracture seen in the figures below in a 14-year-old boy who broke his ankle sliding into a base. He is neurovascularly intact and the skin is intact.

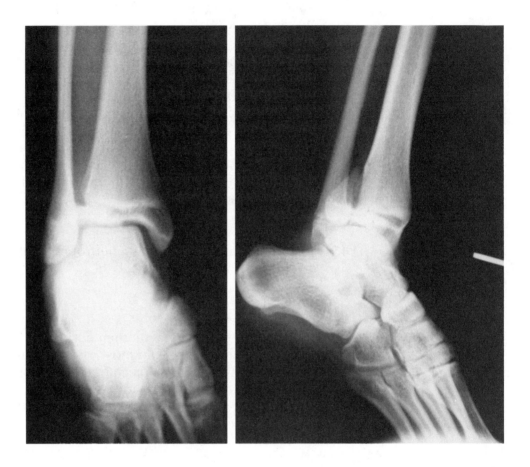

148. Following a closed reduction attempt, the fracture fragments are still separated by 3 mm, but the alignment of the bones is excellent. Is this a satisfactory reduction?

ANSWERS

147. Initial treatment for a triplane fracture consists of closed reduction and immobilization.

148. No. Anything less than an anatomic reduction warrants open reduction and internal fixation.

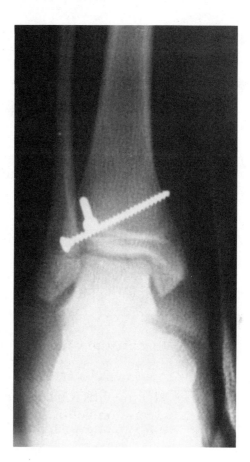

CHAPTER 4

Metabolic Disease

Timothy S. Loth, M.D.

Steven Mardjetko, M.D.

QUESTIONS

1. What orthopedic congenital deformities are associated with Fanconi's syndrome?

2. What orthopedic anomalies are associated with thalassemia major?

3. What is the biochemical abnormality seen in sickle cell disease?

4. What are the x-ray changes in sickle cell disease?

5. Osteomyelitis is a common sequela to sickle cell disease. Differentiate osteomyelitis associated with sickle cell disease from typical osteomyelitis in childhood.

6. What orthopedic problems are associated with fetal alcohol syndrome?

7. A 1-year-old black infant presents with acute pain and swelling of his right thumb. Radiographs reveal cortical scalloping and periosteal elevation. The patient has no systemic symptoms, and blood culture and bone aspirate cultures are negative. Hemoglobin electrophoresis reveals an SS pattern. The most likely diagnosis is:

ANSWERS

1. Anomalies of the thumb, first metacarpal, and hypoplasia of the radius. Others include congenital dislocation of the hip and syndactyly.

2. Osteoporosis and thinned cortices can result in pathologic fractures. The skull demonstrates diploic space widening with hair-on-end appearance. Pathologic fractures result from premature closure of the proximal humeral epiphysis with varus deformity, and spinal cord compression from extramedullary hematopoiesis.

3. Increased Hb S replaces the Hb A due to a single amino acid substitution on the beta chain (position 6, valine by glycine). The mode of transmission is autosomal recessive with 8% of African-Americans carriers of the gene.

4. Osteoporosis, thinning of long bone cortices, ground-glass skull with widened diploic spaces and hair-on-end appearance, decreased vertebral height, discs bulging into the bodies ("Lincoln log" appearance), epiphyseal infarcts (proximal femur and humerus), shaft necrosis, and hand-and-foot syndrome (sickle cell dactylitis) in 6- to 12-month-old infants (can be confused with osteomyelitis).

5. Osteomyelitis associated with sickle cell disease is usually diapyseal, is frequently multifocal, and the etiologic agent is most often salmonella (Epps recently reported staphylococcus to be the most common organism isolated in the United States).

6. Fused joints are frequently seen—radioulnar synostosis, fusion of the cervical spine, coalition of the capitate and hamate. Clinodactyly is also seen.

7. Sickle cell dactylitis. This disorder frequently involves the hands and feet in children under 3 years of age.

QUESTIONS

8. What is the metabolic defect in Gaucher's disease? What are the clinical considerations for management of Gaucher's disease?

9. What is the distal femoral deformity associated with Gaucher's disease?

10. What other orthopedic manifestations are seen in Gaucher's disease?

11. What are matrix vesicles?

12. What are the two sources of electrical potentials in bone?

13. Where do osteoclasts originate from?

14. What is the ruffled border?

15. What stimulates the formation of the ruffled border?

16. What are the zones of the growth plate?

ANSWERS

8. A deficiency of the enzyme β-glucocerebrosidase results in accumulation of glucocerebrosides in the liver, spleen, bone marrow, and sometimes the central nervous system (CNS). Most commonly, it is transmitted by autosomal recessive inheritance. Thrombocytopenia, leukopenia, and anemia result from infiltration of bone marrow. The cortex is thin, eroded by Gaucher's cells which proliferate and fill the marrow space. Patients may complain of bone pain. Vertebral compression fractures may occur. There is increased susceptibility to osteomyelitis which can be difficult to discern from bone infarcts. Avascular necrosis (AVN) must be considered if the patient has hip pain. Enzyme replacement therapy is now available.

ANSWERS

9. Erlenmeyer flask deformity.

10. AVN femoral heads (seen in up to 20% of patients); periosteal new bone and mottled rarefaction of involved bone secondary to marrow infiltration with foam cells.

11. Extracellular, membrane-invested particles that are the initial site of hydroxyapatite crystal formation in newly formed bone matrix, growth plate cartilage, and dental matrix.

12. (1) The piezoelectric effect generated by mechanical stress on bone, and (2) the "regeneration signal," produced in an area subjected to trauma.

13. The osteoclast is a bone marrow–derived cell. Osteoclast progenitors closely resemble monocytes and macrophages.

14. A complex of osteoclast plasma membrane enfoldings found over the portion of bone being resorbed. High levels of acid phosphatase have been identified in this region.

15. Parathyroid hormone (**PTH**) and osteoclast activating factor (**OAF**).

16. (1) The reserve zone, (2) the proliferation zone (chondroblasts actively dividing and synthesizing matrix), and (3) the hypertrophic zone (the chondrocytes enlarge their lacunae). The hypertrophic zone includes the zones of maturation, degeneration, and provisional calcification. In the zone of provisional calcification longitudinal cartilage septa calcify and the chondrocytes die. A zone of invasion has also been described where clasts partially resorb calcified cartilage matrix and osteoblasts form a layer of woven bone on top of the cartilaginous remnants. These trabeculae are the primary spongiosa. Further remodeling in the proximal metaphysis replaces primary spongiosa and cartilage remnants with lamellar bone (secondary spongiosa).

QUESTIONS

17. Where is calcium absorbed in the gut?

18. What effect does PTH have on the kidney?

19. What stimulates phosphate absorption and excretion?

20. Describe the synthesis of 1,25Dihydroxyvitamin D.

21. How does vitamin D affect its major tissue targets (bone, intestine, kidney)?

22. What stimulates and suppresses calcitonin release?

23. What effects does calcitonin have at its target organs (bone, kidney, GI tract)?

24. Which causes osteoporosis? Hyper- or hypothyroidism?

25. What is the differential diagnosis for osteoporosis?

26. What laboratory tests should be ordered initially on patients with osteoporosis?

ANSWERS

17. Calcium is absorbed in the duodenum via active transport, and in the jejunum via facilitated diffusion. Most calcium is absorbed in the jejunum. 1,25-Dihydroxyvitamin D is needed for gut calcium absorption. PTH is unnecessary for this direct effect of vitamin D.

18. It increases resorption of calcium and excretion of phosphate.

19. The major determinant of PO_4 absorption is the availability of PO_4 in the diet. The absorption of PO_4 in the intestine is directly concentration-dependent. PO_4 intestinal absorption is facilitated by 1,25-dihydroxyvitamin D_3. Urinary excretion of PO_4 in healthy adults is directly related to dietary PO_4 intake. Excretion is enhanced by increased PTH levels.

ANSWERS

20. Cholesterol precursors in the skin (7-dehydrocholesterol) and gastrointestinal (GI) tract (ergosterol) are converted by ultraviolet (UV) irradiation to vitamin D_3 (cholecalciferol) and ergocalciferol (vitamin D_2). In the liver, vitamin D_3 is changed to 25-hydroxyvitamin D_3. In the kidney, 25-hydroxyvitamin D_3 is changed to 1,25-dihydroxyvitamin D_3 or 24,25-dihydroxyvitamin D_3. The 1,25-dihydroxy metabolite is the most potent form of vitamin D.

21. Vitamin D acts to increase mobilization of calcium from bone and increase proximal renal tubule resorption of PO_4 and calcium in the kidney. 24-Hydroxylase activity is increased and 1-hydroxylase activity is decreased. In the intestine, vitamin D aids absorption of calcium and PO_4 and stimulates production of calcium-binding protein.

22. Calcitonin release is suppressed by hypocalcemia and stimulated by hypercalcemia.

23. In bone, decreased osteoclastic bone resorption; in kidney, decreased resorption of calcium and PO_4; in gut, increased secretion of sodium, potassium, chloride, and water, and decreased acid secretion. Calcitonin inhibits calcium and PO_4 absorption.

24. Hyperthyroidism.

25. Postmenopausal osteoporosis, hyperparathyroidism, hyperthyroidism, malignancy of medullary cavity (multiple myeloma), osteomalacia, glucocorticoid excess, osteogenesis imperfecta tarda, type I diabetes, rheumatoid arthritis, hemolytic anemia, dietary aberrations (milk intolerance, prolonged low calcium intake, alcoholism, vegetarian diet, GI malabsorption), smoking, drugs (anticoagulants, chronic lithium treatment, chemotherapy, anticonvulsants, chronic PO_4-binding antacids), and inactivity.

26. Serum phosphate, creatinine clearance, urinary hydroxproline, blood urea nitrogen (BUN), urine and serum calcium, thyroid function tests, complete blood count (CBC), and sedimentation rate.

QUESTIONS

27. What are the causes of osteomalacia?

28. What changes are seen in osteomalacia with regard to serum calcium, phosphate, and alkaline phosphatase, and urine phosphate and hydroxyproline?

29. What radiographic findings are consistent with nutritional osteomalacia?

30. What is the histologic hallmark of osteomalacia?

31. What is a common cause of malabsorption osteomalacia and how is it treated?

32. What does increased alkaline phosphate activity indicate in bone?

33. What are the four principal causes of rickets?

34. What is the usual age range during which one sees vitamin D–deficient rickets?

35. What is the basic pathologic disturbance in rickets?

36. What are the abnormalities noted microscopically at the growth plate in rickets?

37. What are the clinical findings in rickets?

ANSWERS

27. Deficiency of vitamin D (post gastrectomy), primary biliary cirrhosis, pancreatic insufficiency, vitamin D–resistant rickets, hypophosphatasia, drug-induced osteomalacia (phenytoin, phosphate-binding antacids, etc.), intestinal malabsorption, acquired and hereditary renal disorders (Fanconi's syndrome).

ANSWERS

28. Decreased or normal serum calcium, usually low serum phosphate, increased alkaline phosphatase; increased urine phosphate, and hydroxyproline.

29. Pseudofractures, Looser's zones, and biconcave ("codfish") vertebrae. Transiliac biopsy reveals widened osteoid seams with sequential tetracycline labeling.

30. Increased width and extent of osteoid seams.

31. Gluten-sensitive enteropathy. Treatment is a gluten-free diet and vitamin D.

32. Increased osteoblastic activity.

33. (1) Vitamin D deficiency, (2) renal tubular insufficiency, (3) chronic renal insufficiency, and (4) hypophosphatasia.

34. Vitamin D–deficient rickets rarely occurs before the sixth month or after the third year of life.

35. Failure of mineralization of osteoid.

36. Failure of deposition of calcium along the mature cartilage columns, disorderly invasion of cartilage by blood vessels, lack of resorption at the zone of provisional calcification, increased thickness of the epiphyseal plate, and disordered columnar arrangement in the zone of maturation. Osteoblastic activity in both endosteal and periosteal tissues is normal, forming abundant osteoid but the osteoid is not calcified and there is no normal lattice formation.

37. Decreased height and weight, muscular weakness, lethargy, and hypotonia; craniotabes (softening and thinning of the skull) and persistent fontanelles; rachitic rosary; thickening of the ankles, knees, and wrists with bone tenderness; bending of the soft bones of the lower extremity with weightbearing, producing tibial varus or valgus deformity and coxa varus; hepatomegaly; poor dentition.

QUESTIONS

38. What radiographic findings are consistent with rickets?

39. How is vitamin D dietary deficiency–induced rickets treated?

40. Which patients with rickets are resistant to vitamin D supplementation?

41. How is hypophosphatemic vitamin D–refractory rickets treated?

42. What is the metabolic defect in hypophosphatasia?

43. What are the microscopic changes seen in hypophosphatasia?

44. What are the clinical changes?

45. What are the laboratory abnormalities seen in hypophosphatasia?

46. How is hypophosphatasia treated?

ANSWERS

38. The epiphyseal plate is thickened and irregular. There is irregularity, cupping, and flaring of the metaphysis and epiphysis, a thinned cortex, and bowed long bones after weightbearing has begun. Looser's lines (pseudofractures) are seen.

39. Prevention. Premature infants require 2,000 IU/day for the first 3 months. Full-term infants require 400 IU/day. Treatment is vitamin D 1,500 to 5,000 units/day for 6 to 10 weeks. Within 2 to 4 weeks radiographs demonstrate evidence of healing.

ANSWERS

40. One of the commonest metabolic bone diseases of children is vitamin D–refractory rickets. Its clinical and radiographic features are the same as for rickets secondary to vitamin D deficiency and it does not respond to the usual dosage of Vitamin D. The problem appears to be diminished resorption of PO_4 in the renal tubules. Serum analysis reveals hypophosphatemia (1–3 mg/dL), increased serum alkaline phosphatase, normal to decreased calcium.

41. Oral phosphates 0.6 to 3.0 g/day and 1,25-dihydroxyvitamin D_3 can facilitate improved growth and healing of rickets.

42. A genetically determined inborn error of metabolism characterized by low alkaline phosphatase, undermineralization of bone and severe rachitic changes, and increased urinary excretion of phosphoethanolamine. The hypophosphatasia seen in infants and children is an autosomal recessive disorder.

43. The same as for rickets. However, histochemical studies of bone alkaline phosphatase activity can distinguish hypophosphatasia from rickets.

44. There are differing presentations depending on the age of onset. The earlier the onset, the more severe the disease manifestations. The childhood variety is characterized by premature loss of the deciduous teeth (usually before the age of 5 years), short stature, and rachitic changes. The prognosis for this variety is variable. It may improve spontaneously but may recur in adulthood. The adult variety presents in middle age with painful, poorly healing, and recurrent metatarsal stress fractures. Patients may also have pain in the hips due to femoral pseudofractures.

45. Decreased alkaline phosphatase (increased in rickets), normal serum phosphate, normal or increased serum calcium, and positive urine phosphoethanolamine.

46. No specific treatment is available.

QUESTIONS

47. Describe the blood chemistry findings (Ca, PO$_4$, alkaline phosphatase, urea, serum pH) for the following: vitamin D–deficiency rickets, hypophosphatemic vitamin D–resistent rickets, renal tubular acidosis, chronic renal failure, hypophosphatasia.

48. Describe the urine findings (glucose, protein, abnormal amino acids) for the following: vitamin D–deficiency rickets, hypophosphatemic vitamin D–resistent rickets, renal tubular acidosis, chronic renal failure, hypophosphatasia.

49. Describe the characteristics of Ehlers-Danlos syndrome.

50. Describe the orthopedic management of Ehlers-Danlos syndrome.

51. Describe the clinical features of Marfan's syndrome.

52. What is the mode of transmission of Marfan's syndrome?

53. Describe congenital contractural arachnodactyly.

ANSWERS

47. Vitamin D–deficiency rickets: normal or low calcium, low PO$_4$, high alkaline phosphatase, normal urea, normal pH; hypophosphatemic vitamin D–resistent rickets: normal calcium, low PO$_4$, high alkaline phosphatase, normal urea, normal pH; renal tubular acidosis: low Ca, low PO$_4$, high alkaline phosphatase, normal urea, acidic pH; chronic renal failure: normal or low calcium, high PO$_4$, high alkaline phosphatase, high urea, acidic pH; hypophosphatasia: normal or high calcium, normal PO$_4$, low alkaline phosphatase, normal or high urea, normal pH.

ANSWERS

48. Vitamin D–deficiency rickets: negative glucose, negative protein, negative amino acids; hypophosphatemic vitamin D–resistent rickets: negative glucose, negative protein, negative amino acids; renal tubular acidosis: negative glucose, positive protein, negative amino acids; chronic renal failure: negative glucose, positive protein, negative amino acids; hypophosphatasia: negative glucose, negative protein, positive aminoaciduria (phosphoethanolamine).

49. Ehlers-Danlos syndrome is usually an autosomal dominant condition characterized by skin that is hyperlax, thin, fragile, and bruisable; pseudotumors form over knees and elbows. Joint hypermobility, hernia, scoliosis, genu recurvatum, and recurrent dislocations of hips, patella, and shoulder occur. Traumatic joint effusions and hemarthrosis can occur secondary to hypermobility.

50. The most common problems are scoliosis and joint dislocation. Scoliosis is managed as idiopathic scoliosis. Joint dislocations (most commonly the patellofemoral and shoulder joints) are managed conservatively.

51. Marfan's syndrome affects the skeleton, heart, and the lens of the eye. Affected persons have tall stature, disproportionate growth of extremities in comparison to the trunk, arachnodactyly, scoliosis, pectus excavatum, protrusio acetabuli, pes valgus, and genu recurvatum; the lens may be superiorly dislocated; cardiovascular defects include heart valve abnormalities, aortic dilatation, and aneurysm.

52. Autosomal dominant.

53. Congenital contractural arachnodactyly is an autosomal dominant disorder that resembles Marfan's syndrome in that arachnodactyly is present. Differentiating it from Marfan's syndrome, however, are congenital peripheral contractures, which improve with growth; ear deformities; absence of heart disease and dislocated ocular lenses.

QUESTIONS

54. Describe homocystinuria.

55. What radiographs should be ordered in the evaluation of a disproportionally short patient?

56. What questions should be asked in the workup of a disproportionately short patient?

57. What is the biochemical defect common to the various forms of osteogenesis imperfecta (OI)?

58. What is the histologic defect seen in OI?

59. What radiographic findings are useful in making the diagnosis of OI?

ANSWERS

54. Homocystinuria is an autosomal recessive disorder characterized by tall stature, arachnodactyly, scoliosis, mental retardation, osteoporosis, fractures, thromboembolic phenomenon, and ectopic lens (inferiorly displaced). Normal intelligence does not rule out this diagnosis. Patients with the clinical features of Marfan's syndrome but no family history should have a urinalysis for homocystine.

55. Lateral skull, anteroposterior (AP) and lateral views of the spine; AP film of the pelvis; one AP and lateral film of one upper and lower extremity with a separate view of one hand; and an AP chest film to include the shoulders and clavicles.

56. Are the skeletal effects generalized or localized? Does any relative have a similar disorder? Was the disorder present at birth? What parts of the skeleton are most affected or deformed? What anatomic areas of the growing skeleton are predominately affected (epiphysis, metaphysis, cortical bone, vertebral bodies)? What portions of the long bones are most shortened (rhizomelic, mesomelic, etc.)? Is there abnormal density of all or parts of bone? Is

ANSWERS

there a combination of skeletal anomalies with other systems involved? Is pain present? (Bone dysplasias are usually not painful, whereas metabolic bone diseases may be.) Is there a history of fractures? Is weakness present?

57. Abnormalities in the structure or synthesis of type I collagen; decreased bone mass and increased bone turnover. Histologically, there is a lack of lamellar bone with abundant woven bone.

58. Inability to make lamellar bone, with the presence of large quantities of woven bone.

59. Osteoporosis; thin cortices; deformity of long bones secondary to fractures; multiple long bone and vertebral fractures; wormian bones in skull (the skull film may be a useful adjunct to evaluation); scoliosis.

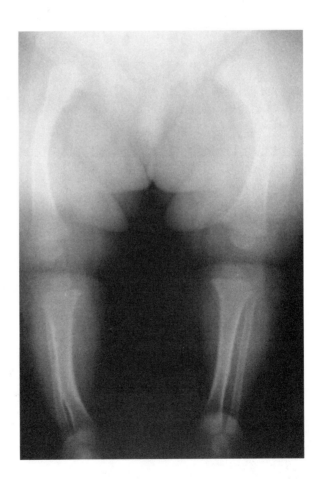

QUESTIONS

60. What orthopedic problems frequently require treatment in OI?

61. The Sillence classification of OI is divided into four types. Describe each.

62. Describe the Shapiro classification of OI.

63. Define osteochondrodysplasia.

64. Define dwarfism.

65. Define rhizomelic, mezomelic, and acromelic dwarfism.

ANSWERS

60. Fractures, bowing of bones, scoliosis.

61. *Type I*, the most common type, is autosomal dominant and characterized by fragile bones, blue sclerae, and hearing loss (in 50% of patients). Growth is least affected. *Type II* is rare, autosomal recessive or autosomal dominant (mutation). Blue sclerae and multiple fractures are found. Death is perinatal. *Type III* is rare, autosomal, recessive, and characterized by twisted, fractured, bowed bones; sclerae are variable in hue, dentinogenesis and hearing loss, are frequent; growth failure is severe. *Type IV* is rare, autosomal dominant. Bone fragility is mild to moderate; sclerae are normal; dentinogenesis is common; short stature is variable.

62. Shapiro's classification is based on when the initial fracture(s) occurred. Those occurring before or at birth are designated as osteogenesis imperfecta congenita (OIC). Patients that sustain fractures after birth are designated osteogenesis imperfecta tarda (OIT). OIC is subdivided based on the appearance of the long bones and ribs at the time of initial fracture. OIC-A patients have short, broad, and crumpled femora and ribs. This group did poorly with 94% mortality and one wheelchair-bound survivor. The OIC-B subgroup has normal bony contours with associated fractures. This group had an 8% early mortality; 59% were in wheelchairs and 33% were ambulatory. The OIT group was subdivided based on whether the initial fracture occurred before or after walking had begun. In OIT-A, the patient experienced the initial fracture before walking. This group was associated with 33% prevalence of wheelchair ambulators and 67% were ambulatory. The OIT-B group, in which fracture occurred after walking had begun, were all ambulatory.

63. Osteochondrodysplasia is a group of disorders characterized by an intrinsic abnormality of growth and remodeling of cartilage and bone.

64. Dwarfism is disproportionate short stature with a standing height below the 3rd percentile for age.

65. Rhizomelic dwarfism is characterized by increased shortening of proximal bone segments; mezomelic dwarfism refers to shortening of the forearms and tibias; acromelic dwarfism refers to involvement of hands and feet.

QUESTIONS

66. Name three common types of short limb dwarfism.

67. What is the most common type of short trunk dwarfism?

68. What is the most common type of short limb dwarfism?

69. What is the mode of inheritance in achondroplasia?

70. Describe the primary defect found in achondroplasia.

71. Describe the primary deformity seen in achondroplasia in the first year of life which demonstrates a tendency to resolution.

72. List the spinal regions where stenosis is frequently encountered in achondroplasia.

73. In an achondroplastic infant, apneic spells and delayed motor milestones have been identified. One possible cause may be:

74. Describe the clinical characteristics and radiographic findings in achondroplasia.

75. What orthopedic problems occur in achondroplasia?

ANSWERS

66. Achondroplasia, hypochondroplasia, and metaphyseal chondrodysplasia.

67. Spondyloepiphyseal dysplasia.

ANSWERS

68. Achondroplasia.

69. Autosomal dominant; 80% of the cases are secondary to random mutation.

70. Abnormal endochondral bone formation.

71. Thoracolumbar kyphosis.

72. At the level of the foramen magnum, frequently in the first year of life, and in the lumbar spine where symptomatic spinal stenosis develops in the third decade.

73. Medulla oblongata compression secondary to foramen magnum stenosis.

74. Marked dwarfing of body height; prominent forehead, saddle nose; disproportionate proximal limb shortening (humerus and femur); "starfish" or trident hands (short, thick divergent digits); prominent buttocks; exaggerated lumbar lordosis; compensatory thoracic kyphosis; bowed legs; short ribs; normal intelligence; waddling gait. On radiograph, the epiphysis is normal, but indented into the metaphysis: the metaphysis is flared; the diaphysis appears normal but short; the pelvic inlet has a "champagne-glass" contour; there is a progressive decrease in interpedicular distance from L1 to L5. As opposed to patients with mucopolysaccharidosis, patients with achondroplasia have extremely short ribs.

75. Thoracolumbar kyphosis. Treatment is to delay sitting in infancy; use a reclining infant's seat to avoid weight transmission to the spine. Bracing is needed if the kyphosis progresses. Spinal stenosis and disc disease occur secondary to the narrowed lordotic lumbar spine. Genu varum is found.

QUESTIONS

76. Describe the typical features of diastrophic dysplasia.

77. What is the incidence of kyphoscoliosis in diastrophic dwarfism?

78. Describe a common deformity of the cervical spine in diastrophic dwarfism.

79. Bilateral clubfoot deformities in diastrophic dysplasia are best treated by:

80. Describe two spinal deformities frequently encountered in metatrophic dysplasia.

81. Describe the clinical features of arthrogryposis.

82. What are the laboratory and x-ray features of postmenopausal osteoporosis?

83. What are the four major diagnoses that can be associated with osteopenia?

84. Where does the body get its source of vitamin D_3 (cholecalciferol) and how is it produced?

85. What are the effects of vitamin D on calcium absorption?

ANSWERS

76. Normal head, micromelia, hitchhiker's thumb, kyphoscoliosis, clubfeet, hip dysplasia, cauliflower ears.

77. 80%.

ANSWERS

78. Cervical kyphosis secondary to hypoplasia of the C3, C4, or C5 vertebrae. Atlantoaxial instability is not common, but can occur.

79. Circumferential release at 1 year of age, which may require talectomy to achieve satisfactory correction.

80. Atlantoaxial instability secondary to odontoid hypoplasia and progressive thoracolumbar kyphoscoliosis.

81. Arthrogryposis is a nonprogressive syndrome of joint contractures and varying degrees of fibrosis of muscles which is present at birth. The upper limbs are internally rotated, the shoulders and elbows are stiff, and there are severe peripheral contractures. The lower limbs are externally rotated. The hips and knees are stiff. Clubfoot is common. Intelligence is normal.

82. The x-ray features are decreased bone and sparing of skull. Laboratory tests (calcium, phosphate, alkaline phosphatase, etc.) are normal.

83. (1) osteoporosis (all laboratory tests are normal except for occasional abnormalities; in triiodothyronine [T_3], thyroxine [T_4], or glucose); (2) osteomalacia; (3) myeloma (90% have an abnormal erythrocyte sedimentation rate [ESR], 80%–90% have abnormal serum protein electrophoresis; (4) hyperparathyroidism (abnormal calcium, phosphate, alkaline phosphatase values). Ninety-eight percent of osteopenias fall into one of these differential diagnoses. The laboratory evaluation approach to osteopenia is (1) bone mass determination with quantitative CT scan or dual photon absorptiometer (DPA); (2) CBC, ESR, urinalysis, calcium, phosphate, alkaline phosphatase, BUN, glucose, serum immunoelectrophoresis, aspartate aminotransferase (AST, SGOT) T_3 and T_4; (3) sometimes a bone biopsy is helpful.

84. Vitamin D_3 is formed through the effect of UV light on 7-dehydrocholesterol.

85. Increased GI absorption of calcium; increased renal calcium absorption, and increased calcium mobilization from bone.

QUESTIONS

86. What effects does PTH have on calcium absorption?

87. What role does PTH play in PO_4 diuresis?

88. What is normal total serum calcium? What is normal phosphate?

89. What are normal urine phosphate and calcium values?

90. What orthopedic problems can be seen in babies of diabetic mothers?

91. What is said to be the pathognomonic radiographic finding in hyperparathyroidism?

92. What is the major skeletal manifestation of Cushing's disease?

93. What laboratory tests are helpful in the evaluation of pathologic fractures?

94. Of the above-described laboratory tests, what abnormalities are seen in postmenopausal osteoporosis?

95. What changes are seen in serum calcium, phosphate, alkaline phosphatase, and urine calcium, phosphate, and hydroxyproline in primary hyperparathyroidism?

96. What changes are seen in serum calcium, phosphate, alkaline phosphatase, and BUN in renal osteodystrophy?

97. What changes are seen in serum calcium, phosphate, alkaline phosphatase, BUN, and urine hydroxyproline levels in Paget's disease?

98. Which cells make PTH?

ANSWERS

86. PTH does all of the above, as noted for vitamin D, and increases 1,25-vitamin D synthesis and osteolysis (osteoclast stimulation).

87. PTH induces PO_4 diuresis by decreasing the renal reabsorption of PO_4 while mobilizing PO_4 and calcium from bone.

88. Normal serum calcium value is 8.8 to 10.8 mg/dL. Normal serum phosphate is 3.0 to 4.5 mg/100 dL.

89. Normal urine phosphate is 340 to 1,000 mg/day. Normal urine calcium is 400 mg/day.

90. Sacral agenesis (caudal regression syndrome).

91. Subperiosteal resorption of the distal end of the clavicle.

92. Osteoporosis.

93. Serum calcium, phosphate, and alkaline phosphatase, ESR, CBC, BUN, PTH; urine calcium, phosphorus, hydroxyproline, protein; urine and serum protein electrophoresis for suspected myelomas.

94. None.

95. Increased serum calcium, alkaline phosphatase, and decreased or normal phosphate; increased urine calcium, phosphate, and hydroxyproline.

96. Decreased serum calcium; increased phosphate, alkaline phosphatase, and BUN.

97. Normal calcium, phosphate, and BUN; increased alkaline phosphatase and urine hydroxyproline.

98. Chief cells in the parathyroid gland.

QUESTIONS

99. Where is active PTH inactivated?

100. What are the effects of PTH on kidney, bone, and the GI tract?

101. Where is calcitonin secreted?

102. What effects do PTH and calcitonin have on serum calcium and phosphate?

103. What effect does calcitonin have on bone, kidney, and the GI tract?

104. What effect does vitamin D have on serum calcium and phosphate?

105. What is pseudohypoparathyroidism?

106. What are the somatic manifestations of pseudohypoparathyroidism?

107. How do you treat pseudohypoparathyroidism?

108. What is pseudopseudohypoparathyroidism?

109. What are the radiographic features of cretinism (hypothyroidism)?

ANSWERS

99. Predominantly in the liver and kidney.

100. Kidney: increased calcium resorption, increased PO_4 excretion; bone: increased calcium released through increased osteoclastic activity; GI tract: increased calcium absorption indirectly by activation of 1,25-dihroxyvitamin D_3 in the kidney.

ANSWERS

101. C cells in the perifollicular areas of the thyroid.

102. PTH increases serum calcium, decreases phosphate. Calcitonin decreases serum calcium and phosphate.

103. Bone: inhibits bone resorption; Kidney: increased urinary excretion of calcium, PO_4, and other cations; GI tract: inhibits calcium and PO_4 absorption.

104. Vitamin D increases serum calcium and phosphate through increased bone release; increases intestinal absorption of calcium and PO_4, and increases kidney PO_4 and calcium absorption.

105. The basic biochemical defect in pseudohypoparathyroidism is a peripheral unresponsiveness to PTH at the renal tubule. Uninhibited resorption of PO_4 in the renal tubule causes hyperphosphatemia and a reciprocal depression of serum calcium. Secondary hyperparathyroidism may occur secondary to depressed serum calcium levels. These patients have elevated PTH levels.

106. Short stature, short fourth and fifth metacarpals, and ectopic bone in subcutaneous tissue and ligamentous structures. Radiographs, of physes in children resemble rickets because of hypocalcemia.

107. Increased oral calcium intake and administer a phosphate binder (such as aluminum hydroxide) to bind PO_4 in the gut.

108. The physical appearance is the same as in pseudohypoparathyroid patients, but there is no evidence of resistance to PTH. Pseudopseudohypoparathyroid patients are normocalcemic.

109. Retarded endochondral growth; complete absence of epiphyseal ossification centers in the carpal region; transverse sclerotic bands in the metaphyses of tubular bones of the hands secondary to deficiency of osteoclastic remodeling. The distal femoral ossification center, which should be present at birth, is absent.

QUESTIONS

110. Congenital hypothyroidism frequently presents with a delay in the usual ossification sequence. In a newborn, which radiograph would be most helpful in evaluating this delay?

111. What is the differential diagnosis for femoral heads that have a Perthes-like radiographic appearance?

112. What are the radiographic changes in sarcoidosis?

113. What are the microscopic features of sarcoidosis?

114. What are the mucopolysaccharidoses?

115. Name three MPS molecules.

116. Describe the clinical and biochemical aspects of Hurler syndrome.

117. Hurler syndrome, or mucopolysaccharidosis type II, follows what mode of inheritance?

118. Describe Scheie's syndrome.

ANSWERS

110. The knee film may reveal absence of the distal femoral epiphysis ossification center which should normally be present at birth.

111. Morquio's syndrome, cretinism, Gaucher's disease, infection, multiple epiphyseal dysplasia, hemophilia, juvenile rheumatoid arthritis (JRA), lymphoma, neoplasm, residuals of CDH, sickle cell disease, spondyloepiphyseal dysplasia, synovitis, posttraumatic AVN.

ANSWERS

112. Manifestations are present most frequently in the bones of the hands and feet and appear as punched-out lytic areas in the middle and distal phalanges. There is also a reticular trabecular pattern in these bones. Advanced disease can lead to pathologic fractures. Lower thoracolumbar vertebral lesions consist of lytic areas with a sclerotic margin.

113. Tubercles, noncaseating granulomas, or epithelioid cells surrounded by granulomatous infiltrate. Langhans' giant cells are seen in the centers of some tubercles. The presence of Schaumann's bodies—amorphous hyalinized eosinophilic bodies in the cytoplasm of Langhans' giant cells—is pathognomonic.

114. The mucopolysaccharidoses are recessively inherited lysosomal storage diseases in which mucopolysaccharide (MPS) accumulates as a result of a deficiency of specific degradative enzymes. They are characterized by accumulation of MPS in connective tissue, variable skeletal dysplasia, and excessive urinary excretion of MPS.

115. Dermatan sulfate (DS), heparin sulfate (HS), keratan sulfate (KS).

116. Hurler syndrome is the most common mucopolysaccharidosis. There is excessive urinary excretion of DS and HS and a deficiency of α-L-iduronidase. The baby appears normal in the first few months of life with a gradual change to an enlarged head, with a scaphocephalic skull. Hurler syndrome is further characterized by thoracolumbar kyphosis, hepatosplenomegaly, corneal clouding, umbilical hernia, and ocular hypertelorism. Survival past 10 years is rare. Tubular bones have an expanded diaphysis. Stature may be normal.

117. X-linked recessive (all other mucopolysaccharidoses have autosomal recessive inheritance).

118. Scheie's syndrome is the same biochemical abnormality as Hurler syndrome. Clinical signs are dense corneal clouding; glaucoma; clawhand deformity; carpal tunnel syndrome, stiff joints; normal height; normal intelligence.

QUESTIONS

119. Describe Hunter's syndrome.

120. Describe Morquio syndrome (chondro-osteodystrophy).

121. Morquio syndrome presents a phenotype reminiscent of which osteochondrodysplasia?

122. Which mucopolysaccharidosis stores dermatan sulfate?

123. What characteristic abnormalities are seen on hand radiographs of mucopolysaccharidosis patients (Morquio, Hunter's, and Hurler)?

124. What are the negative prognostic factors for surgical treatment of unicameral bone cyst?

125. Osteopetrosis, or marble bone disease, is characterized by generalized increase in medullary radiodensity. Describe the usual histologic findings and effective treatment.

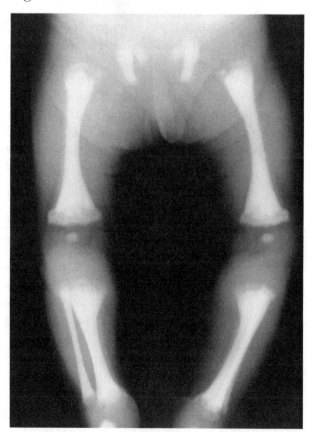

ANSWERS

119. Hunter's syndrome is an X-linked recessive disorder. It is similar to Hurler syndrome except for the absence of corneal clouding, and a less severe course. The same biochemical abnormalities—DS and HS urinary excretion—are present: Onset is later than Hurler syndrome; mental retardation is less severe, and the clinical phenotype is milder.

120. Morquio syndrome is characterized by abnormal degradation of KS. The clinical picture develops by age 3 to 4 years: flatfeet; genu valgum; waddling gait disturbance; chest deformity (pectus carinatum); enlarged wrists, ankles, knees, shoulders and elbows due to hypertrophy of bone ends; joint hypermobility; dwarfism (striking, primarily due to short trunk); platyspondylia with dorsolumbar kyphosis; flexion contracture of hips; atlantoaxial subluxation secondary to odontoid hypoplasia; corneal opacities and hearing deficits are common.

121. Spondyloepiphyseal dysplasia congenita.

122. Maroteaux-Lamy syndrome.

123. Bullet-shaped phalanges, delay in ossification of carpal bones, tapered bases of the metacarpals. In Morquio syndrome there is central constriction of the phalanges and metacarpals.

124. The prognosis in patients less than 10 years old and with active lesions (within 1 cm of the epiphysis) is worse than in other patients. Curettage and grafting in these patients leads to a higher recurrence rate.

125. There is a failure of osteoclastic and chondroclastic resorption secondary to deficient or abnormally functioning osteoclasts. In the severe form of this disorder, bone marrow transplant from an HLA-compatible donor can ameliorate this condition.

QUESTIONS

126. Describe the most appropriate treatment for Caffey's disease.

127. What are the clinical features of the autosomal recessive form of osteopetrosis?

128. What are the features of the autosomal dominant form of osteopetrosis?

129. How are congenital lues and Caffey's disease differentiated on radiograph?

130. What spinal radiographic finding differentiates multiple epiphyseal dysplasia from most mucopolysaccharidoses?

131. What is the clinical presentation for the Schmid type of metaphyseal chondrodysplasia?

132. What is the cellular defect in metaphyseal dysplasia and what are the radiographic abnormalities produced?

133. What causes osteosclerotic bands near the metaphysis in lead or bismuth poisoning (or growth arrest lines as in nephritis)?

ANSWERS

126. The majority of patients recover spontaneously, but if symptoms persist, steroids appear to reduce discomfort.

127. This form is "malignant." Features are failure to thrive; hepatosplenomegaly, lymphadenopathy; cranial nerve palsies (II, III, VII) because the cranial foramina do not widen fully; infections of all varieties (because marrow production of white blood cells is depressed); osteomyelitis (mandibular involvement is frequent secondary to dental caries); retardation of skeletal growth; occasional mental retardation; anemia. Survival beyond the first decade

ANSWERS

is rare. The skeletal lesions are caused by a markedly decreased rate of cartilage and bone resorption. Decreased osteoclastic activity is the underlying problem. Bone marrow transplants have helped some of these patients.

128.   The autosomal dominant form is discovered in late childhood and adolescence. It is characterized by increased bone density, dental caries, cranial palsies, rarely anemia or marrow dysfunction, coxa vara, flask shape at the ends of long bones. It is usually asymptomatic. Healing of fractures of both varieties of osteopetrosis is at a normal rate. Patients have more fractures than the rest of the population. Nonoperative treatment of fractures is recommended.

129.   Scapular, clavicular, and mandibular involvement in Caffey's disease is very common but rarely seen in syphilis. In radiographs of Caffey's disease there is no lytic involvement of the metaphysis, as is seen in lues and scurvy. Radiographic changes in Caffey's disease do not become evident for 4 to 6 weeks after the clinical onset of soft tissue edema.

130.   Lack of platyspondylia in multiple epiphyseal dysplasia.

131.   Short stature and coxa vara characterize this disorder. At birth the children appear normal and skeletal changes appear with weight-bearing at about ages 3 to 5. One also sees a waddling gait with lateral bowing of the femora and genu varum. The dwarfing is moderate. There is no involvement of the skull, spine, or thorax. Radiographs demonstrate cupping of the metaphyses, splaying, and irregularity.

132.   The apparent fragmentation of metaphyseal bone seen on radiograph is secondary to the sporadic and irregular appearance of hypertrophic cartilage and irregular appearance of hypertrophic cartilage extending as elongated tongues well down into the metaphyseal bone. The cartilage formed in the hypertrophic zone does not undergo normal degeneration, which leads to this defect. Epiphyses appear normal; skull and spine are normal. Physeal lines are widened, suggesting rickets, but the diaphyseal bone is of normal density.

133.   A specific toxoid effect on osteoclasts which results in failure of bone resorption during toxic exposure.

QUESTIONS

134. What is diaphyseal aclasis?

135. What are the clinical and radiographic features of Engelmann's disease (progressive diaphyseal dysplasia)?

136. Describe the clinical and radiographic findings in spondyloepiphyseal dysplasia congenita.

137. How are spondyloepiphyseal dysplasia and multiple epiphyseal dysplasia differentiated from achondroplasia on clinical examination?

138. What are the findings seen in spondyloepiphyseal dysplasia on lateral spinal film?

139. Which inherited condition is characterized by aplasia of the clavicles, a generalized disturbance of bone growth, and dental abnormalities?

140. Describe the heritable condition in which bilateral hip and knee dislocations are common.

141. True or false? Hypochondroplasia represents a milder form of achondroplasia.

ANSWERS

134. Also known as multiple hereditary exostosis, this autosomal dominant condition is characterized by multiple cartilaginous and bony exostoses in the metaphyseal region of long bones.

ANSWERS

135. Children present with a limping, broad-based, waddling gait, leg pain and muscle wasting; enlarged head, prominent forehead; thin limbs secondary to reduced muscle mass; thick bones; normal height. Radiographic findings are cortical hyperostosis of long-bone diaphyses usually ending abruptly at the metaphysis; normal epiphyses and metaphyses. Engelmann's disease is similar to osteopetrosis with increased density of bones but does not affect the metaphysis, as does osteopetrosis. Another differentiation from osteopetrosis is absence of anemia and pathologic fractures.

136. The clinical findings are short-trunk dwarfism with cleft palate, myopia, and retinal detachment; commonly a barrel chest with pectus carinatum; increased lumbar lordosis; normal hand and foot size relative to shortened proximal and middle segments of limbs; generalized muscle weakness and easy fatigability; coxa vara; stiff elbows, hips, and knees. Radiographic findings are delayed appearance of ossification centers; platyspondylia with posterior vertebral wedging. Findings on lateral spinal films are odontoid hypoplasia and os odontoidium.

137. The head and face are normal in **SED** and **MED**.

138. Platyspondylia of the thoracolumbar spine with secondary shortening of the trunk and resultant horizontal arrangement of the ribs; central anterior beaking of lumbar vertebrae; dysplastic odontoid, which may cause atlantoaxial instability; irregular vertebral end plates with multiple disk invaginations into the bodies.

139. Cleidocranial dysostosis.

140. Larsen's syndrome.

141. False. Hypochondroplasia represents a genetically distinct entity.

QUESTIONS

143. What are the primary criteria for the diagnosis of hypochondroplasia?

144. Multiple epiphyseal dysplasia is transmitted by what mode of inheritance?

145. What is the most common presentation of a patient with multiple epiphyseal dysplasia?

146. What angular deformities are typical in multiple epiphyseal dysplasia?

147. Describe features of chondroectodermal dysplasia (Ellis–van Creveld syndrome).

148. True or false? AVN of the femoral head may occur in association with multiple epiphyseal dysplasia.

149. What features are characteristic of chondrodysplasia punctata?

150. Prader-Willi syndrome is characterized by severe morbid obesity secondary to an insatiable appetite, hypogenitalia, mental deficiency, and short stature. Recently, an interstitial deletion in the long arm of chromosome 15 has been identified as a common finding in Prader-Willi syndrome patients. What is the most common orthopedic problem found in these patients?

151. Describe the clinical appearance and radiographic findings of Kniest dysplasia.

ANSWERS

143. Narrowed lumbar interpedicular distance, short broad iliac crest, short broad femoral necks, mild metaphyseal flaring, mild brachydactyly, normal facial features.

ANSWERS

144. Autosomal dominant.

145. Complaints of lower extremity joint pain.

146. Genu valgum, genu varum, and ankle valgus deformities.

147. Short stature secondary to distal limb deficiencies (short tibia and forearms); short pedicles; scalloping of posterior vertebral borders; postaxial polydactyly, hypoplastic spoon-shaped nails; dysplastic or absent teeth; heart septal defect; normal head and face; genu valgum in adolescence; disproportionally short fibula. The pattern of limb shortening worsens the farther out from the spine one looks (i.e., the phalanges are shortened the most). Intelligence is usually normal. Cone epiphyses in the middle phalanges of the hand, the hypoplastic proximal radius, and distal ulna, and sometimes radial head dislocation are seen.

148. True. Occasionally, superimposed unilateral and asymmetric Perthes-like changes have been seen in association with the irregular ossification of multiple epiphyseal dysplasia.

149. Short-limb dwarfism, congenital cataracts, mental retardation in those severely affected, coxa vara, congenital scoliosis, C1–2 instability. Radiographic findings are "butterfly vertebrae" on lateral view (separate anterior and posterior centers of ossification separated by wide translucent coronal clefts), and stippling of the epiphyses, carpal bones, and pelvis.

150. Scoliosis has been reported to occur in 50% to 80% of these children. Because of their severe obesity, bracing is not plausible and surgical stabilization is indicated if the magnitude of the curvature warrants.

151. Short trunk and rhizomelic dwarfism with short limbs that have enlarged joints. Contractures of the elbows, hips, and knees develop by 1 year of age. Patients have normal intelligence. Severe myopia, retinal detachment, and cleft palate are frequent. Thoracic kyphoscoliosis, platyspondylia, odontoid hypoplasia, and clubfeet are found.

QUESTIONS

152. Name two dwarfing conditions that are frequently not recognized until the age of 2 to 3 years.

153. Name three dwarfing conditions in which interpedicular narrowing can be identified on an AP lumbar radiograph.

154. Describe the most common mode of inheritance of spondyloepiphyseal dysplasia tarda.

155. Which dwarfing conditions are occasionally referred to the orthopedic surgeon with a diagnosis of bilateral Perthes' disease?

156. What is Trevor's disease?

157. What are the most common sites of involvement of this disorder?

158. At what age does this condition present?

159. Histologic evaluation of Trevor's disease appears to be most closely associated with what other common benign osseous process?

160. What are the zones of cartilage in a joint?

161. What is the composition of the cartilage matrix?

162. What is the most superficial layer of articular cartilage?

163. What type of collagen makes up the largest percentage in hyaline cartilage?

164. What is the composition of proteoglycan?

ANSWERS

152. Hypochondroplasia and pseudoachondroplasia.

153. (1) Achondroplasia, (2) hypochondroplasia, (3) diastrophic dwarfism.

154. X-linked recessive.

155. Spondyloepiphyseal dysplasia tarda and multiple epiphyseal dysplasia.

156. Dysplasia epiphysealis hemimelia.

157. The medial aspect of the distal femur, the distal tibial epiphysis, and the talus.

158. Diagnosis is usually made in the first year of life.

159. Osteochondroma.

160. Starting from the joint surface and moving toward subchondral bone, they are: (1) the tangential zone—cells are flat and parallel to surface; (2) the transitional zone—random arrangement of chondrocytes; (3) the radial zone—short columns perpendicular to the surface; (4) the calcified zone—cells are pyknotic.

161. Water, collagen, proteoglycan.

162. Lamina splendens.

163. Type II.

164. Core protein to which up to 150 chains of glycosaminoglycans (chondroitin sulfate or keratan sulfate) are linked.

QUESTIONS

165. The compressive stiffness of cartilage is directly proportional to

166. How much water (%) is in normal cartilage matrix?

167. What is the coefficient of friction in a synovial joint? How does this compare with the artificial joint?

168. With which HLA antigen is rheumatoid arthritis associated?

169. This 45-week-old child was born at 28 weeks of life. Intravenous hyperalimentation has been required to maintain nutritional status. Clinical examination reveals enlargement of multiple joints. The upper extremity radiograph is shown here. What is the most likely diagnosis?

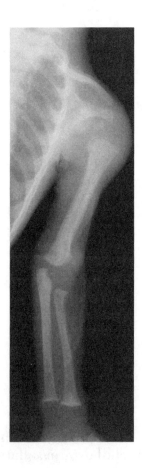

ANSWERS

165. Proteoglycan-hyaluronate aggregate integrity and aggregate water content.

166. 70%.

167. 0.002. The best artificial joint has a coefficient which is 30 times higher.

168. HLA-DR4.

169. Neonatal rickets. The causes of this disorder are myriad. Inadequate dietary calcium, phosphate, vitamin D, and hepatic and renal insufficiency can all contribute to the clinical picture. The underlying cause must be treated.

QUESTIONS

170. A 4-year-old boy with a normal facial appearance demonstrates short trunk dwarfism. A lateral radiograph of the spine and a standing AP radiograph of the lower extremity are shown here. What is the likely diagnosis?

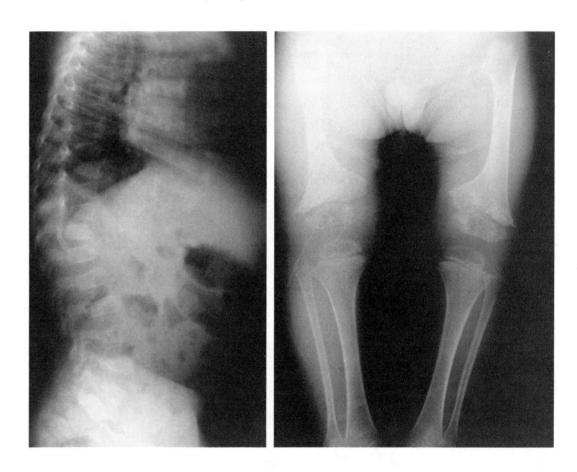

ANSWERS

170. Spondyloepiphyseal dysplasia. The lateral spinal radiograph reveals small misshapen vertebral bodies, with a mild thoracolumbar kyphosis. Odontoid hypoplasia with mild C1–2 instability, and abnormality of the epiphysis, physis, and metaphysis are noted at both the hip and knee levels.

QUESTIONS

171. Fill in the chart listing the serologic and urine profiles for the listed conditions.

	Serum Calcium	Phosphate	Alkaline Phosphatase	Parathyroid Hormone	1,25-Dihyroxyvitamin D$_3$	Urine Calcium
Example:						
Vitamin D deficiency	Normal to low	Low	High	High	Variable	Low
Osteomalacic conditions						
Vitamin D–dependent rickets						
Vitamin D–resistant rickets						
Osteoporotic conditions						
Hyperthyroidism						
Hypercortisolism						
Postmenopausal osteoporosis						
Multiple myeloma						
Others						
Paget's disease						
Primary hyperparathyroidism						
Renal failure						

ANSWERS

171.

	Serum Calcium	Phosphate	Alkaline Phosphatase	Parathyroid Hormone	1,25-Dihydroxyvitamin D	Urine Calcium
Osteomalacic conditions						
Vitamin D–dependent rickets	Normal to low	Low	High	Normal to high	Variable	Normal to low
Vitamin D–resistant rickets	Normal	Low	High	Normal	Normal to Low	Normal
Osteoporotic conditions						
Hyperthyroidism	Normal to high	Normal	Normal to high	Normal to low	Normal to low	Normal to high
Hypercortisolism	Normal	Normal	Normal	Normal to high	Normal to high	Normal to high
Postmenopausal osteoporosis	Normal	Normal	Normal	Normal	Normal	Normal
Multiple myeloma	Normal to high	Normal	Normal to high	Normal to low	Normal to low	High
Others						
Paget's disease	Normal	Normal	High	Normal	Normal	Normal to high°
Primary hyperparathyroidism	High	Low	Normal to high	High	Normal to high	Normal to high
Renal failure	Normal to low	High	Normal to high	High	Low	Normal

°Elevated urine hydroxyproline.

QUESTIONS

172. Duchenne's muscular dystrophy is an X-linked recessive disorder. What laboratory study presently identifies approximately 80% of female carriers?

173. Proteus syndrome may be confused with neurofibromatosis because similar features are noted. What distinguishes this disorder?

174. A child has been placed on prolonged bed rest following surgical management of spinal osteomyelitis. Approximately 4 weeks following surgery the patient develops a diffuse abdominal syndrome and constipation. Lethargy is followed by obtunded mental status. The most likely diagnosis is

175. A 3-year-old child presents to an urban medical center with a non-displaced toddler's fracture. An incidental finding on the radiograph is a broad sclerotic band of metaphyseal bone adjacent to the growth plates. Which laboratory tests could help define the cause of these radiodense bands?

176. Describe the bony changes occasionally associated with leukemia.

177. Hemophilia A (factor VIII deficiency) and hemophilia B (factor IX deficiency) represent the majority of bleeding disorders noted in childhood. How are these conditions inherited?

178. What is the life expectancy of a human immunodeficiency virus (HIV)–negative hemophilic patient using recombinant factor replacement in a self-administered home program?

179. In hemophilia, what levels of factor activity are found with mild, moderate, moderately severe, and severe disease?

180. Below what level do spontaneous bleeds occur after minor or unrecognized trauma?

181. Describe the orthopedic management of acute hemarthrosis in a hemophilic patient.

ANSWERS

172. Serum creatinine phosphokinase (CPK) levels may be elevated. Three serial measurements of serum CPK are recommended since the elevation may be variable and mild.

173. Hemihypertrophy, partial gigantism of hands or feet, skin nevi, subcutaneous tumors, and skull hyperostosis, but no cafe-au-lait spots and no neurofibromas are encountered.

174. Immobilization-induced hypercalcemia.

175. The CBC would reveal anemia with markedly microcytic indices and a serum lead level determination would demonstrate significant elevation above normal (>25 μg/dL).

176. Osteolytic lesions involving the metaphysis are noted in approximately two thirds of patients. Leukemia lines, radiolucent lines adjacent to the physis, are commonly noted. Diffuse periosteal elevation involving the whole bone is occasionally noted.

177. Both conditions are X-linked recessive.

178. Life expectancy is close to that of the general population.

179. Mild—25% to 50% of normal; moderate—5% to 25% of normal; moderately severe—1% to 5% of normal; severe—less than 1% of normal.

180. 5%.

181. The patient and family should self-administer appropriate factor replacements; splint the joint in a compressive dressing for several days; aspirate if the joint is markedly distended; and in 3 to 7 days begin physical therapy for range of motion.

QUESTIONS

182. What are the orthopedic manifestations of hemophilia?

183. Describe the radiographic changes noted in the knee affected by hemophilic arthropathy.

184. The two joints most frequently involved with hemophilic arthropathy are

185. A patient with hemophilia presents with a right hip flexion contracture, numbness along the anteromedial aspect of the right leg, and a quadriceps paresis with muscle power of three-fifths. Attempts to extend the hip cause increasing pain with radiation down the anterior thigh and into the anteromedial leg. The most likely diagnosis in this patient is:

186. At the present time the most effective means of preventing significant bone and soft tissue bleeds is:

187. In the hemophilia patient scheduled to undergo elective surgery, factor VIII replacement during the operation should be maintained at:

188. Synovectomy of the knee can be considered in a joint in which chronic and recurrent bleeding has occurred over a period of 6 months, and which is unresponsive to medical management. What are the likely benefits and sequelae of this procedure?

189. An infant is born with osteogenesis imperfecta. The extremities are markedly shortened and deformed. The femora are widened and crumpled. There is obvious posterior bowing. The chest film reveals a bell-shaped rib cage with multiple fractured ribs. Caput membraniceum is noted. What is this patient's prognosis for walking? For survival?

ANSWERS

182. Hemarthrosis, soft tissue bleeding, and the sequelae of these hemorrhages: nerve palsy, pseudotumor, myositis ossificans, chronic hemophilic arthropathy, and subacute hemophilic arthropathy.

183. Widening of the distal femoral epiphysis, squaring of the inferior pole of the patella, flattening of the distal femoral condyles, and widening of the intercondylar notch.

184. The knee and the ankle.

185. Spontaneous hemorrhage into the iliopsoas muscle with secondary femoral nerve compression. The most appropriate treatment includes factor replacement and rest followed by mobilization of the hip and knee. Complete resolution of the femoral nerve deficit may be anticipated.

186. Immediate self-infusion of clotting factor as soon as a bleed is suspected.

187. 100% activity. This can be continued for 3 to 5 days while physiotherapy is administered. Levels of 50% can be maintained for an additional 7 to 10 days. Prior to surgery a factor VIII kinetics study should be performed to rule out the possibility of an inhibitor, and to aid in dosage determination.

188. Subsequent decrease in bleeding episodes can be expected. If synovectomy is carried out prior to development of significant degenerative changes, some protective and lasting effect against joint destruction may be attained. Synovectomy, especially open synovectomy, does little to improve, and may actually worsen, joint motion.

189. This clearly represents an osteogenesis imperfecta congenita type A (Shapiro). The vast majority of these patients die in the first few years of life. Those that survive will be wheelchair-bound.

QUESTIONS

190. A 3-year-old child is referred from a general orthopedist who has treated the child for three lower extremity fractures involving the femur. All fractures healed in appropriate time. A diagnosis of osteogenesis imperfecta is made. Radiographs reveal long bones of normal shape, width, and length. Mild cortical thinning and minimal osteopenia are recognized. Chest radiograph reveals no obvious rib fractures. The father also has a history of multiple fractures prior to the age of 10. What is this patient's chance of survival? For independent ambulation?

ANSWERS

190. This child represents osteogenesis imperfecta tarda type B (Shapiro). Fractures are noted after walking age. The children survive into adulthood and reproduce. The incidence of fractures appears to decrease with age. Seventy-six percent of patients have a positive family history suggestive of an autosomal dominant pattern. These children are independent ambulators.

CHAPTER 5

Spine

J. Kenneth Burkus, M.D.

QUESTIONS

1. In the midcervical spine a central disc herniation with midline osteophytes is most reliably treated by what surgical approach?

2. A 65-year-old man with progressive cervical myelopathy from cervical stenosis unresponsive to conservative management is referred to you. Lateral radiographs show a reversal of the normal cervical lordosis and the patient has a 15-degree midcervical kyphosis. The local kyphosis does not change on lateral flexion-extension radiographs. What surgical procedure would you recommend?

3. A 35-year-old man has complaints of sensory dysesthesia along the ulnar border of his right hand. Physical examination demonstrates ipsilateral motor weakness in the hand intrinsic muscles. A lateral disc herniation at the C7–T1 level was demonstrated on magnetic resonance imaging (MRI) scans and computed tomograph (CT)–myelogram without any foraminal osteophytes. His symptoms persist despite 6 weeks of conservative treatment. What surgical procedure would you recommend?

4. What are the indications for the surgical treatment of a patient with an os odontoideum?

5. What surgical procedure is recommended for patients with a symptomatic os odontoideum?

6. What region of the spine is most commonly involved in juvenile rheumatoid arthritis?

ANSWERS

1. An anterior approach is best for central disc herniations in the midcervical spine. Posterior excision of cervical disc herniations are best reserved for lateral disc herniations without associated osteophytes. Anterior decompression of the cervical cord does not involve retraction or manipulation of the neural elements. Excision of midline disc herniations and osteophytes has been associated with postoperative neurologic deficits from posterior approaches to the cervical spine.

2. Posterior laminectomy and decompression is contraindicated in patients with preoperative cervical kyphosis. The patient is a candidate for anterior decompression and fusion.

3. A posterior disc excision can be safely performed for isolated unilateral disc herniations without associated osteophytes. The posterior "keyhole" foraminotomy is most often used for lateral disc excisions at the extremes of the cervical spine (C2–3 or C7–T1 levels).

4. Objective neurologic deficit, incapacitating pain, atlantodens interval (ADI) greater than 10 mm (the ADI is the interval between the anterior ring of C1 and the dens); space available for the cord (SAC) less than 13 mm.

5. A posterior C1–2 fusion with autogenous bone grafting. Anterior C2 screws are contraindicated in these longstanding, hypotrophic bony abnormalities.

6. The cervical spine; the thoracic and lumbar spine are rarely involved.

QUESTIONS

7. What clinical problems are associated with diffuse idiopathic skeletal hyperostosis (DISH) involving the cervical spine?

8. What percentage of patients with established pseudarthroses following anterior interbody fusion of the cervical spine have symptoms of neck pain or radiating arm pain?

9. What are the treatment options for patients with neck pain and *referred* arm pain with an established pseudarthrosis in the mid-cervical spine following anterior discectomy and interbody fusion?

10. At what age does the synchondrosis between the dens and the body of C2 fuse?

11. Where are the joints of Luschka located?

12. What neurologic structure is most likely injured during a right-sided anterior approach to the cervical spine?

13. What are the symptoms associated with an injury to the recurrent laryngeal nerve?

14. What structure is at risk for injury from a left-sided anterior approach to the lower cervical spine?

15. Chassaignac's (carotid) tubercle is found at what level in the cervical spine?

16. A patient with a C6–7 unilateral disc herniation will demonstrate weakness in which muscle groups?

17. What is the cause of os odontoideum?

18. A patient with a C4–5 unilateral disc herniation will demonstrate weakness in which muscle groups?

ANSWERS

7. Limitation of range of motion and dysphagia. Anterior osteophytes can compress the esophagus against the trachea. The bridging osteophytes limit motion across the involved disc spaces.

8. Approximately 50% of pseudarthroses following anterior interbody fusions are associated with symptoms of neck or arm pain. Half are asymptomatic.

9. Surgical treatment options include posterior spinous process wiring and fusion at the level of the pseudarthrosis or revision of the anterior interbody fusion.

10. Usually by age 7 years.

11. The uncovertebral joints of Luschka are the articulations in the cervical spine between the uncus (an osseous prominence along the lateral margin of the cephalad vertebral end plate) and the caudal surface of the adjacent vertebral body.

12. The recurrent laryngeal nerve.

13. A hoarse, scratchy voice from unilateral paralysis of the vocal cord.

14. The thoracic duct.

15. The C6 level.

16. A C7 radiculopathy produces weakness in the triceps and finger extensors.

17. An os odontoideum is not a congenital malformation; it results from an injury to the dens.

18. Deltoid and biceps; the C5 root is injured.

QUESTIONS

19. A patient with a C4–5 unilateral disc herniation will demonstrate dysesthesia in what part of the upper extremity?

20. A patient with a C6 radiculopathy will demonstrate weakness in which muscle groups?

21. A patient with a C6 radiculopathy will demonstrate sensory changes in what part of the upper extremity?

22. On palpation of the neck, the cricoid cartilage is at what level of the cervical spine?

23. How much rotation occurs at the atlantoaxial (C1–2) joint in comparison to the rest of the cervical spine?

24. What are the treatment options for patients with neck pain, radiating arm pain, and a persistent objective neurologic deficit with an established pseudarthrosis in the midcervical spine following anterior discectomy and interbody fusion?

25. Is a posterior stabilization procedure necessary following a unilateral keyhole foraminotomy in a patient with normal spinal kinematics?

26. What is the incidence of thoracic disc herniations?

27. What segment of the population is most commonly affected by thoracic disc herniation?

28. At what levels do most thoracic disc herniations occur?

ANSWERS

19. Along the lateral border of the shoulder; the C5 root is compressed.

20. Biceps, brachioradialis, and wrist extensors.

21. The thumb and index finger.

22. The C6 level.

23. Approximately 50%.

24. Posterior nerve root decompression through a keyhole foraminotomy followed by spinous process wiring and fusion at the level of the pseudarthrosis. A second option is anterior revision of the anterior interbody fusion and root decompression and repeat interbody fusion.

25. A unilateral foraminotomy does not destabilize the cervical spine. A fusion may be indicated if the patient demonstrated preoperative instability at the decompressed motion segment (i.e., translation >3.5 mm or angulation >11 degrees) or a preoperative fixed kyphotic deformity.

26. The incidence is less than 0.3% of the population; they account for less than 1.0% of all surgical disc procedures.

27. Both males and females are equally affected; thoracic disc herniations occur most commonly in the fourth through sixth decades of life.

28. Any thoracic level may be involved but they occur most frequently between T9 and T12.

QUESTIONS

29. What are the physical findings associated with thoracic disc herniations?

30. What other disease processes can mimic the signs and symptoms of thoracic disc herniations?

31. What are the treatment options for thoracic disc herniations?

32. In patients with DISH, the flowing osteophytes are absent from which portion of the spine?

33. What are the types of lumbar disc herniations?

34. What is the incidence of cauda equina syndrome in lumbar disc disease?

35. What are the major anatomic features of the lumbar spine?

ANSWERS

29. Neurologic deficits vary and depend on the level of the herniation, the size of the spinal canal, and the size, position, and composition of the disc. Approximately half of these patients have lower extremity weakness. Long track signs including spasticity, hyper-reflexia, and abnormal Babinski response are commonly found. Approximately one third of patients will have some bladder or bowel dysfunction.

ANSWERS

30. Demyelinating diseases (multiple sclerosis, amyotrophic lateral sclerosis), spinal cord tumors or infarction, transverse myelitis, angina pectoris, intercostal neuritis, and pleuritis.

31. Observation, posterior transpedicular decompression, posterolateral costotransversectomy decompression, anterior transthoracic decompression, and fusion.

32. The osteophytes are not found along the left side of the mid- to lower thoracic spine. Their absence is thought to be secondary to pulsations from the descending aorta.

33. Radial bulging (intact annulus), disc protrusion (intact posterior longitudinal ligament, PLL), disc extrusion (ruptured PLL), and disc sequestration (migration away from the disc space).

34. It is seen in 0.2% of patients with herniated lumbar discs; it is associated with massive central disc herniations, saddle anesthesia, and bladder and bowel dysfunction.

35. The vertebral bodies are connected by the intervertebral discs and the neural arches are joined by the facet joints. Each vertebra has three functional components: (1) the vertebral bodies, designed to bear weight; (2) the neural arches, designed to protect the neural elements; and (3) the bony processes (spinous and transverse), designed as outriggers to increase the efficiency of muscle action. The disc surface of the vertebral body demonstrates, on its periphery, a ring of cortical bone. This ring acts as the anchoring site for the attachment of the fibers of the annulus. The cartilaginous plate lies within the confines of the ring. Intervertebral discs are complicated structures both anatomically and physiologically. They are constructed in a manner similar to a car tire, with a fibrous outer casing, the annulus, containing a gelatinous inner tube, the nucleus pulposus. Fibers of the annulus are divided into three main groups consisting of concentric fibrous rings surrounding the nucleus pulposus. The anterior fibers of the annulus are strongly reinforced by the powerful anterior longitudinal ligament. The posterior longitudinal ligament only gives weak reinforcement to the posterior fibers of the annulus, which may contribute to disc herniations occurring posteriorly.

QUESTIONS

36. What is the primary function of the annulus fibrosus?

37. What are the five categories of low back pain?

38. What is viscerogenic low back pain?

39. What is vascular back pain?

40. What is neurogenic back pain?

41. What is psychogenic back pain?

42. What is spondylogenic back pain?

43. What are the radiographic differences between a vertebral body tumor and osteomyelitis?

44. What are the radiographic signs of segmental instability due to disc degeneration?

ANSWERS

36. The annulus serves to stabilize the spine preventing abnormal translation of one vertebral body relative to the other. It also serves in a shock-absorbing capacity through the loading of the fibers as transmitted largely through the nucleus pulposus. This function of the annulus is compared to the hoops around a barrel.

37. (1) Viscerogenic pain, (2) neurogenic pain, (3) vascular pain, (4) psychogenic pain, and (5) spondylogenic pain.

38. This back pain is described from the kidneys or pelvisacral lesions of the lesser sac or retroperitoneal tumors. This type of pain is neither aggravated by activity nor relieved by rest. This differentiates it from back pain which is a result of spinal disorders.

ANSWERS

39. This results from aneurysms or peripheral vascular disease. Intermittent claudication tends to be associated with these problems. These symptoms are sometimes mimicked by spinal stenosis. Spinal stenosis–type pain, however, is not relieved by standing still. Both conditions are aggravated by walking short distances. Pain due to abdominal aneurysms tends not to be associated with activities which would normally worsen spinal pain. This pain tends to be deep-seated and is usually unrelated to activity.

40. Neurogenic back pain is most commonly caused by neurofibromas, neurilemmoma, ependymoma, cysts, and tumors arising from nerve roots in the lumbar spine. Symptoms are similar to disc herniation. Unlike disc herniation, these patients describe night pain, which may cause them to get out of bed to obtain relief.

41. Pain resulting from nonorganic causes. Purely psychogenic back pain is uncommon. One must rule out organic causes prior to making this diagnosis.

42. Spondylogenic back pain is derived from the spinal column, sacro-iliac joint, or from changes occurring in the soft tissues. It is aggravated by activities and relieved by rest.

43. The radiologic evidence of spinal infection typically lags 4 weeks or more behind the clinical manifestations. Rarefaction of the vertebral end plates with involvement of the adjacent vertebrae and narrowing of the disc spaces is first seen. Spinal radiographs demonstrate erosion of the contiguous vertebral bodies. Later there is sclerosis and reactive bone formation. With neoplasms the disc space is generally spared. This contrasts with disc space infection wherein the disc space is the first area destroyed.

44. Lateral flexion-extension radiographs of the spine can demonstrate this abnormal motion provided the patient is not in so much pain that splinting of the spine occurs. Also indicative of segmental instability is the traction spur seen about 1 to 2 mm above the vertebral body edge, projecting horizontally. The third sign is gas in the disc.

QUESTIONS

45. What is end-stage degenerative disc disease?

46. How does degenerative disc disease lead to nerve root compression?

47. What are the differences between prolapsed, extruded, and sequestrated intervertebral disc herniations?

48. A midlateral disc herniation at the L4–5 level most frequently compresses which nerve root?

49. A midlateral disc herniation at the L5–S1 level most frequently produces compression of which nerve root?

50. Under what circumstances would an L5 nerve root be compressed by an L5–S1 disc herniation?

51. Massive central sequestration involving several roots of the cauda equina with bowel and bladder paralysis is most commonly seen with what level of disc herniation?

52. What is adhesive radiculitis?

53. What are the three major regions of spinal stenosis?

54. What is spinal claudication?

ANSWERS

45. Disc space narrowing occurs with overriding and subluxation of the posterior joints. Posterior joints assume a posture of hyperextension. As the facet joints assume a position of extreme extension, there is no cushioning effect at these joints, and the extension strains of daily living push the joints past their physiologically permitted limits and produce pain. Repeated trauma to the posterior joints leads to subluxation and degenerative osteoarthritis.

ANSWERS

46. Through disc protrusion (disc herniation), bony root entrapment (lateral recess stenosis, subarticular stenosis), and redundant ligamentous entrapment (central stenosis from the ligamentum flavum).

47. In prolapsed intervertebral discs, the nuclear material is confined by a few of the outermost fibers of the annulus. Prominence of the annulus is noted at surgery with the demonstration of nuclear material upon incision of the remaining fibers of the annulus. An extruded intervertebral disc demonstrates nuclear material which has blown out through the annulus and has been restrained by the posterior longitudinal ligament. Sequestrated intervertebral disc herniations consist of free fragments in the spinal canal.

48. L5.

49. S1.

50. A lateral disc protrusion could compress the exiting L5 nerve root in the neuroforamina.

51. L4–5.

52. The nerve roots are bound down by fibrotic tissue in association with some cases of degeneration. A persistent nagging pain results because nerve roots are tethered, unable to slide normally, producing constant pain with activity.

53. The central, subarticular, and lateral recess.

54. This is intermittent claudication which is symptomatic more frequently in the thigh than in the calf. It becomes progressively severe with walking, but, standing still does not relieve the pain, in contrast to vascular insufficiency. Recumbency (lumbar flexion) tends to improve the patient's symptoms.

QUESTIONS

55. What objective neurologic deficits are most commonly found with a L5–S1 disc herniation?

56. What are the clinical findings associated with an L4–5 herniated disc?

57. What are the physical findings associated with L4 nerve root compression?

58. What is the Patrick test?

59. A 10-year-old girl is referred by a local school nurse for evaluation of a spinal deformity (Tanner stage I). A radiograph demonstrates a 26-degree right thoracic scoliosis. She has had no prior spinal radiographs. How will you treat the patient?

60. An 11-year-old (Tanner stage II) boy is referred for evaluation of a spinal deformity. He has had no prior radiographs. A radiograph on the day of the clinic visit demonstrates a 31-degree thoracic scoliosis. How will you treat the patient?

61. A 14-year-old girl (Tanner stage IV) with 34-degree left lumbar scoliosis is referred. She is 18 months postmenarche. The spinal radiographs shows that she has a Risser stage 4 curvature. How will you treat her?

62. What is the inheritance pattern for lumbar hemivertebra?

63. What is the inheritance pattern for idiopathic adolescent scoliosis?

ANSWERS

55. There is weakness in toe standing with decreased ankle jerk reflex. Sensation is decreased to the outer aspect of the foot and leg.

ANSWERS

56. This would produce a deficit most frequently in the L5 nerve root, which would produce weakness in the extensor hallucis longus, and sensory changes in the dorsum of the foot.

57. This might be seen with an L3–4 herniated disc. Weakness would be seen in the anterior tibial muscle, and the patellar reflex might be depressed. Sensory changes would be noted along the medial side of the leg.

58. A test to detect a pathologic condition in the hip as well as the sacroiliac (SI) joint. With the patient in a supine position, the foot of the involved side is placed on the opposite knee. This places the hip into a flexed, abducted, externally rotated position. Inguinal pain generally indicates a hip disorder. In this position the SI joint can be stressed by placing one hand on the flexed knee joint and the other on the anterosuperior iliac spine of the opposite side of the pelvis, and pressing down simultaneously. A complaint of increased pain indicates an SI joint disorder.

59. Only one out of four patients with scoliosis curvatures between 25 and 30 degrees will progress. The patient should be followed closely at 4-month intervals for curvature progression. If the curvature progresses 5 degrees or more, the girl should be braced.

60. Skeletally immature patients with a curvature in the 30-degree range should be treated with a brace immediately. Without treatment, the majority of these patients will demonstrate progression of their curvature patterns.

61. The patient should be followed in approximately 6 months. She is not a candidate for bracing. Only patients with at least 9 months of growth remaining should be started in a bracing program.

62. Isolated congenital spinal deformities are spontaneous occurrences without a specific genetic inheritance pattern.

63. There are at least three recessive autosomal alleles in the inheritance pattern for adolescent idiopathic scoliosis.

QUESTIONS

64. A 15-year-old soccer player has acute onset of low back pain which radiates into his posterior thighs but not below his knees. On physical examination he has tight hamstrings but no objective neurologic deficits. Radiographs demonstrate a grade 1 isthmic lytic spondylolisthesis. How would you treat this patient?

65. A 9-year-old girl with a 1-year history of intermittent low back pain is referred. She is a member of the gymnastic team. She has no objective neurologic deficits and no limitation in motion of her lumbosacral spine. Radiographs demonstrated a 55% spondylolisthesis of L5 on the sacrum. What is your treatment plan?

66. A 10-year-old girl is seen with a 21-degree left thoracic scoliosis. She has had no prior radiographs. What is your treatment plan?

67. A 6-year-old girl with a myelomeningocele at the L1 level has a 25-degree thoracolumbar scoliosis. Over a 2-month period her curvature has increased to 55 degrees. What is your treatment plan?

68. A 3-year-old boy is seen in clinic with an isolated anterior vertebral failure of formation at a single level and a kyphosis that has progressed from 38 degrees to 45 degrees over a 6-month period of observation. What is your treatment plan?

69. What are the five types of spondylolisthesis?

70. How should children with symptomatic and asymptomatic grade 1 spondylolisthesis be treated?

ANSWERS

64. With a lumbosacral orthosis and restriction of vigorous physical activity for 3 months. Once he is pain-free he may resume all physical activities.

65. The patient is a surgical candidate. Slips of greater than 50% are at risk for progression of the deformity.

ANSWERS

66. MRI of the entire spinal cord. Left thoracic scoliosis is associated with an occult neuromuscular etiology such as spinal cord tumors and fistulas.

67. The patient needs to be evaluated for hydrocephalus, syringomyelia, and a tethered cord syndrome. Acute increase in scoliosis curvatures in myelodysplastic patients has been associated with ventricular shunt malfunction and hydrocephalus. If no hydrocephalus is present, syringomyelia or spinal cord tethering should be ruled out.

68. Bracing is ineffective in cases of congenital kyphosis secondary to failures of formation. Patients with less than 55 degrees of kyphosis and less than 5 years old respond well to posterior spinal fusion without instrumentation.

69. Dysplastic spondylolisthesis (type I) is secondary congenital malformation of the sacrum or neural arch of L5, which allows forward slippage of L5 on the sacrum. Isthmic spondylolisthesis (type II) is the most common form; it involves the pars as a lysis or elongation of the bone. Separation or dissolution of the pars allows forward slippage; elongation of the pars may be secondary to healing of repeated microfractures. Degenerative spondylolisthesis (type III) results from loss of the ligamentous integrity of the annulus fibrosis and the posterior facet joints. This is associated with the normal aging process of lumbar spinal motion segments. Traumatic spondylolisthesis (type IV) results from an acute fracture of the pars and requires casting. Pathologic spondylolisthesis (type V) results from bone tumors involving the pars.

70. If they are asymptomatic, do not treat but perhaps follow with lateral spinal films every 6 months until age 15, then every 1 to 2 years until age 20. If symptomatic (mild to moderate symptoms) treatment is conservative—decrease in activities, anti-inflammatory drugs, analgesics, bed rest, hamstring stretching, and occasionally a cast for 6 weeks to 3 months. No surgery is performed unless conservative treatment is not helpful for 6 months to 1 year. Patients with recent fracture of the pars require a cast for 3 to 6 months, which often leads to healing.

QUESTIONS

71. What are the indications for surgery in spondylolisthesis?

72. How are childhood grade 1 and 2 spondylolistheses treated surgically?

73. What advantages does the Wiltse muscle-splitting approach have over a midline approach to the lumbosacral spine for posterolateral fusions?

74. An unrestrained passenger involved in a motor vehicle accident sustained a closed head injury. The CT scan of the head also demonstrated a Jefferson fracture. How can you ascertain if the injury is stable and how should the fracture be treated?

75. A clay shoveler's fracture should be treated with what form of orthosis?

76. What are the anatomic structures that compose the anterior column in Denis' "three-column theory" of spinal fractures?

77. What are the anatomic structures that compose the middle column in Denis' three-column theory of spinal fractures?

78. What are the anatomic structures that compose the posterior column in Denis' three-column theory of spinal fractures?

79. A flexion distraction injury occurs at the thoracolumbar junction. The patient is intact neurologically; radiographs show that the disc, the facet joint capsule, and the interspinous ligament have been disrupted. The local kyphosis is 33 degrees. How should the patient be treated?

ANSWERS

71. Greater than 50% slippage, persistent symptoms after an adequate trial of conservative treatment, neurologic findings, documented progression, postural deformity, abnormal gait secondary to hamstring tightness.

72. In situ posterolateral fusion.

73. It provides direct access to the transverse processes and sacral ala. It does not destabilize the spine by disrupting the midline ligamentous structures.

74. An increase in the ADI of more than 4 mm is consistent with injury to the transverse ligament and an unstable fracture pattern. Combined lateral mass of C1 overhang over the C2 facet joints of more than 7 mm on the anteroposterior (AP) open mouth view of the dens is also consistent with a transverse ligament tear and an unstable fracture pattern. Unstable C1 injuries are best treated with a halo orthosis.

75. A clay shoveler's fracture is an avulsion fracture through the posterior spinous process of C6 or C7. These are stable spinal injuries that need be treated only symptomatically with a soft cervical collar.

76. The anterior longitudinal ligament, anterior half of the annulus fibrosus, and anterior half of the vertebral body.

77. The posterior longitudinal ligament, posterior half of the annulus fibrosus, and posterior half of the vertebral body.

78. The facet joints, ligamentum flavum, and interspinous ligament.

79. This is a purely ligamentous injury. The patient should undergo open reduction of the facet joint dislocation and posterior compression instrumentation and fusion.

QUESTIONS

80. What patterns of occipital condyle fractures occur and how are they treated?

81. What are the most common clinical findings associated with occipitoatlantal dislocations?

82. What is the accepted measurement for ADI?

83. What cervical vertebral level is involved in a Jefferson fracture?

84. What is the mechanism of injury involved in a Jefferson fracture of the cervical spine?

85. What is the recommended treatment for Jefferson fractures?

86. How are odontoid process fractures treated?

87. What are the prognostic factors in the healing of type 2 dens fractures?

88. How is the hangman's fracture treated?

ANSWERS

80. There are three types: type 1 is an impacted condyle fracture; type 2 is a condyle fracture associated with a basal skull fracture; type 3 is an avulsion fracture of a condyle. They are treated with a SOMI or halo orthosis.

ANSWERS

81. These injuries are usually fatal with anterior displacement of the skull on the atlas.

82. A normal ADI is 3 to 4 mm; 5 mm or greater is abnormal.

83. The C1 vertebral body (atlas).

84. A Jefferson fracture is a four-part fracture of the ring of the atlas and results from axial loading of the occiput on the cervical spine.

85. Initial halo traction until muscle spasms diminish and pain subsides, then a halo plaster cast for 6 to 8 weeks and a cervical brace for 6 to 8 weeks. Four months after fracture, if there is no displacement on flexion-extension films and the patient has no pain, bracing is discontinued.

86. *Type 1* is an avulsion, or oblique fracture through the upper part of the odontoid process. It is treated with a cervical orthosis. *Type 2* is a fracture through the isthmus at the junction of the odontoid process and the body. Fractures in persons less than 40 years old that are nondisplaced have a union rate of 60% to 80%. Patients over 50 with a displacement of more than 4 mm have a 20% to 40% healing rate with immobilization. Treatment is a halo cast for 12 weeks. Sometimes C1–2 fusion is necessary. Others advocate open reduction with internal fixation, but there is a high associated complication rate. *Type 3*, fracture into the upper body of C2, is treated with a cervical orthosis if there is no displacement, and with a halo cast, if there is displacement.

87. The prognosis of healing of type 2 dens fractures depends on the age of the patient, the amount of initial displacement and angulation, and timing of diagnosis and initiation of treatment.

88. With a halo body jacket until union occurs in 10 to 12 weeks. This fracture will heal even in displaced positions. If nonunion occurs it may be treated with a posterior C1–2 arthrodesis or anterior C2–3 arthrodesis.

QUESTIONS

89. What are some possible observations and findings in the initial evaluation of a cervical spine injury?

90. Describe the neurologic examination for sensation in cervical spine injuries.

91. What are the sensory areas associated with C2, C3, C4, C5, C6, C7, C8, and T1?

92. What muscles are associated with C4, C5, C6, C7, C8, and T1?

93. What are acceptable measurements for the C2–3 prevertebral space and the C4–5 soft tissue shadow?

94. Describe the laboratory work that should be done on a cervical spine–injured patient upon arrival in the emergency room.

95. Describe the two classifications of neurologic injuries in the cervical spine.

96. What are the four types of incomplete spinal cord lesions?

ANSWERS

89. Observe voluntary movements of the extremities. Palpate the neck. Hypotension in the range of 90/50 mm Hg is not uncommon in quadriplegic patients secondary to temporary generalized sympathectomy. This should not be confused with hemorrhagic shock since treatment is much different. Excessive fluids do not raise blood pressure in neurogenic shock and may cause a serious overload of fluid. The pulse rate is usually normal (70–90 bpm). Look for associated injuries.

90. Sensation is evaluated by pin prick and light touch in the anterior column. Deep pressure, vibration, and position sense are used in examination of the posterior column.

91. C2, the back of the scalp; C3, the anterior neck; C4, the anterior clavicles to the second rib interspace; C5, the deltoid area; C6, the radial forearm, thumb, and index, and middle fingers; C7, the ring and small fingers; C8, the ulnar border of the hand and forearm; T1, the medial arm.

92. C4, diaphragmatic muscle, trapezius, sternocleidomastoid; C5, deltoid and biceps; C6, extensor carpi radialis brevis and longus; C7, pronator teres, flexor carpi radialis, triceps, finger extensors; C8, flexor digitorum superficialis and profundus; T1, intrinsic muscles of the hand.

93. C2–3 prevertebral space: 3 mm; C4–5 soft tissue shadow: 8–10mm.

94. Hematocrit (Hct), blood urea nitrogen (BUN), arterial blood gases (ABG), vital capacity, and urine output. A preoperative tracheostomy should be considered if vital capacity is less than 1,000 mL or less than 20% of predicted normal.

95. (1) Root injury: these are peripheral nerve injuries, which can recover somewhat. (2) Spinal cord injury: any sparing distal to the injury constitutes an incomplete lesion, and recovery varying from minimal to full is possible. Complete spinal cord injury demonstrates no function below the level of the injury.

96. (1) Brown-Séquard, (2) central cord, (3) anterior cord, and (4) posterior cord syndromes.

QUESTIONS

97. Describe the clinical features and prognosis for each type of incomplete lesion.

98. What complications are associated with early care of quadriplegia?

99. When is a urethral catheter placed in a spinal cord–injured patient?

100. How often should you turn a spinal cord–injured patient?

101. What steps can be taken to prevent pulmonary complications in the spinal cord–injured patient?

102. How is the bladder managed in quadriplegia?

103. What is the bowel program in quadriplegia?

ANSWERS

97. (1) Brown-Séquard syndrome, injury to the lateral half of the spinal cord causes ipsilateral muscle paralysis and contralateral loss of pain and temperature sensation. The prognosis for partial recovery is good. Most patients are able to ambulate and control bowel and bladder once recovery is complete. (2) The central cord lesion is the most common incomplete syndrome. It is usually caused by extension injury to an osteoarthritic spine. On radiograph there is no fracture or dislocation. However, there is almost complete flaccid quadriplegia. The cause is cord compression by anterior osteophytes and the posterior ligamentum flavum, resulting in severe flaccid lower motor neuron paralysis of the fingers, hands, and arms. Damage to the central portion of the corticospinal and spinothalamic tracts in white matter causes upper motor neuron spastic paralysis of the trunk and lower extremities. Sacral sparing is present when careful examination is performed. Sacral tracts, positioned on the periphery of the cord, are usually spared from injury. The prognosis is fair. Progressive return of motor and sensory function to the lower extremities and trunk can occur. However, there is poor recovery of hand function. Patients ambulate with a spastic gait. (3) The anterior cord syndrome is characterized

ANSWERS

by complete motor paralysis and sensory anesthesia, with the exception of dorsal column sparing, providing deep pressure and proprioception. The prognosis is good if recovery progresses during the first 24 hours. After 24 hours, if sacral motor function or sensation has not returned, the prognosis is poor; less than 10% of patients make a functional recovery. (4) In the posterior cord syndrome, there is loss of deep pressure, deep pain, and proprioception, but with intact motor function, and pain and temperature sensation. Patients walk with a slapping gait similar to that in tabes dorsalis. This is a rare syndrome.

98. Respiratory insufficiency and pneumonia, pressure ulceration, gastrointestinal bleeding, urinary retention with bladder distention and calculus formation, joint contracture, skeletal osteoporosis, psychologic withdrawal.

99. A urethral catheter is placed for the first 24 to 48 hours. These patients have low blood pressure and demonstrate a sympathectomy-type picture. Urine output is usually low and therefore intravenous (IV) and oral fluids should be restricted during the first 24 to 48 hours. When urinary diuresis occurs at 36 to 48 hours, oral and IV fluids can be administered accordingly. The paralyzed bladder should be treated with intermittent catheterization.

100. Every 2 hours for skin care or use a side-to-side rotating bed.

101. Intermittent positive pressure breathing several times daily to maintain full expansion of the lungs with proper humidification is essential. Tracheostomy must be done if secretions cannot be cleared by nasal or oral suctioning. Pulmonary edema and right congestive heart failure may occur during the first week secondary to excessive fluid overload.

102. Catheterization for 24 to 40 hours followed by an intermittent catheterization program to develop automatic reflex emptying of the bladder. Consult a urologist.

103. Reflex emptying of the bowels with a suppository is the goal of bowel training. Every 2 to 3 days a glycerine or bisacodyl (Dulcolax) suppository is introduced, occasionally with digital stimulation. Stool softeners are given p.r.n.

QUESTIONS

104. A patient sustained an L3 fracture-dislocation with loss of sensory and motor function below the L3 level. What type of neurologic injury did the patient sustain?

105. An 8-year-old boy sustained a complete spinal cord lesion at the T2 level. What are his chances of developing scoliosis?

106. What is spinal shock?

107. What is the significance of spinal shock?

108. What is sacral sparing?

109. What is the significance of sacral sparing in patients with spinal cord injuries?

110. What is the bulbocavernosus reflex?

111. What is the significance of the bulbocavernosus reflex?

112. If a patient with a T8 spinal cord lesion has return of distal spinal reflexes (i.e., the bulbocavernosus reflex) and has no return of any distal voluntary motor or sensory function, what are his or her chances of having any significant functional recovery?

ANSWERS

104. The patient sustained an injury to the cauda equina. Below the L1 level, lumbar and sacral nerve roots are injured; the spinal cord ends above this level with the conus medullaris. A spinal cord injury produces an upper motor neuron spastic paralysis while a cauda equina lesion produces a flaccid paralysis. The lumbar and sacral root injuries may demonstrate progressive recovery whereas complete cord injuries do not.

ANSWERS

105. All patients that are skeletally immature at the time of such injury develop a neuromuscular scoliosis.

106. Spinal shock is that period of time immediately following spinal cord injury when the reflex activity of the entire spinal cord is depressed. In spinal shock, the reflex arcs below the level of the spinal cord injury are absent. An example of this is loss of the bulbocavernosus reflex in patients with a cervical spinal cord injury. The bulbocavernosus reflex is a sacral nerve root reflex and inferior to the cervical cord injury. This reflex is often absent following cervical cord injury. This absence of reflexes below the cord injury is spinal shock. Spinal shock usually lasts less than 24 hours. Return of reflex activity below the level of injury indicates the end of spinal shock.

107. The diagnosis of a complete or incomplete spinal cord injury cannot be made until the patient is out of spinal shock.

108. Sacral sparing is the presence of any voluntary control of the anal sphincter or toe flexor muscles or the presence of any perianal (saddle) sensation.

109. The presence of sacral sparing indicates the transmission of neural signals across the proximal level of the spinal cord injury. Preservation of distal spinal cord functioning indicates that the patient has a partial spinal cord injury and may demonstrate some neurologic recovery.

110. The bulbocavernosus reflex is a spinal reflex in which there is anal sphincter contraction following glans penis or clitoris compression.

111. Its absence indicates spinal shock. Its return indicates the end of spinal shock. With return of the bulbocavernosus reflex and the end of spinal shock, if the patient has no motor or sensory function below the level of injury or no sacral sparing, the spinal cord lesion is complete.

112. Patients with complete spinal cord injuries heralded by the return of distal spinal reflexes show no significant functional recovery.

QUESTIONS

113. What partial spinal cord injury has the best prognosis for functional recovery?

114. A 70-year-old man fell at home and struck his forehead on a night stand. He was brought directly to the emergency room. On physical examination the patient demonstrated flaccid paralysis of the upper extremities, spastic involvement of the lower extremities, and intact sacral sensation and motor function. No fractures were seen on radiographs; radiographs did demonstrate degenerative changes in the midcervical spine. What type of spinal cord injury pattern does the patient have?

115. If no fractures are present, what is the mechanism of injury to the spinal cord?

116. Why are the upper extremities involved more than the lower extremities?

117. What is the patient's prognosis for recovery?

118. A 30-year-old man is stabbed in the back at the midthoracic level with an ice pick. In the emergency room he is noted to have no motor strength but preservation of sensation in his left leg and motor preservation without sensation in his right leg. What type of spinal cord injury did the patient sustain and which portion of the cord was injured?

119. What is his prognosis for neurologic recovery?

120. A patient with a C5–6 fracture-dislocation who demonstrated significant root recovery will need what rehabilitative appliances?

121. A patient sustained a C3–4 injury and has a C3 functional level. What rehabilitative appliance and apparatus is the patient a candidate for?

ANSWERS

113. Ninety percent of patients with Brown-Séquard syndrome make functional recovery.

114. Central cord syndrome.

115. When the cervical spine is acutely hyperextended, the cervical cord is pinched between anterior bony spurs and posterior infolded ligamentum flavum. This causes an ischemic insult to the central gray matter of the spinal cord.

116. Within the corticospinal and spinothalamic tracts the upper extremity neural elements are positioned centrally and the lower extremity neural elements are more peripherally placed.

117. Fifty percent recover some function. Flaccid paralysis in the upper extremities has a poor prognosis secondary to central gray matter necrosis.

118. The patient has a Brown-Séquard syndrome (spinal cord hemitransection). This unilateral injury to the spinal cord results in loss of ipsilateral motor function and contralateral loss of sensation. The left half of the cord was injured.

119. Ninety percent of patients make functional recovery.

120. A C6 quadriplegia patient will have voluntary wrist extension. He or she can be independent with sliding board transfers from bed to chair and be able to propel a manual wheelchair with quadriplegic pegs on the wheel rim. He or she will require a wrist-driven flexor-hinge splint for prehension and may develop independent living including feeding and personal hygiene.

121. A patient with C3-level quadriplegia will have head and neck control but will require a respirator, at least at night. He or she will have loss of phrenic nerve function and is a candidate for an internal phrenic pacemaker. The patient may be able to propel an electric wheelchair with a chin-controlled device.

QUESTIONS

122. A patient with C5-level quadriplegia will have what functioning muscle groups and will need what type of upper extremity orthoses?

123. What type of ambulatory patterns are expected from patients with thoracic-level paraplegia?

124. What type of ambulatory status and orthoses may be expected for a patient with L3-level paraplegia?

125. What is autonomic dysreflexia?

126. What is the incidence of pyogenic osteomyelitis involving the spine?

127. What is the most common location of pyogenic osteomyelitis in the·spine?

128. What is the most common organism found in pyogenic vertebral osteomyelitis?

129. What are the most common radiographic findings associated with pyogenic osteomyelitis?

130. What is the cause of postoperative disc space infections?

131. What is the incidence of postoperative disc space infections?

ANSWERS

122. A patient with C5 quadriplegia will demonstrate voluntary shoulder abduction and elbow flexion; he or she will be unable to move the wrist or hand and will be dependent for transfers, feeding, and hygiene. The patient may use an arm-control electric wheelchair and will require mobile arm supports and an externally powered hand splint for prehension.

ANSWERS

123. Patients with thoracic-level paraplegia may stand in parallel bars and are independent wheelchair ambulators.

124. Patients with L3 paraplegia have voluntary knee extension and can be expected to become community ambulators with KAFOs or AFOs.

125. Autonomic dysreflexia is associated with cervical cord lesions. Stimulation of the sympathetic nervous system in the thoracic region may result from bladder irritation or distention. Stimulation of the thoracic sympathetics causes peripheral arterial constriction and elevated systemic blood pressure. The rise in blood pressure stimulates the carotid sinus to slow the heart rate. The parasympathetics cannot modulate the sympathetic response because of the cervical cord injury. As a result, blood pressure can continue to rise and heart rate to fall. The patient complains of headache and presents with systolic pressures of 200 to 300 mm Hg and bradycardia. Treatment is through removal of the thoracic sympathetic stimulus and usually responds to simple bladder drainage.

126. Spinal involvement is less than 1% of all cases of osteomyelitis.

127. Pyogenic osteomyelitis most commonly occurs in the lumbar spine followed by the thoracic and cervical spine.

128. Staphylococcus. There is an increasing frequency of gram-negative organisms; *Pseudomonas* infections are associated with IV drug users.

129. Absence of bony or disc changes for 4 to 6 weeks; enlarged paravertebral soft tissue density or mass; loss of the psoas margin; disc space narrowing and vertebral end-plate erosions; vertebral body destruction and collapse; reactive bone formation.

130. Direct inoculation of disc space during surgery.

131. Less than 2% of discectomies; they can also occur with percutaneous nuclectomy.

QUESTIONS

132. What is the most common organism in postoperative disc space infections?

133. What is the usual clinical presentation of a disc space infection following discectomy?

134. What is the treatment of postoperative disc space infections?

135. What are risk factors for the development of osteomyelitis of the spine?

136. What is the role of chemotherapy in the surgical treatment of granulomatous infections of the spine?

137. Is skin testing for suspected granulomatous infections of the spine adequate for making the diagnosis?

138. What is spinal dysraphism?

139. What are the physical findings associated with spinal dysraphism?

140. What are some common forms of spinal dysraphism?

141. What are the radiographic findings associated with diastematomyelia?

142. What are the two morphologic patterns of congenital spinal deformities?

ANSWERS

132. *Staphylococcus.* Gram-negative organisms have been reported; there is great difficulty in obtaining positive cultures.

ANSWERS

133. There is typically initial relief of the preoperative pain followed 1 to 8 weeks later by severe backache associated with excruciating pain out of proportion to the objective findings. A few patients demonstrate symptoms consistent with infection. Some do, however, run an afebrile course. The erythrocyte sedimentation rate (ESR) is usually elevated. Radiographic changes include narrowing of the disc space approximately 4 to 6 weeks postoperatively. This narrowing occurs much earlier than usual following discectomy and is typically more pronounced. Later, the vertebral end plates become blurred. Over half of these patients progress to interbody fusion. Diagnosis is confirmed through needle biopsy.

134. Biopsy, IV antibiotics, and immobilization; surgical debridement is rarely indicated.

135. Age, diabetes, history of genitourinary manipulation, IV drug use.

136. Chemotherapy should be started 1 to 2 weeks prior to surgical debridement of the spine and continued postoperatively.

137. No. Biopsy of the lesion must be carried out to establish the cause of the lesion and provide adequate material for culture and sensitivity.

138. A congenital malformation of the neural axis.

139. Skin changes include a hairy patch or lipoma over the spine, asymmetry in calf or thigh circumferences, asymmetry in foot dimensions.

140. Diastematomyelia, tight filum terminale, myelomeningocele, Arnold-Chiari malformation, spinal cord syrinx.

141. Widening of the pedicles, midline bony abnormality, decreased disc space height.

142. Failure of formation, failure of segmentation, or both. The last is most common.

QUESTIONS

143. Which pattern of congenital deformity has the worst prognosis for development of a frontal plane spinal deformity (i.e., scoliosis)?

144. Which pattern of congenital deformity has the worst prognosis for developing a sagittal plane deformity (i.e., kyphosis)?

145. What is the "crankshaft phenomenon?"

146. How can the crankshaft phenomenon be avoided?

147. What is the role of bracing in the treatment of patients with congenital kyphosis?

148. What is the role of bracing in the treatment of patients with congenital scoliosis?

149. What is the genetic inheritance pattern of isolated congenital abnormalities in the thoracic and lumbar spine?

150. What other systemic abnormalities are associated with congenital spinal deformities?

151. What is infantile idiopathic scoliosis?

152. What is the sex ratio of patients affected by infantile idiopathic scoliosis?

153. Where do most of the curvatures occur in patients with infantile idiopathic scoliosis?

ANSWERS

143. Unilateral unsegmented bar associated with a contralateral hemivertebra.

144. Anterior failure of formation (hemivertebra).

145. Progression of the spinal deformity despite a solid posterior arthrodesis. Progression occurs through rotation of the spinal column. This results from the continued anterior growth of the spinal column which is tethered by the posterior fusion.

146. By performing an anterior arthrodesis across the apex of the deformity at the same time as the posterior arthrodesis.

147. Bracing is not effective in controlling the progression of the spinal deformity resulting from congenital kyphosis.

148. Bracing may help in the treatment of long flexible curvatures. A brace may help to control curvatures that are compensatory to the congenital curvature. A brace is rarely the definitive therapy but it may allow for additional spinal growth prior to surgery.

149. There is no specific inheritance pattern; they are isolated occurrences without a genetic predisposition.

150. Congenital heart defects (10%), congenital urogenital defects (20%), limb abnormalities, anal atresia, Sprengel's deformity, hearing deficits, and facial asymmetry.

151. A lateral curvature of the spine which is identified in a patient less than 3 years of age.

152. The majority (52% to 58%) are males.

153. In the thoracic spine.

QUESTIONS

154. How do infantile idiopathic scoliosis curvature patterns differ from those in adolescent idiopathic scoliosis?

155. What are the prognostic factors related to progression in infantile idiopathic scoliosis?

156. What is Mehta's angle?

157. How do you assess the phase of the ribs in patients with infantile idiopathic scoliosis?

158. What percentage of patients with idiopathic infantile scoliosis have progressive curvatures and require treatment?

159. What are the treatment options for patients with progressive infantile idiopathic scoliosis?

160. What are the radiographic findings associated with progression of the spinal deformity in patients with infantile idiopathic scoliosis?

161. A 3½-year-old boy has failure of formation of the L1 vertebral body. The local sagittal plane kyphosis between T12 and L2 has progressed from 27 degrees to 39 degrees over a 12-month period. He is intact neurologically and there is no scoliosis. How would you treat this patient?

162. A 6-year-old girl has an anterior failure of formation (hemivertebra) at T11. The local kyphosis between T10 and L1 has increased from 56 degrees to 62 degrees over 18 months. She is neurologically intact and has no scoliosis. How would you treat this patient?

163. A 2-year-old girl has a unilateral unsegmented bar and a contralateral convex hemiverterba at the thoracolumbar junction. The scoliosis has increased from 35 degrees to 48 degrees over the past year. How would you treat the patient?

ANSWERS

154. The curvature patterns have a left apex in the thoracic spine and do not have compensatory curvatures.

155. Apical rib-vertebra angle difference and apical rib phase.

156. The apical rib-vertebral angle difference.

157. Assessing the amount of overlap of the apical ribs over the apical vertebral body.

158. Approximately 10%.

159. Observation, bracing, subcutaneous rodding, spinal fusion.

160. A rib-vertebral angle difference of more than 20 degrees and phase-2 rib and vertebral body overlap.

161. Posterior spinal fusion.

162. Anterior and posterior spinal fusion. Patients with kyphosis of more than 55 degrees and patients older than 5 years require that posterior arthrodesis be supplemented with an anterior fusion.

163. Anterior and posterior spinal fusion. The posterior fusion needs to be supplemented with the anterior arthrodesis to prevent the crankshaft phenomenon.

QUESTIONS

164. When can a combined anterior and posterior convex hemiepiphy-seodesis and hemiarthrodesis be successfully used in congenital scoliosis?

165. What is juvenile idiopathic scoliosis?

166. What percentage of patients with neurofibromatosis have bony lesions of the vertebral bodies?

167. What is the "cast syndrome?"

168. What causes cast syndrome?

169. How is cast syndrome treated?

170. What are two patterns of scoliosis seen in patients with neurofibromatosis?

171. What percentage of patients with Friedreich's ataxia develop scoliosis?

172. A 14-year-old girl with osteogenesis imperfecta has a 46-degree scoliosis which has progressed from 40 degrees in 9 months. What are your treatment options?

173. What is adolescent idiopathic scoliosis?

174. An underarm orthosis can be utilized in which thoracic idiopathic curvature patterns?

175. In what curvature pattern are underarm braces in the treatment of idiopathic scoliosis least effective?

ANSWERS

164. The patient must have documented curvature progression, the curvature must be less than 60 degrees, the curvature must involve six vertebral segments or less, and the patient must be age 5 years old or younger.

165. A lateral spinal curvature that is first identified between ages 3 and 10 years.

166. Approximately 50%.

167. Compression of the duodenum and restriction of gastric contents outflow follow spinal deformity correction.

168. Compression of the duodenum between the superior mesenteric artery and the aorta.

169. Removal of the cast, gastric decompression with a nasogastric tube, lateral decubitus position of the patient, IV hyperalimentation.

170. Idiopathic and dysplastic.

171. Over 90%.

172. Posterior spinal fusion with segmental instrumentation.

173. Lateral curvature of the spinal column identified between age 10 years and skeletal maturity.

174. Curve patterns with an apex at T7 or below.

175. Curves with an apex at or above T6.

QUESTIONS

176. A 21-year-old man sustained a lap belt flexion-distraction injury to his thoracolumbar spine. Lateral radiographs show that the transverse fracture line extends through all three columns of the spine and involves the posterior spinous process, the pedicles, and the vertebral body. The local kyphosis is 8 degrees. What is your treatment plan?

177. A 31-year-old man sustained an L3 burst fracture during a fall while rock climbing. After a 48-hour period of observation he shows no change in his neurologic status. On physical examination, he has no perianal sensation, no voluntary bladder function, weak quadriceps, and trace motor function in all muscle groups below the knee. A CT scan shows that the spinal canal is compromised by 80% from retropulsed bone fragments. There is no lamina fracture. What is your treatment plan?

178. What type of curvature pattern is associated with syringomyelia?

179. In what age group is a grade 2 spondylolisthesis most likely to progress?

180. Is a patient's sex a risk factor for progression of spondylolisthesis?

181. A 12-year-old girl has intermittent low back pain which always resolves spontaneously. She has never complained of radiating leg pain. A standing lateral radiograph of the lumbosacral spine demonstrates a spondylolisthesis at L5 and S1. The sagittal translation is 55% and the slip angle is 42 degrees. How would you treat this patient?

182. What are the radiographic risk factors for progression of spondylolisthesis?

183. What are the indications for in situ repair of the pars interarticularis defect?

184. What is the incidence of spondylolysis?

ANSWERS

176. This is a bony Chance fracture. The patient does not have a significant sagittal plane deformity. The fracture can be treated with a hyperextension body cast.

177. The patient requires spinal canal decompression and stabilization. The decompression can be carried out either posterolaterally or anteriorly. The spinal column can be stabilized with short segmental spinal fixation posteriorly or anteriorly.

178. Apex left thoracic curve.

179. Spondylolisthesis is most likely to progress during the adolescent growth spurt.

180. Yes. Females are at greater risk for progression than males.

181. She is a candidate for a posterior spinal fusion from L4 to the sacrum followed by extension and reduction with pantaloon spica cast immobilization. The patient is at risk for progression of the deformity because of her sex, the magnitude of the deformity, and her age.

182. Dysplastic spondylolisthesis, domed-shaped sacrum, sagittal translation greater than 50%, and slip angle greater than 40 degrees.

183. No sagittal translation (spondylolysis only), vertebral involvement of L1 to L4 (L5 should be fused to the sacrum), age less than 30 years.

184. In white males it is 5% to 6%; in white females it is 2% to 3%. In blacks it is less than 3%. In Eskimos it is approximately 50%.

QUESTIONS

185. What is the role of bracing in patients with osteogenesis imperfecta and progressive thoracic scoliosis?

186. What percentage of patients with Duchenne muscular dystrophy will develop scoliosis?

187. What is the natural history of scoliosis in patients with Duchenne muscular dystrophy?

188. What cranial nerve is most commonly injured with halo traction?

189. How can one identify a sixth cranial nerve palsy?

190. What is the artery of Adamkiewicz?

191. Where does the artery of Adamkiewicz arise from?

ANSWERS

185. Spinal bracing for progressive scoliosis in patients with osteogenesis imperfecta is not advised, is without benefit, and has several complications associated with it. Bracing these children often results in further chest wall deformity and does not prevent progression of the curvatures.

186. Approximately 80%.

187. The curves progress relentlessly, especially once the child loses ability to ambulate.

188. The sixth cranial nerve (abducens).

189. Loss of lateral gaze.

190. The segmental artery which represents the main blood supply to the thoracic T4–9 portion of the spinal cord; it is also referred to as the arterioradicularis magnum.

191. It arises from an intercostal or lumbar artery, generally at the level of T8 to L2 on the left.

QUESTIONS

192. A 22-year-old man injured his back in a work-related lifting accident 2 weeks prior to presenting as an outpatient. He complains of back pain which radiates down his right posterior thigh to the lateral border of the foot. The referring family practice physician has ordered a CT scan (see Figure). Physical examination shows that the patient has a positive straight leg raise at 45 degrees and a diminished Achilles reflex. There is no motor weakness. What is your treatment plan?

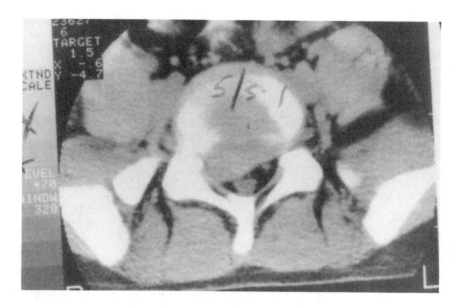

193. The patient's pain has increased in intensity and is exacerbated with all physical therapy treatment modalities at 8 weeks following the injury. What is your treatment plan?

194. While awaiting surgery, the patient vigorously sneezes and notes the acute onset of bilateral radiating leg pain and perianal anesthesia. He also has difficulty emptying his bladder. What is your treatment plan?

ANSWERS

192. The CT scan shows a right-sided L5–S1 disc herniation. The right S1 nerve root is posteriorly displaced. However, the patient has had symptoms for only 2 weeks. Initial treatment to reduce the acute painful symptoms should involve low back modalities such as moist heat, traction, reduction of activities, and nonsteroidal anti-inflammatory agents. Physical therapy and back rehabilitation exercises are instituted when the patient can tolerate increased activity levels.

193. The patient is a surgical candidate; he has failed a 6-week trial of conservative therapy. The large extruded disc fragment precludes the use of chymopapain or percutaneous nuclectomy. A standard unilateral discectomy or microdiscectomy are the surgical options.

194. The patient has developed the clinical symptoms of cauda equina syndrome. The patient should be treated with an open discectomy as soon as possible.

QUESTIONS

195. A 37-year-old man has a 3-month history of radiating anterior chest pain. He is referred from an internist who has excluded cardiac or pulmonary disease. The patient also complains of diffuse leg weakness and ambulates with a wide-based gait. On physical examination, you note clonus in the lower extremities and hyperreflexia. An MRI scan of the thoracic spine is shown in the figure. What is your treatment plan?

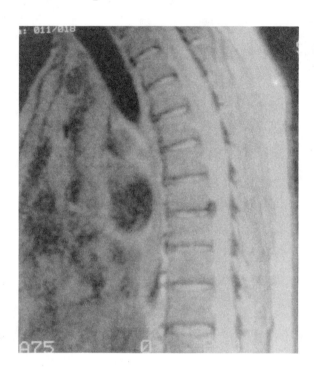

ANSWERS

195. The MRI scan shows central disc herniation in the midthoracic spine. The extruded, desiccated disc fragment appears dark on this T1-weighted image. The patient's symptoms and physical examination are consistent with spinal cord compression. The patient requires a discectomy and spinal cord decompression. The discectomy can be safely performed through either an anterior or anterolateral approach. The disc herniation appears to be centrally located and cannot be safely excised through a posterior approach. The central herniation cannot be exposed through the posterior approach without manipulating the spinal cord.

QUESTIONS

196. A 9-year-old premenarcheal girl has noted an increased hump in her back at the thoracolumbar junction. The progressive deformity is not painful and she denies any leg pain or weakness. A lateral radiograph of the thoracolumbar spine demonstrates a local kyphosis of 62 degrees. A lateral chest film taken 1 year ago demonstrated a 54-degree local kyphosis. A sagittal MRI scan is shown here. What is your treatment plan?

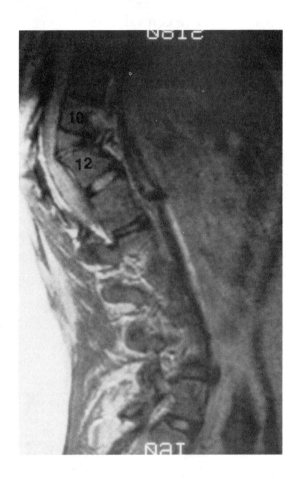

ANSWERS

196. The MRI scan shows a T11 hemivertebra. There is no evidence of any spinal dysraphism and the spinal cord is normal. The patient has shown documented progression of the local kyphosis of more than 5 degrees. The deformity is likely to continue to progress until she reaches skeletal maturity. She is a candidate for an anterior and posterior spinal fusion. The deformity is too big (>55 degrees) and the patient is too old (>5 years) to be a candidate for a posterior fusion alone.

QUESTIONS

197. An 11-year-old boy has undergone a posterior spinal fusion with instrumentation for thoracolumbar kyphosis. On the third day postoperatively, the patient started to vomit a greenish-colored liquid. On physical examination, he has abdominal distention and hypoactive bowel sounds. A gastrointestinal upper (GI) series is performed and is shown in the Figure. What is your treatment plan?

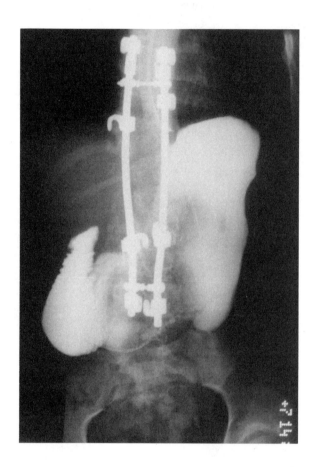

ANSWERS

197. The upper GI series shows a distended stomach with an obstruction at the upper third of the duodenum. This is the cast syndrome. The duodenum is obstructed as it travels between the superior mesenteric artery and the aorta. Treatment involves gastric decompression with nasogastric suction and hyperalimentation. Any restrictive cast should be removed and the patient should be placed in the lateral decubitus position.

QUESTIONS

198. A 68-year-old man has a 3-month history of low back pain and bilateral radiating leg pain. His leg pain is worse than his back pain. The leg pain radiates down his posterior thigh and involves his calf and foot bilaterally. The patient reports that his leg pain is exacerbated by walking and relieved by sitting and bending forward. The patient has already tried a course of physical therapy and a course of epidural and oral steroids. A myelogram of the patient's lumbar spine is shown in the figure. What is your treatment plan?

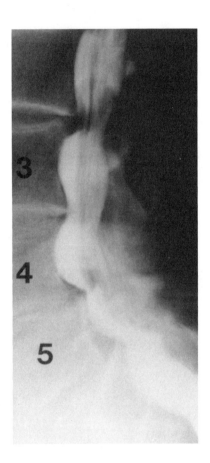

ANSWERS

198. The lateral myelogram shows multiple levels of narrowing of the spinal canal. At the L2–3 level, there is retrolisthesis of L2 on L3, disc space narrowing, and decreased sagittal diameter of the spinal canal. At L3–4 there is diffuse spondylosis but no significant narrowing of the spinal canal. At L4–5, there is a grade 1 degenerative spondylolisthesis associated with a severe narrowing of the spinal canal and a high-grade block of the myelographic dye. At L5–S1, there is some narrowing of the spinal canal consistent with spinal stenosis. The patient has failed a conservative treatment regimen. He now requires surgery. Treatment would involve multilevel posterior decompression laminectomies and posterolateral fusion between L4 and L5. The fusion must be performed because of the degenerative spondylolisthesis.

CHAPTER 6

Upper Extremity

David Strege, M.D.

QUESTIONS

1. At 5 weeks' gestational age, which of the long bones is likely to be ossified?

2. At what age does the medial epiphysis of the clavicle close?

3. What is the clinical significance of the age of medial clavicle epiphyseal closure?

4. Avascular necrosis of the medial end of the clavicle is known by what eponym?

5. What is the differential diagnosis of nontraumatic sternoclavicular joint pain?

6. Describe the two types of sternoclavicular joint dislocations and the significance of each.

ANSWERS

1. Earliest bone ossification is noted in the fifth intrauterine week. The clavicle is the first of the long bones to ossify.

2. The medial epiphysis of the clavicle is the last epiphysis of the long bones to appear in the body, occurring between the ages of 18 and 20 years. This epiphysis is also the last to close, which occurs at the age of 23 to 25 years.

3. Since the medial epiphysis of the clavicle does not close until the age of 23 to 25 years, this becomes clinically important when considering injuries in the region of the sternoclavicular joint. Because of this late closure most injuries to the sternoclavicular joint in patients under the age of 25 are likely to be physeal fractures and not true sternoclavicular joint dislocations, as would be true for those older than 25 years. If a true physeal fracture does exist, with healing one can expect remodeling to occur and aggressive attempts at anatomic reduction are not warranted. The treatment of choice for these displaced physeal injuries is attempted closed reduction, placement of a figure-8 clavicle strap, and then to allow for remodeling.

4. Friedreich's disease.

5. Avascular necrosis of the medial end of the clavicle (Friedreich's disease), condensing osteitis of the medial clavicle epiphysis, Paget's disease, sternoclavicular hyperostosis, Tietze's syndrome, spontaneous subluxation or dislocation, osteoarthritis, septic arthritis, or any of the rheumatologic arthropathies (rheumatoid arthritis, gout, psoriasis, etc.)

6. Sternoclavicular joint dislocations may occur anteriorly or posteriorly. Anterior dislocations are far more common and are associated with relatively few complications. The morbidity related to posterior dislocations is, however, much greater owing to impingement on mediastinal structures.

QUESTIONS

7. What physical findings are commonly seen with posterior dislocations of the sternoclavicular joint?

8. How is the diagnosis of sternoclavicular joint dislocation made?

9. Describe the closed reduction maneuver for posterior dislocations of the sternoclavicular joint.

10. How are anterior dislocations of the sternoclavicular joints treated?

11. What are the indications for open reduction of the sternoclavicular joint in cases of dislocation?

12. When should transarticular fixation pins be used for the treatment of sternoclavicular joint dislocations?

ANSWERS

7. Venous congestion of the neck or upper extremity, breathing difficulties, shortness of breath, choking, arterial insufficiency of the ipsilateral upper extremity, difficulties in swallowing, a tight feeling in the throat, pneumothorax, or thoracic outlet syndrome. When compared with anterior dislocations, posterior dislocations of the sternoclavicular joint frequently are associated with more pain and less prominence at the sternoclavicular joint.

8. The diagnosis and especially distinguishing anterior from posterior dislocation can be quite difficult by physical examination alone. Radiographs are usually necessary. Owing to the overlap of spine, ribs, sternum, clavicle, and soft tissue shadows of structures at the level of the mediastinum, anteroposterior (AP) views of the chest or shoulder are usually not helpful in making this diagnosis. Special radiographic views are necessary. A serendipity view of the sternoclavicular joints can assist in making this diagnosis. This view involves positioning the patient supine and orientating the x-ray tube with a 40-degree cephalic tilt to the horizontal plane. Tomograms or computed tomography (CT) scan may also be necessary to make this diagnosis.

ANSWERS

9. The patient is placed supine with a 3- to 4-in. bolster positioned posteriorly between the scapulae. Gentle traction is applied to the affected extremity with the arm abducted in line with the clavicle. As traction is increased the arm is brought into slight extension. A gentle downward push on the clavicle may be necessary to dislodge it from behind the sternum. If this is unsuccessful, the anterior chest wall should be surgically prepared and a sterile towel clip used to grasp the proximal clavicle and lift it, reducing the dislocation. After closed reduction these dislocations tend to be stable and can be treated with a figure-8 clavicle strap.

10. They are treated simply with attempted closed reduction. After closed reduction the sternoclavicular joint tends to be unstable and recurrence of the dislocation is likely. However, since there is minimal morbidity resulting from anterior dislocation of the sternoclavicular joint, the treatment of choice is "skillful neglect." Open reduction is generally not recommended owing to the overall poor results and the likelihood of changing a small, painless, bony prominence into a painful unsightly scar and persistent unstable sternoclavicular joint.

11. Indications are relatively limited. Owing to the severity of complications resulting from posterior dislocations and the rare failure of closed reduction, open reduction is then recommended. Anterior dislocations require operative intervention only in the rare case when chronic dislocation continues to be symptomatic after 6 to 12 months or painful traumatic arthritis results in this joint. In this case the treatment of choice is sternoclavicular joint arthroplasty including resection of the medial segment of the clavicle.

12. Because of the complications seen with the use of transarticular fixation pins across the sternoclavicular joint, the use of this type of fixation is generally not recommended and is condemned by most. Migration of complete or fractured fixation pins into the heart, lungs, and great vessels have caused significant morbidity and even death.

QUESTIONS

13. An 18-year-old man has only local tenderness after sustaining posterior displacement of the medial clavicle in a high school football game. Attempts at closed reduction were unsuccessful. How should this patient be managed?

14. What is the most common musculoskeletal birth injury?

15. A newborn baby is noted to have a "bump" on the right midclavicle. Radiographs demonstrate discontinuity of the clavicular shaft. What is the differential diagnosis of this finding?

16. The neurovascular structures of the superior thorax are protected by what structure in cases of midshaft clavicle fractures?

17. A 4-year-old child with a midshaft clavicle fracture is seen in the emergency room. How is this managed?

18. What are the indications for operative management of an adult with a clavicle shaft fracture?

ANSWERS

13. Posterior displacement of the medial clavicle in an 18-year-old man is more than likely due to physeal fracture resulting from late closure of the medial clavicular physis rather than posterior dislocation of the sternoclavicular joint. Radiographic documentation of this particular injury can be difficult as the medial epiphysis does not begin to ossify until approximately the 18th year. Therefore, after attempted closed reduction, if the patient has no significant symptoms related to compression of the vital structures within the mediastinum, these injuries should be allowed to heal. Remodeling frequently corrects any deformity with time.

14. Fracture of the clavicle.

ANSWERS

15. Discontinuity of the clavicle shaft in a newborn is most commonly due to a clavicle fracture. However, other diagnoses must be considered. Clavicle fracture must be suspected with a history of trauma, tenderness over the bump, pain with passive motion of the involved upper extremity, crepitance at the site of irregularity, and pseudoparalysis with decreased activity of the involved upper extremity. Congenital pseudoarthrosis of the clavicle should be suspected when there is no history of trauma, no tenderness, an enlarged pseudarthrosis site, and especially if the occurrence is in the right clavicle. Cleidocranial synostosis involves the absence of all or part of the clavicle without the formation of a lump. This is a hereditary abnormality of membranous bone and this diagnosis should be considered when other skeletal abnormalities, including skull deformities, smallness of the facial bones, scoliosis, deficiencies of the pelvis, or abnormal epiphyses in the hands and feet, are present.

16. The medial and lateral cord of the brachial plexus as well as the subclavian vessels are at risk for injury with midshaft clavicle fractures. Owing to their interposed position, these structures are somewhat protected by the subclavius muscle and clavipectoral fascia.

17. Closed clavicle fractures in children are treated simply with a figure-8 bandage or sling and swath. Attempts at maintaining closed reduction of these fractures can frequently be difficult, frustrating, and are usually unnecessary in view of the rapidity of healing of these fractures as well as the potential for remodeling.

18. (1) Neurovascular compromise; (2) open fractures requiring debridement; (3) severe displacement with tenting of the skin that is unreducible by closed means; (4) floating shoulder (displaced clavicle fracture and unstable scapular fracture); (5) a patient who is unable to tolerate closed immobilization (seizure disorder, Parkinson's disease); (6) painful nonunion; (7) the rare case in which a healed clavicle fracture has resulted in a bony prominence and the patient is willing to trade a surgical scar for removal of the bony prominence.

QUESTIONS

19. How are distal clavicle fractures frequently classified?

20. Which of the distal clavicle fractures require open reduction and fixation?

21. A 26-year-old moderately obese woman sustains a closed midshaft humerus fracture after a motor vehicle accident. After attempted closed reduction and placement of a coaptation splint, postreduction radiographs revealed a transverse fracture of the midshaft of the humerus with 1-cm overlap and 25 degrees of varus angulation. How should treatment proceed?

22. A 42-year-old man sustains a closed fracture of the distal third of the humeral shaft after a fall from a ladder. Immediate evaluation reveals an ipsilateral wrist drop. Closed reduction of the fracture results in satisfactory fracture alignment without bayonet apposition but there is no immediate change in neurologic status. How should this patient be managed?

23. After fracture of a humeral supracondylar process, a patient may demonstrate paresthesias at what anatomic location?

24. A patient sustains a grade III open humerus fracture with segmental radial nerve loss. What management plan should be recommended?

ANSWERS

19. Neer has classified distal clavicle fractures into three types. In type I, the coracoclavicular and acromioclavicular ligaments are intact. In type II, the medial clavicular segment is detached from the coracoclavicular ligament, resulting in significant displacement. In type III, there is fracture into the acromioclavicular joint but no disruption of the acromioclavicular or coracoclavicular ligaments.

ANSWERS

20. The type II fracture of the distal clavicle tends to be unstable and it is difficult to maintain reduction by closed means. These usually require open reduction and internal fixation, commonly with the use of an intermedullary fixation pin.

21. No further attempts at reduction are necessary. The patient should be followed closely in her coaptation splint. The majority of humeral shaft fractures can be treated by closed means. Owing to the soft tissue bulk surrounding the humerus, a fair amount of angulation and shortening of fractures is well tolerated. Acceptable reduction is less than 25 degrees of anterior angulation and less than 30 degrees of varus angulation. Bayonet shortening is considered acceptable if less than 1 in.

22. Because of the close proximity of the radial nerve to the humeral shaft in distal third humeral fractures, radial nerve injuries are probably the most common complication of these fractures. Holstein and Lewis are credited with describing this relationship in these fractures. As the majority of these radial nerve palsies (approximately 90%) are neuropraxias, in cases of radial nerve injury after closed fractures, resolution of radial nerve palsy would be expected with time. Appropriate management would be to wait at least 3 to 4 months until clinical or electromyographic (EMG) evidence of muscle reinnervation should have occurred before considering nerve exploration.

23. Median nerve distribution of the hand.

24. Early nerve grafting of the radial nerve is appropriate. Additionally, early tendon transfers should be considered owing to the long time required for nerve recovery as well as the relatively poor long-term results from nerve graft procedures. Tendon transfers for radial nerve palsy should restore thumb, finger, and wrist extension. An example is the Green tendon transfers, in which the pronator teres is transferred to the extensor carpi radialis brevis, the palmaris longus to the extensor pollicis longus, and the flexor carpi ulnaris to the extensor digitorum communis.

QUESTIONS

25. A 25-year-old obese man sustained multiple trauma with a closed head injury as the result of a motor vehicle accident. He is noted to frequently thrash violently in bed. Among other orthopedic injuries he has a closed transverse fracture of the humeral shaft. There is no apparent peripheral nerve injury. How should this fracture be managed?

26. What anatomic structures define the quadrangular space in the shoulder and what important structures pass through it?

27. Injury of the axillary nerve results in what functional deficits?

28. The rotator cuff of the shoulder is composed of which muscles?

29. Which muscles insert on the greater and lesser tuberosities of the proximal humerus?

30. What is the predominant vascular supply to the humeral head?

31. What is the distal extent of the lateral surgical approach to the shoulder?

ANSWERS

25. Because of the high rate of success of closed treatment and immobilization of closed humeral shaft fractures, operative intervention is rarely required. However, open reduction and internal fixation is, at times, necessary. In the case of the uncooperative patient, the treatment of closed humeral shaft fracture with hanging cast or coaptation splint is unlikely to maintain adequate reduction. In this case, when the patient is medically stable and cleared for surgery and after other orthopedic injuries have been addressed, management of the humerus fracture would be internal fixation by means of intramedullary rod or dynamic compression plate.

ANSWERS

26. The boundaries of the quadrangular space, viewed from posteriorly, are the teres minor superiorly, the teres major inferiorly, the long head of the triceps medially, and the surgical neck of the humerus laterally. The contents of the quadrangular space include the axillary nerve, and the posterior circumflex humeral artery.

27. (1) Weakness of shoulder abduction, extension, and forward flexion due to paralysis of the anterior, middle, and posterior deltoid muscle; (2) weakness of shoulder external rotation due to paralysis of the teres minor; and (3) decreased sensation in a variable region over the lower one half of the deltoid due to loss of the cutaneous sensory branch of the axillary nerve, the superolateral brachial cutaneous nerve.

28. Subscapularis, supraspinatus, infraspinatus, and teres minor.

29. The greater and lesser tuberosities of the proximal humerus are separated by the bicipital groove through which passes the tendon of the long head of the biceps. The supraspinatus, infraspinatus, and teres minor insert into the greater tuberosity. The subscapularis inserts into the lesser tuberosity.

30. The ascending branch of the anterior humeral circumflex artery terminates in a tortuous vessel called the arcuate artery. This supplies the majority of the humeral head. Smaller contributions come from the posterior humeral circumflex artery and from the rotator cuff muscles through their tendinous osseous anastomoses.

31. The axillary nerve leaves the quadrangular space, winds around the proximal humerus, and enters the deep surface of the deltoid. Extension of the lateral surgical approach to the shoulder by splitting the fibers of the deltoid greater than 5 cm beyond the tip of the acromion risks injury to the axillary nerve and denervation of the deltoid.

QUESTIONS

32. How are fractures of the proximal humerus classified?

33. A 31-year-old man sustains injury to his shoulder after a fall off his bicycle. Radiographs of the shoulder reveal a surgical neck fracture of the proximal humerus with 30 degrees of angulation. How should this fracture be managed?

34. A 67-year-old woman tripped and injured her right shoulder. Radiographs demonstrate a displaced four-part humerus fracture. What is the treatment of choice?

35. A 50-year-old rancher is thrown off his horse injuring his shoulder. Radiographs of the shoulder reveal a displaced greater tuberosity fracture of the proximal humerus. What other structure is necessarily injured and how is this treated?

36. A 34-year-old sustains a greater tuberosity three-part proximal humerus fracture as a result of a skiing injury. In what direction is the articular surface of the humeral head positioned and what is the treatment of choice?

37. Describe the ligaments that stabilize the acromioclavicular joint.

38. Horizontal stability of the acromioclavicular joint is controlled by which ligaments?

ANSWERS

32. The most common classification is the Neer four-part classification. Displaced fractures of the proximal humerus occur through the anatomic neck, the surgical neck, the greater tuberosity, and the lesser tuberosity. A single displaced fragment through one of these fracture sites, or any combination of fracture fragments through multiple fracture sites, is classified as a two-part, three-part, or four-part fracture. These fractures may be further defined if anterior or posterior dislocation is an element of the fracture.

ANSWERS

33. In the Neer classification, this fracture would be classified as a two-part fracture of the surgical neck. Fragments are considered displaced if there is greater than 1-cm separation or more than 45 degress of angulation between fragments. Since there is only 30 degrees of angulation in this case, it would be considered a minimally displaced fracture. Therefore, reduction is not necessary and treatment should consist of a period of sling-and-swathe immobilization and early mobilization.

34. In the Neer-classification, a displaced four-part proximal humerus fracture involves fragmentation of the lesser tuberosity, greater tuberosity, and humeral head. These fractures tend to occur in the elderly, osteoporotic person. Overall results of fixation of these fractures have been poor owing to poor fixation of osteopenic bone, malunion, and a high incidence of avascular necrosis. The treatment of choice is prosthetic humeral head replacement.

35. Displaced greater tuberosity fractures must have an accompanying rotator cuff tear. Owing to soft tissue attachments, these are unlikely to be amenable to closed reduction. Therefore, open reduction of the fracture fragment and repair of the rotator cuff is the treatment of choice.

36. As the lesser tuberosity remains attached to the humeral head, the subscapularis tendon insertion will internally rotate the humeral head so that the articular surface faces posteriorly. These fractures are unstable and are unlikely to be reduced closed. Therefore, open reduction and internal fixation is the treatment of choice.

37. The acromioclavicular joint is a diarthrodial joint with a fibrocartilaginous intraarticular disc. It is stabilized by two sets of ligaments. The acromioclavicular joint capsular ligaments are the superior, inferior, anterior, and posterior ligaments, of which the superior is the strongest. Additionally, the coracoclavicular ligament provides support to the acromioclavicular joint. The coracoclavicular ligament is a strong ligament composed of two components, the conoid and the trapezoid.

38. The acromioclavicular ligaments control horizontal stability. Vertical stability is controlled by the coracoclavicular ligaments.

QUESTIONS

39. Rockwood classifies acromioclavicular joint injuries into six types. What are they?

40. What is the treatment of choice for acromioclavicular joint injuries by type?

41. How should sternoclavicular injuries be treated?

42. What can be done for unreduced chronic symptomatic anterior or posterior sternoclavicular dislocations?

43. What is the treatment for spontaneous anterior and posterior dislocation of the sternoclavicular joint?

44. The site for safe aspiration of the elbow joint is defined by what anatomic landmarks?

45. The mobile wad of Henry is composed of which muscles?

46. What is the normal carrying angle of the elbow?

47. Bifurcation of the brachial artery occurs at what level?

ANSWERS

39. *Type I:* sprain of the acromioclavicular ligament with no disruption of the acromioclavicular or coracoclavicular ligaments (no instability); *Type II:* acromioclavicular ligament disruption leading to horizontal acromioclavicular instability (subluxation); *Type III:* "classic" acromioclavicular dislocation with disruption of the acromioclavicular and coracoclavicular ligaments; *Type IV:* posterior dislocation of the acromioclavicular joint (into or through the trapezius); *Type V:* superior dislocation of the acromioclavicular joint with severe displacement; *Type VI:* inferior dislocation of the acromioclavicular joint.

ANSWERS

40. *Types I* and *II:* symptomatic treatment with sling and early range-of-motion exercises; *Type III:* for patients older than 25, and non-laborers, only symptomatic treatment is required. For heavy laborer or those less than 25 years of age, operative repair with some type of internal fixation (commonly a coracoclavicular screw); *Types IV, V,* and *VI:* attempted closed reduction. If reduced, treat as type III. If unreduced, proceed to open reduction and internal fixation.

41. Type I injuries are treated with ice, a sling for 3 to 5 days, and then return to daily activities. Type II injuries are reduced and placed in a figure-8 clavicle strap, or the arm is supported in a sling for 1 to 2 weeks followed by gradual use of the arm. In type III injuries, closed reduction can be performed for anterior or posterior dislocation and a figure-8 clavicle strap worn by the patient for 4 weeks. Anterior dislocations are usually unstable and the deformity is accepted since this is less risky than the potential problems of operative repair and internal fixation. A sling is worn for 2 weeks and then range-of-motion exercises are begun when the patient is comfortable.

42. Resection of the medial 1 in. of clavicle.

43. "Skillful neglect" (Rockwood). Immobilize until comfortable, then begin active range-of-motion exercises.

44. Elbow joint aspirations are safely performed laterally within the triangle formed by the lateral epicondyle of the humerus, the radial head, and the tip of the olecranon.

45. The brachioradialis, extensor carpi radialis longus, and extensor carpi radialis brevis muscles.

46. The angle formed by the intersection of the long axis of the humerus and the axis of the ulna with the elbow in a full extension is a measure of the carrying angle of the elbow. Normally, the carrying angle measures 10 degrees valgus in males and 13 degrees valgus in females.

47. The brachial artery bifurcates into the ulnar and radial arteries within the proximal forearm at the level of the radial head.

QUESTIONS

48. Describe the relationship of the median nerve to the brachial artery in the arm.

49. What functional arc of motion at the elbow is considered necessary for most daily activities?

50. A 20-year-old woman falls while playing volleyball, landing on her left elbow. She complains of poorly localized elbow pain. Radiographs demonstrate no evidence of fracture or dislocation but an anterior fat pad is noted. What is the significance of this finding?

51. The posterolateral (Kocher) surgical exposure approaches the elbow joint through which intramuscular interval and potentially puts which nerve at risk for injury?

52. How can injury to this nerve be avoided when using the posterolateral (Kocher) approach to the elbow?

53. In the anterolateral surgical exposure of the elbow a nerve is encountered at the muscular interval between the biceps tendon and the brachialis muscle. What is this nerve? Where does it originate? What is its function?

54. How are supracondylar distal humerus fractures distinguished from transcondylar distal humerus fractures?

ANSWERS

48. In the upper arm the median nerve lies lateral to the brachial artery. In the midarm the nerve crosses anterior to the artery as it crosses the intramuscular septum so that in the distal arm the nerve lies medial to the brachial artery.

49. The normal range of motion at the elbow is from 0 to 145 degrees of flexion. However most daily activities can be carried out within a functional arc of 30 to 130 degrees. Additionally, normal pronation of 75 degrees and supination of 85 degrees is well beyond the functional arc of 50 degrees of pronation and 50 degrees of supination necessary to carry out most daily activities.

ANSWERS

50. A fat pad sign is a radiolucent stripe found within the soft tissue shadow of extremity radiographs and is due to the low radiodensity of adipose tissue. At the elbow, anterior and posterior fat pads are most easily seen on the lateral projection. These fat pads are intracapsular but extrasynovial. The anterior fat pad is normally visible anterior to the coronoid fossa of the humerus. The posterior fat pad is normally obscured on the lateral view owing to its position within the olecranon fossa. If the posterior fat pad is viewed or the anterior fat pad is enlarged, an intraarticular abnormality is suspected due to increased intraarticular fluid collections from inflammation or hemarthrosis after trauma. In the present example, if no posterior fact pad is viewed, the presence of an anterior fat pad is probably a normal finding.

51. The posterolateral (Kocher) approach exposes the elbow joint through the interval between the anconeus and extensor carpi ulnaris muscles. The posterior interosseous nerve is at risk for injury in this dissection as it passes within the substance of the supinator muscle at the level of the radial tuberosity and continues to wind around the shaft of the radius as it passes distally to the dorsum of the forearm.

52. Distal extension of this exposure must be limited and care taken not to dissect beyond the level of the radial neck. Also, as approximately 1 cm of radial nerve translation can occur with forearm pronation and supination, pronation of the forearm will position the posterior interosseous nerve farthest away from the surgical field.

53. The lateral antebrachial cutaneous nerve becomes superficial at the anterolateral aspect of the elbow between the biceps tendon and the brachialis muscle. It provides sensory innervation to the lateral aspect of the forearm. It is a continuation of the musculocutaneous nerve originating from the C5–8 nerve roots and the lateral cord of the brachial plexus.

54. Both are rare in the adult. When the transverse fracture line extends through the olecranon fossa of the distal humerus, this is considered a transcondylar distal humerus fracture. Supracondylar humerus fractures are within the distal humeral metaphysis proximal to the olecranon fossa.

QUESTIONS

55. How is a nondisplaced transcondylar distal humerus fracture treated?

56. How are supracondylar humerus fractures classified?

57. What structure(s) most likely prevents satisfactory closed reduction of the displaced extension-type supracondylar humerus fracture?

58. How are displaced, closed extension-type supracondylar humerus fractures treated?

59. How are T and Y intracondylar distal humerus fractures classified?

60. A 72-year-old woman slips and falls on an icy parking lot, landing on her elbow. Radiographs of the swollen elbow reveal an extensively comminuted T intracondylar humerus fracture. How should this fracture be managed?

ANSWERS

55. Immobilization for 1 to 2 weeks in a long arm posterior splint followed by early active range-of-motion exercises monitored closely radiographically for signs of displacement.

56. Supracondylar humerus fractures are of two types: (1) The extension type is more common and occurs as a result of a fall on the outstretched arm. The distal humeral fragment is displaced posteriorly and proximally secondary to the pull of the triceps. (2) The flexion type results from direct trauma against the posterior aspect of the flexed elbow. The distal fragment lies anterior to the humerus and is flexed at the elbow.

57. Attempts at closed reduction can be impeded by the brachialis muscle interposed at the fracture site or by the proximal humerus fracture fragment buttonholed through brachialis muscle such that an attempted closed reduction maneuver with application of longitudinal traction may further tighten the muscle around the protruding fragment.

ANSWERS

58. After careful neurovascular assessment of the involved upper extremity and with adequate anesthesia and muscle relaxation, closed reduction of the supracondylar humerus fracture can be attempted. Longitudinal traction is applied to the arm with the elbow extended. This overcomes the proximal pull of the triceps and biceps and unlocks the fracture fragments. The thumb positioned posteriorly is used to manipulate the distal humerus fragment forward and reduced as the elbow is flexed to maintain stable reduction. The elbow should then be immobilized (4–6 weeks) in maximal flexion but 10 degrees short of where the radial pulse disappears to allow for swelling. The forearm position is controversial but placing the forearm in pronation may prevent displacement due to the unopposed pull of the pronator teres at the elbow. If the fracture remains unstable after closed reduction or if excessive flexion is required to maintain reduction such that the radial pulse is lost, percutaneous pinning with two crossed or two laterally placed Kirschner wires may be necessary. Open reduction with plate and screw fixation and early mobilization has also been recommended.

59. Riseborough and Radin have classified these fractures into four types based upon their radiographic appearance. *Type I:* undisplaced; *type II:* displacement between the capitellum and the trochlea but without appreciable fracture fragment rotation; *type III:* displacement of the capitellum and trochlea with rotational deformity; *type IV:* severe comminution of the articular surface with wide separation between the humeral condyles.

60. Owing to poor results with open reduction and internal fixation of extensively comminuted and osteopenic bone of the elderly, closed treatment with either olecranon traction or the "bag of bones" technique is recommended. In the latter, the elbow is placed in maximum flexion within the limits dictated by swelling and circulatory compromise. The arm is placed in a collar and cuff with the elbow hanging free so that gravity can be used to obtain ligamentotaxis and possible fracture reduction. At 2 weeks motion is begun in flexion at the elbow. The sling is gradually loosened in order to increase flexion motion and the sling is discarded at 6 weeks. In the younger population with better-quality bone, these fractures are treated with open reduction and internal fixation.

QUESTIONS

61. A 28-year-old man was thrown from his automobile and landed on his elbow. He sustained a closed displaced T intracondylar distal humerus fracture with minimal comminution. How should this fracture be managed?

62. How are condylar fractures of the distal humerus classified?

63. What complications may result from malunion of type II lateral condyle fractures?

64. How are displaced condylar humerus fractures treated?

65. How are displaced capitellar fractures of the elbow managed?

66. How are radial head fractures classified?

67. What is the treatment of choice for type I radial head fractures?

ANSWERS

61. Open reduction and internal fixation. This is accomplished by first obtaining anatomic reduction of the articular surface of the distal humerus and maintaining this reduction with Kirschner wires or lag screw fixation. Dual plate fixation is then recommended to reduce the distal humerus fracture to the proximal humerus. Semi-tubular plates or reconstruction plates may be used and should be placed with the plates orientated perpendicularly.

62. Milch has classified condylar fractures of the distal humerus into two types. *Lateral condyle* type I involves the capitellum through the capitellotrochlear sulcus. Type II involves the capitellum and the lateral lip of the trochlea through the trochlear sulcus. *Medial condyle* type I involves the medial lip of the trochlea. Type II involves the entire trochlea through the capitellotrochlear sulcus. Type II fractures are considered fracture dislocations because the ulna remains articulated with the displaced fracture fragment.

ANSWERS

63. Joint incongruity may result in early posttraumatic arthritis, loss of motion, or joint instability. Malunion may also result in a cubitus valgus deformity with tardy ulnar nerve palsy and cosmetic disfigurement.

64. Because of the unstable nature of condylar fractures, displaced type I and II fractures are treated by open reduction and internal fixation with anatomic restoration of the articular surface. Screw fixation is followed by early range-of-motion exercises at 5 to 10 days. Depending on the stability of fixation, splinting is usually recommended between exercise periods for 3 to 6 weeks.

65. Capitellar fractures of the distal humerus are purely intraarticular fractures occurring in the coronal plane with no soft tissue attachments. These are to be distinguished from lateral condylar fractures which occur in the sagittal plane and possess some soft tissue attachment. Most fractures of the capitellum involve a large osseous portion of the capitellum (type I). Less commonly, the capitellar fragment has very little subchondral bone attached (type II) or is comminuted. Owing to involvement of the articular surface of the elbow joint, displaced capitellar fractures require operative intervention. Open reduction and internal fixation with Kirschner wires, small fixation screws, or Herbert screws should be attempted for type I capitellar fractures. Type II or comminuted fractures require excision of these small fragments. Early range-of-motion exercises should be instituted within the first week of surgery with either open reduction or excision of the capitellar fragment.

66. Radial head fractures are classified into four types: *type I:* nondisplaced; *type II:* marginal fracture with displacement; *type III:* comminuted fracture involving the entire radial head; *type IV:* any radial head fracture with simultaneous elbow dislocation.

67. Joint aspiration and instilling local anesthetic in the joint will substantially reduce the patient's acute pain. The involved extremity is placed in a sling or splinted for 5 to 7 days, at which time early range-of-motion exercises should be initiated.

QUESTIONS

68. What is the treatment of choice for type II radial head fractures?

69. What is the treatment of choice for type III radial head fractures?

70. At what level should the radial head be excised when treating radial head fractures by radial head excision?

71. After initiating postinjury elbow rehabilitation, why is passive manipulation and stretching generally not recommended?

72. After surgical excision of the radial head, how much proximal radial migration can be expected?

73. A 24-year-old man undergoes radial head excision at the time of injury for a comminuted radial head fracture involving the entire radial head. The patient regains excellent range of motion of the right elbow, but his postoperative course is complicated by increasing ipsilateral wrist pain. What is the likely cause of this wrist pain?

74. A patient with an elbow injury demonstrates radiographic evidence of comminuted radial head fracture and fracture of the coronoid process. What is the significance of this injury and how is it treated?

ANSWERS

68. The treatment of these fractures is controversial. However, the following guidelines generally apply. Marginal fractures with less than 2 mm displacement and involving less than one third of the head with no mechanical block to elbow or forearm motion can be treated as a type I fracture, placing the arm in a sling and initiating early range-of-motion exercises. If displacement is greater than 2 mm and involves greater than 30% of the radial head or involves mechanical block to elbow or forearm motion, operative intervention is recommended. In the young patient with a large fragment, open reduction and internal fixation with Kirschner wires or fixation screws is recommended. If anatomic reduction and fixation is not possible, or in the older patient, radial head excision is the treatment of choice.

ANSWERS

69. Radial head excision. In order to minimize the risk of formation of heterotopic ossification, most recommend early excision of the radial head within 24 hours from the time of injury followed by early active range-of-motion exercises within 3 to 5 days postoperatively.

70. The level most commonly recommended is that of the annular ligament.

71. There is a high risk of heterotopic bone formation and subsequent ankylosis.

72. Under normal circumstances, where there is no compromise of the distal radioulnar ligamentous support, only approximately 2 mm of proximal radial migration should be expected.

73. The association of radial head fracture with disruption of the distal radioulnar joint is called Essex-Lopresti injury. Disruption of the interosseous membrane of the forearm as well as the ligamentous support of the distal radioulnar joint is believed to occur concurrently with the radial head fracture. This ligamentous disruption after radial head excision allows greater than normal proximal radius migration. With time this results in an increasing ulnar positive variance with subsequent subluxation of the distal radioulnar joint and increasingly painful ulnar abutment at the wrist. Various treatment alternatives have been advised for this problem, including Silastic radial head replacement, radiocapitellar joint replacement, tightening of the interosseous membrane, ulnar shortening, ulnar head excision, and radioulnar synostosis. At this time there is no ideal solution.

74. Combined fractures of the radial head and coronoid process tend to be very unstable and may be associated with medial or lateral collateral ligament disruption. This requires open reduction and fixation of the coronoid process fracture or reattachment of the brachialis to the proximal ulna as well as repair of torn medial or lateral collateral ligaments. If salvage of the radial head is not possible due to comminution, prosthetic radial head replacement is usually necessary to maintain stability at the elbow.

QUESTIONS

75. In what position should the elbow be immobilized for a nondisplaced fracture of the olecranon?

76. An 18-year-old man sustains a displaced transverse fracture of the olecranon. How should this be treated?

77. What portion of the olecranon can be safely excised without producing instability at the elbow?

78. A 73-year-old woman trips and falls, landing on her left elbow. She sustains a comminuted fracture of her olecranon. What is the treatment of choice?

79. A 20-year-old man injured his elbow while playing hockey. Radiographs reveal an ossicle formation posteriorly, just proximal to and separated from the olecranon apophysis by a radiolucent line. What is this ossicle and how is this injury treated?

80. A patient is seen in the emergency room and found to have an acute posterior dislocation of the elbow. How should this be treated?

ANSWERS

75. Immobilization should be at 45 degrees of flexion. Immobilization in full extension should be avoided because of the likelihood of loss of flexion after immobilization. Immobilization beyond 45 degrees risks displacing the fracture. Cast immobilization should be maintained for 3 weeks followed by protected range-of-motion exercises. Flexion beyond 90 degrees should be avoided until the fracture has healed at 6 to 8 weeks.

ANSWERS

76. This is probably best treated using the AO tension band wiring technique using figure-8 stainless steel wire over longitudinally placed parallel intramedullary Kirschner wires.

77. Excision of the olecranon may be the treatment of choice for certain olecranon fractures, especially fractures involving extensive comminution, small avulsion fractures, or fractures in the very elderly, osteoporotic population. If the distal surface of the semilunar notch of the ulna, as well as the coronoid process, remains intact, as much as 80% of the olecranon may be excised without producing instability of the elbow.

78. If the coronoid process and distal surface of the semilunar notch of the olecranon remain intact, the treatment of choice in an elderly person with osteopenic bone would be excision of the olecranon. If comminution were minimal and bone quality good, then plate and screw fixation using a one-third tubular plate is appropriate.

79. This ossicle occurs within the triceps tendon near its insertion and is considered a true sesamoid bone. It is called a patella cubiti. It is rare and although it may fracture, this injury can be treated symptomatically.

80. After initial examination and assessment of the neurovascular function of the involved upper extremity and after administration of appropriate sedation or general anesthetic, closed reduction should be attempted. Most reduction maneuvers involve application of countertraction to the arm as traction is applied to the wrist and forearm. Medial or lateral displacement is corrected first. As distal traction is continued, anterior pressure is directed on the olecranon and the elbow is gradually flexed. This unlocks the coronoid out of the olecranon fossa. Most authors recommend avoiding hyperextension maneuvers owing to the potential for injury to the brachialis muscle and for heterotopic ossification. If after several attempts closed reduction cannot be accomplished, proceed with open reduction. After reduction is accomplished, the elbow is brought through a full range of motion and the neurovascular status again assessed.

QUESTIONS

81. After successful closed reduction of a posterior dislocation of the elbow, how should postreduction care and rehabilitation proceed?

82. What is the most common nerve injury seen after elbow dislocation?

83. Immediately after closed reduction of a posterior elbow dislocation, the elbow is noted to have an apparent mechanical block when attempting to take the elbow through a range of motion. What is the most likely cause of this block?

84. What are the most common sites of involvement of heterotopic ossification after elbow dislocation?

85. Four months after elbow dislocation a patient is noted to have a 60-degree flexion contracture with radiographic evidence of mild heterotopic ossification in the anterior capsule. How should treatment proceed?

86. A patient is noted to have a 30-degree flexion contracture at the elbow 12 months after elbow dislocation. The patient has undergone extensive physical therapy including dynamic splinting prior to this time. How should management proceed?

87. A 3% to 5% incidence of ectopic bone formation is noted to occur after fractures or dislocations about the elbow. What are the risk factors that increase the likelihood of ectopic bone formation?

ANSWERS

81. The elbow should be splinted at 90 degrees of flexion. The splint is removed within a few days and early active range-of-motion exercises are begun. A removable elbow splint may be used for comfort between exercise periods during the first 1 to 2 weeks. Passive motion and stretching are avoided during the early rehabilitation period.

82. Injuries to the median, radial, and ulnar nerves at the time of elbow dislocation are relatively common. Therefore, careful neu-

ANSWERS

rovascular assessment of the involved extremities is important before and after attempted reduction maneuvers. Most commonly, the ulnar nerve is injured resulting from valgus stress at the time of dislocation. Injury to the radial nerve is least commonly reported.

83. Although more common in children and adolescents after posterior elbow dislocation and reduction, this block is most likely caused by entrapment of a medial epicondyle fracture fragment. Most commonly these fracture fragments are noted on postreduction radiographs lying at the level of the joint. While closed reduction maneuvers have been described, most medial epicondyle avulsion fractures require open reduction and internal fixation. If a fracture fragment remains undetected, it may lead to significant posttraumatic arthritis.

84. The medial and lateral collateral ligaments, the anterior capsule, and the brachialis muscle.

85. Surgical intervention should be delayed until the osseous elements are completely mature. While this is believed to occur at 9 to 12 months after time of injury, there is no reliable means of predicting tissue maturation. Radioactive isotope scanning has not been shown to be completely reliable as an indicator of tissue maturation. This patient would most likely benefit from physical therapy including heat, ultrasound, dynamic splinting, and gentle active assisted stretching exercises.

86. Since the results of surgical release in obtaining extension beyond 30 degrees are unpredictable, the general recommendation is to refrain from surgery for flexion contractures of less than 45 degrees. Additionally, as the functional range of motion is 30 to 130 degress in flexion, a lack of the last 30 degrees of full extension does not tend to be an overwhelming functional deficit. In this case no further treatment need be offered.

87. Head injury increases the likelihood of ectopic bone formation to 89%. Dislocation combined with fracture about the elbow, frequent manipulation in reduction attempts, delayed reduction, and delayed motion at the elbow all increase the likelihood of ectopic bone formation. Injuries in the younger patient population decrease the likelihood of ectopic bone formation.

QUESTIONS

88. After elbow fracture or dislocation, what measures can be taken to prevent ectopic ossification in patients at high risk for this to occur?

89. How are coronoid process fractures of the proximal ulna classified?

90. How are coronoid process fractures of the proximal ulna treated?

91. What is the functional loss resulting from distal biceps tendon rupture and how should this problem be managed acutely?

92. What is the recommended surgical approach for surgical repair of distal biceps tendon rupture?

93. Lateral epicondylitis is the most common cause of lateral elbow pain. What other entities should be considered before making this diagnosis?

ANSWERS

88. Three treatment options are available. (1) Indomethacin is most generally recommended because of its effectiveness in clinical trials and because it is well tolerated with relatively few side effects. The recommended dosage is 25 mg. t.i.d. beginning as soon after the injury or surgery as possible. (2) Radiation has been utilized in the past to retard ectopic bone formation but its efficacy in the elbow joint has never been demonstrated and the risks of delay in wound healing for wounds within the radiation portal and other dangers of radiation must be considered. (3) Diphosphonates have been shown experimentally to decrease calcification of ectopic bone formation but have not been demonstrated to inhibit bone induction. Therefore, their effectiveness has been questioned.

ANSWERS

89. Coronoid process fractures of the proximal ulna are classified by Regan and Morrey into three types. A type I fracture involves avulsion of the tip of the coronoid process, type II is a fracture involving less than 50% of the coronoid process, and type III is a fracture involving greater than 50% of the coronoid process.

90. Type I fractures are usually stable and can be treated with 2 to 3 weeks of immobilization followed by early active range-of-motion exercises. Type II fractures, if stable, are treated as type I fractures, if unstable, treatment is open reduction and internal fixation. Type III fractures tend to be unstable and should be treated with open reduction and internal fixation followed by cast immobilization for 3 weeks or hinged cast bracing allowing limited early elbow range of motion.

91. If left untreated, distal biceps tendon ruptures result in approximately 40% loss of strength of both flexion and supination at the elbow. Therefore the treatment of choice is surgical repair of the complete biceps tendon rupture distally within 7 to 10 days of injury. However, as other muscles surrounding the elbow are available to assume the function of the biceps muscle, surgical repair in the elderly patient, in whom demands on the upper extremity are minimal, may not be warranted.

92. Boyd and Anderson have described a two-incision technique intended to minimize the risk of injury to the neurovascular structures within the antecubital fossa, especially the radial nerve. An anterior approach is used to identify and mobilize the biceps tendon stump. Heavy sutures are then placed within the tendon stump, which are passed between the radius and ulna to a second posterolateral incision. Through the second incision, the proximal radius is exposed and a window made within the radius into which the biceps tendon is attached. All dissection is carried out extraperiosteally to avoid the potential complication of proximal radioulnar synostosis.

93. Injury or fracture of the radial head or capitellum, lateral elbow instability, and radial tunnel syndrome.

QUESTIONS

94. What is the pathologic process and the specific anatomic site of involvement of lateral epicondylitis?

95. How is lateral epicondylitis treated?

96. What structures at the elbow are most susceptible to injury in the throwing athlete?

97. What are the radiographic and physical findings associated with "Little Leaguer's elbow?"

98. How is Little Leaguer's elbow treated?

99. Before attempting elbow arthrodesis, what other upper extremity functions should be taken into consideration?

100. What is the optimal position for elbow arthrodesis?

ANSWERS

94. *Lateral epicondylitis* is the term frequently used to describe an overuse syndrome resulting in lateral elbow pain. This results in a tendinitis occurring at the origin of the extensor carpi radialis brevis tendon. The pathologic findings consist of replacement of normal tendon collagen fibers with tissue composed of fibroblasts and vascular granulation-like tissue described by Nirschl as "angiofibroblastic proliferation."

95. Symptoms usually respond to nonsurgical treatment. Rarely is surgical intervention necessary. Intital management should consist of rest and refraining from activities that aggravate the condition; use of aspirin or nonsteroidal anti-inflammatory medication, and physical therapy modalities (heat, ultrasound, cortisone phonophoresis) followed by aggressive strengthening exercises. This may be supplemented with wrist cock-up or lateral elbow counterforce bracing. If there is no response to this treatment, consideration should be given to local corticosteroid injection. In the rare case, where

ANSWERS

symptoms continue to persist after nonsurgical management, surgical intervention should be considered. This involves excision of the abnormal angiofibroblastic tissue at the origin of the extensor carpi radialis brevis muscle.

96. Repetitive valgus stress occurs at the elbow of the throwing athlete. The primary stabilizer to valgus stress is the relatively strong anterior oblique medial collateral ligament and the secondary restraint to valgus stress is the radiocapitellar articulation at the elbow. With repetitive valgus stress there is attenuation or incompetence of the medial collateral ligament and secondary injury to the radiocapitellar joint.

97. Little Leaguer's elbow, a condition seen in young, throwing athletes, is manifested by progressive medial elbow pain, especially with throwing. Owing to the repetitive valgus stress of throwing as well as the strong pull of the flexor muscles off the medial epicondyle, this condition is thought to be due to a subtle stress fracture through the physis of the medial epicondyle. On physical examination there is point tenderness over the medial epicondyle as well as an elbow flexion contracture, frequently greater than 15 degrees. Radiographic findings, if present, consist of subtle widening or even fragmentation of the epiphyseal line of the medial epicondyle when compared with the opposite normal elbow.

98. Treatment is always nonoperative. Most patients respond to a period of rest and refraining from the aggravating activity for a period of 2 to 3 weeks. This should be followed by supervised physical therapy with progressive strengthening and reconditioning before returning to throwing activities.

99. The function of the shoulder and elbow is to position the hand in space. When considering elbow arthrodesis, satisfactory motion of the shoulder is absolutely essential or the patient will loose his or her ability to position the hand. Bilateral elbow arthrodesis should not be considered because the functional limitation is too great.

100. In the patient with satisfactory motion at the elbow and wrist, arthrodesis at 90 degrees of flexion will optimize functioning. With adaptive motion at the neck, shoulder, and wrist, the hand can reach the mouth and writing can also be done comfortably.

QUESTIONS

101. What is a "safe interval" in the posterior surgical approach to the shoulder?

102. What anatomic structures are responsible for impingement tendinitis of the shoulder?

103. Why is the supraspinatus tendon most commonly involved in impingement tendinitis and rotator cuff tears?

104. What is the function of the rotator cuff?

105. Neer has classified impingement tendinitis into three stages. What are these stages?

106. How do the Neer stages of impingement tendinitis differ by history and physical examination?

ANSWERS

101. After the deltoid muscle is detached from the spine of the scapula, the safe interval is entered between the infraspinatus and teres minor muscles. Proceeding through this internervous plane prevents injury to the suprascapular nerve innervating the infraspinatus superiorly and the axillary nerve innervating the teres minor inferiorly.

102. Structures which cause narrowing of the subacromial space. Bony changes and osteophyte formation tend to occur on the anteroinferior surface of the acromion, along the coracoacromial ligament, especially as it inserts into the anteromedial portion of the acromion, and also in the acromioclavicular joint.

103. Involvement of the supraspinatus tendon in impingement tendinitis and rotator cuff tears is probably related to the vascularity of this tendon. The area of the tendon just proximal to the site of insertion tends to be hypovascular, a "watershed zone." Vascular filling within this area is dependent upon shoulder positioning. With the arm in an adducted position, the tendon is compressed over the humeral head and vascular filling is prevented. With the

ANSWERS

arm in abduction, compression of the tendon across the humeral head is decreased and vascular filling occurs. Hypovascularity, in addition to mechanical impingement of the supraspinatus tendon at this site, can then result in inflammation as well as impaired ability to heal and repair small tears within the rotator cuff.

104. The rotator cuff serves multiple functions. It assists with shoulder abduction, internal rotation (assisted by the subscapularis), and external rotation (provided by the infraspinatus and teres minor muscles). The rotator cuff additionally serves to stabilize the glenohumeral joint by depressing the humeral head in the glenoid fossa. When portions of the rotator cuff are selectively contracted, these muscles can serve to resist displacing forces, thereby preventing shoulder subluxation and dislocation.

105. Stage I is edema and hemorrhage, stage II is fibrosis and tendinitis, and stage III is tendon degeneration and rupture.

106. Stage I can occur at any age, but most frequently under age 25. An aching shoulder pain is brought on by activities involving the upper extremity. Positive physical findings include tenderness over the greater tuberosity and anterior acromion; painful motion of the shoulder, especially in abduction, which is increased with resistance at 90 degress of abduction; and a positive impingement sign. The biceps tendon is also frequently involved and can be demonstrated by tenderness over the biceps tendon and pain elicited with resisted forward flexion of the humerus with the forearm in supination and extension at the elbow (straight arm raising test). Stage I is a reversible lesion. Stage II usually occurs between the ages of 25 and 40. Shoulder discomfort occurs not only with strenuous activities but also with activities of daily living and at night. Pain has occurred over a prolonged period of time. Signs are similar to those noted in stage I, but increased shoulder stiffness and tenderness over the acromioclavicular joint are more commonly found in stage II. Because of repeated insults, the supraspinatus tendon, the biceps tendon, and the subacromial bursa become thickened and fibrotic making this lesion irreversible. Stage III usually occurs after the age of 40. The usual history is prolonged and recurrent shoulder problems with pain occuring at night and with work-related activities. Signs are similar to stages I and II, but shoulder weakness is significant (especially with shoulder abduction and external rotation). Infraspinatus and supraspinatus muscle wasting may also be noted.

QUESTIONS

107. What is an impingement sign?

108. What is an impingement test?

109. What radiographic findings are consistent with impingement tendinitis and rotator cuff tear of the shoulder?

110. What is the diagnostic study of choice to demonstrate rotator cuff tears?

111. An 18-year-old high school shortstop has a 3-week history of considerable discomfort in his dominant right shoulder after baseball games or prolonged practice. There has been no history of trauma and no night pain. On examination the patient has full active motion of the shoulder with tenderness over the greater tuberosity of the humerus and a positive impingement sign. Radiographs of the right shoulder are negative. How should this patient be managed?

ANSWERS

107. An impingement sign is demonstrated by having the patient place the affected arm in neutral rotation, while the examiner forcibly forward flexes the humerus. This causes the greater tuberosity of the humerus to be jammed against the undersurface of the acromion. Eliciting pain with this maneuver is a positive impingement sign. A less reliable but commonly used maneuver to demonstrate impingement is performed with the patient's humerus at 90 degrees of forward flexion and forcibly internally rotating the shoulder. Once again this causes the greater tuberosity to be driven further underneath the acromion and produces pain in the case of impingement tendinitis.

ANSWERS

108. After a positive impingement sign has been elicited, 10 mL of 1% lidocaine is injected into the subacromial bursa of the shoulder. If a local anesthetic relieves the pain of the repeated impingement sign, this further confirms the diagnosis of impingement tendinitis.

109. The findings on plain radiographs of the shoulder are subtle. Frequently the glenohumeral joint appears normal. Osteophyte formation is noted over the anteroinferior surface of the acromion and at the acromioclavicular joint with cystic degeneration at the greater tuberosity of the humerus. The space between the humeral head and the acromion is also frequently narrowed in large rotator cuff tears because the rotator cuff has lost its ability to function as a humeral head depressor. Less than 7 mm of space between the humeral head and the acromion is suggestive of a rotator cuff tear.

110. While ultrasonography and MRI are used in some centers, these methods require considerable experience, which leads to variability in diagnosis. The gold standard for diagnosis of full-thickness rotator cuff tears is the shoulder arthrogram. The escape of dye into the subacromial or subdeltoid space after injection of the glenohumeral joint demonstrates a full-thickness rotator cuff tear. The accuracy of this study is 95% to 100%. While the size of the rotator cuff tear cannot be demonstrated by routine shoulder arthrogram, supplementation with double contrast arthrogram or arthrotomogram may assist in defining the size.

111. This patient's symptoms and signs are consistent with impingement tendinitis and would be classified as stage I in Neer's classification. These are reversible lesions and generally respond to nonoperative treatment. This would include a period of rest, refraining from aggravating activities (i.e., baseball) anti-inflammatory medications, and physical therapy modalities followed by progressive shoulder rehabilitation after pain has subsided.

QUESTIONS

112. A 62-year-old woman presents with a 6-month history of increasing shoulder discomfort. Pain occurs with any activity involving use of the affected extremity as well as at night. There has been no history of trauma. On examination there is tenderness over the lateral acromion and anteriorly over the biceps tendon. Active range of motion is full, but there is significant weakness, especially with abduction and external rotation. The impingement sign is positive. Radiographs demonstrate a normal glenohumeral joint with small subacromial osteophyte formation. How should management of this patient proceed?

113. A 38-year-old woman has a 9-month history of persistent shoulder pain. The pain limits her work-related activities. There has been no specific trauma. She maintains full active range of motion of the shoulder with a positive impingement sign. The patient has undergone 4 months of conservative treatment measures for impingement tendinitis without significant improvement. Radiographs of the right shoulder demonstrate minimal osteophyte formation in the subacromial region. Shoulder arthrogram is negative. How should this patient be managed?

114. A 42-year-old man falls down several steps injuring his shoulder. He is unable to abduct his shoulder beyond 30 degrees actively, but maintains full passive range of motion. Plain radiographs of the shoulder are negative for fracture or dislocation. How should this patient be managed?

115. When acromioplasty is selected for treatment of impingement tendinitis, what part and how much of the acromion is resected?

ANSWERS

112. This patient demonstrates stage III of Neer's classification for impingement tendinitis with possible chronic rotator cuff tear. A trial of conservative treatment measures should be initiated including rest, anti-inflammatory medications, and physiotherapy. If these measures fail and pain persists, an arthrogram should be performed to demonstrate suspected rotator cuff tear. Treatment should proceed with surgical subacromial decompression (acromioplasty and resection of the coracoacromial ligament) with repair of the rotator cuff tear, if present.

113. This patient demonstrates impingement tendinitis of the shoulder without rotator cuff tear which is resistant to conservative treatment. Since pain is interfering with her activities, surgical intervention with subacromial decompression (acromioplasty and coracoacromial ligament resention) is warranted. Simple coracoacromial resection alone may relieve pain, but tends to be short-lived so that this procedure along with acromioplasty is generally recommended.

114. Suspicion of an acute rotator cuff tear should be confirmed with a shoulder arthrogram to demonstrate that weakness of abduction is not due to other causes of abduction weakness (i.e., suprascapular nerve palsy). In a very active person with acute rotator cuff tear, the treatment of choice is surgical repair.

115. Since the anterior portion of the undersurface of the acromion is the actual site of impingement, the anteroinferior portion of the acromion should be resected. This is accomplished by resecting a wedge-shaped piece of bone from the undersurface of the acromion measuring approximately 9 mm anteriorly and approximately 2 cm in length. At the time of acromioplasty the coracoacromial ligament should always be resected. Additionally, the acromioclavicular joint should be resected if it is noted to be arthritic and symptomatic or if this joint is enlarged by periarticular osteophytes and is causing further impingement on the supraspinatus tendon.

QUESTIONS

116. A 53-year-old farmer felt a "pop" in his shoulder while attempting to lift a bag of seed. He is noted to have a bulge ("Popeye arm") in the anterior aspect of his right arm. How should this patient be managed?

117. Is glenohumeral joint stability dependent on the surrounding musculature?

118. What is the most common type of anterior dislocation of the shoulder?

119. What is meant by luxatio erecta?

120. What is the most common type of posterior dislocation of the shoulder?

121. What is the most common mechanism of action causing anterior dislocation of the shoulder?

122. What is the most common mechanism of action causing posterior dislocation of the shoulder?

ANSWERS

116. This patient has a rupture of the proximal long head of the biceps tendon. Because of the high association of proximal biceps tendon rupture with impingment tendinitis and rotator cuff tears, shoulder examination for signs of impingement as well as a shoulder arthrogram should be performed. In an active patient, the biceps tendon should be repaired by suturing it to the intertubercular groove of the humerus. The intraarticular portion of the biceps tendon should be excised and acromioplasty and repair of the rotator cuff tear, if present, should be performed. While disability related to biceps tendon rupture is minimal, attention to shoulder impingement and rotator cuff tear is of importance with this tendon rupture.

ANSWERS

117. In the resting state and with minimal loads across the joint, glenohumeral joint stability does not depend upon the surrounding musculature. Passive joint stability is provided by ligamentous and capsular restraints, the concavity of the glenoid surface and its labrum, negative intraarticular pressure produced by a finite joint volume, and by the adhesive and cohesive properties of the joint fluid. The stability provided by these passive restraints is noted in the anesthetized and paralyzed patient whose shoulder stability is maintained, as well as in the fresh cadaveric specimen in which the glenohumeral articulation is also maintained. When larger loads are placed across the glenohumeral joint, dynamic stability is provided by the surrounding musculature.

118. Subcoracoid dislocation. Subglenoid, subclavicular, and intrathoracic anterior dislocations are less common.

119. Luxatio erecta is an inferior dislocation of the shoulder with the humeral head located in a subglenoid position such that the superior articular surface of the humeral head is directed inferiorly. This places the humerus in a severely abducted position.

120. Posterior dislocations of the shoulder are defined by the position of the humeral head. The subacromial posterior dislocation occurs most commonly and is noted by the position of the humeral head behind the glenoid and beneath the acromion. Subglenoid and subspinous posterior dislocations occur less frequently.

121. Anterior dislocations of the shoulder are most commonly the result of an indirect force with the arm axially loaded in an abducted, extended, and externally rotated position.

122. A posterior dislocation of the shoulder is most commonly the result of axial loading of the arm in an adducted, flexed, and internally rotated postition.

QUESTIONS

123. Why are electric shock and convulsive seizures more likely to be associated with posterior dislocations of the shoulder?

124. In examination of the shoulder, what is the significance of an apprehension sign and how is it elicited?

125. A 72-year-old obese woman, complains of shoulder pain after a fall. She holds the affected extremity in the "sling position" with the forearm across the abdomen. She resists attempts to abduct the shoulder because it causes pain. The neurovascular status of the upper extremity and the remainder of the physical examination are otherwise normal. An AP radiograph of the shoulder is read as negative. How should this patient be managed?

126. AP radiographs of the shoulder in the case of subacromial posterior dislocation may appear quite normal. What subtle radiographic signs suggest posterior dislocation in this radiograph?

127. What is a Hill-Sachs lesion and how is it best demonstrated radiographically?

ANSWERS

123. Electric shock and convulsive seizures result in violent contracture of all of the muscle groups surrounding the shoulder. When this occurs the stronger internal rotators (pectoralis major, lattissimus dorsi, and subscapularis muscles) simply overwhelm the weaker external rotators (teres minor and infraspinatus muscles) resulting in posterior dislocation of the shoulder.

124. A positive apprehension sign is one in which manipulation of the shoulder elicits apprehension or a sensation that the shoulder is about to dislocate. This suggests shoulder instability. In the most common apprehension test, or crank test, to demonstrate anterior shoulder instability, the examiner holds the patient's arm in 90

ANSWERS

degrees of abduction and applies progressive external rotation to the arm while stabilizing the posterior shoulder with the opposite hand. Similarly, posterior instability can be tested with the jerk test, in which the examiner axially loads the humerus while grasping the elbow and placing the arm in 90 degrees of forward flexion and internal rotation. With continued axial loading the arm is moved horizontally across the body into an adducted position. This may produce a jerk as the humeral head subluxates posteriorly over the posterior glenoid rim. Additonally, this frequently elicits apprehension on the part of the patient. While pain may be elicited with these maneuvers, the presence of pain alone without signs of apprehension does not demonstrate instability and other conditions should be considered.

125. The physical findings of posterior dislocation are minimal, especially in the obese patient. Additionally, a single AP radiograph is inadequate for examination of the shoulder after trauma. Subacromial posterior dislocation may appear deceptively normal on the AP radiograph. Additional views (axillary or transcapular) are necessary in determination of shoulder dislocations.

126. Posterior dislocation places the humerus in an internally rotated position. Thus the normal profile of the neck of humerus is not seen on the AP view. In the normal shoulder, overlap between the glenoid and the humeral head creates an elliptic shadow and the humeral head fills the majority of the glenoid cavity. With posterior dislocation, this shadow is lost and the humeral head no longer fills the majority of the glenoid cavity. A "trough line," or longitudinal radiodense line formed within the humeral head, representing an impaction fracture of the anterior humeral head, may be demonstrated with posterior dislocation. Additionally, posterior dislocation is suggested if there is greater than 6 mm of space between the anterior rim of the glenoid and the humeral head.

127. The Hill-Sachs lesion is a compression fracture of the posterolateral aspect of the humeral head resulting from anterior dislocation of the shoulder. Radiographic views used to demonstrate the Hill-Sachs lesion are the Stryker notch or Hill-Sachs view. In the Stryker notch view the x-ray cassette is placed under the shoulder of the supine patient. The palm of the hand of the affected extremity is placed behind the head, the elbow is placed straight upward, and the x-ray beam is centered over the coracoid process tilting 10 degrees cephalad. In the Hill-Sachs view an AP radiograph of the shoulder is made with the humerus in extreme internal rotation.

QUESTIONS

128. What is a Bankart lesion and what is its significance?

129. What is the West Point view and what is its significance?

130. How frequently are rotator cuff tears seen associated with anterior dislocations of the shoulder?

131. A patient has sustained an anterior dislocation of the shoulder which is easily reduced. After reduction the patient is noted to have significant weakness on shoulder abduction. Sensation over the lateral aspect of the shoulder and arm is normal. The remainder of the neurovascular examination is negative and postreduction radiographs of the shoulder are negative. What is the likely cause of the abduction weakness and how should this be managed?

132. After shoulder dislocation, what factors place the patient at risk for recurrence?

ANSWERS

128. A Bankart lesion is an avulsion of the capsule and glenoid labrum off of the anterior rim of the glenoid resulting from traumatic anterior dislocation of the shoulder. The importance of this lesion is that it may contribute to shoulder instability resulting in recurrent dislocation. While the Bankart lesion is probably not the only "essential" lesion leading to recurrent anterior dislocation, this lesion, combined with a posterolateral defect in the humeral head (Hill-Sachs lesion) and erosion or fracture of the anterior rim of the glenoid, is responsible for anterior instability of the shoulder.

ANSWERS

129. The West Point axillary view of the shoulder is most commonly used to detect fractures or defects of the anteroinferior rim of the glenoid resulting in anterior dislocations of the shoulder. This view is obtained with the patient prone, with x-ray cassette placed under the involved shoulder, and the involved extremity placed on a 7.5-cm pad. After the head and neck are turned away from the involved shoulder, the x-ray beam is directed toward the axilla, raised 25 degrees off the horizontal, and aimed 25 degrees toward the patient's midline.

130. Rotator cuff tears are thought to occur relatively frequently after anterior dislocations of the shoulder. The incidence increases with increasing age of the patient, exceeding 30% after age 40 years and 80% after age 60.

131. Injury to the axillary nerve is the most common nerve injury after anterior dislocation of the shoulder. This is thought to occur with an overall incidence of approximately 30% and occurs more often in the elderly population. With axillary nerve injury cutaneous sensation over the lateral shoulder is frequently normal and therefore sensory examination is an unreliable indicator of injury. After anterior dislocation of the shoulder these nerve injuries are most often traction neuropraxias and should simply be treated by observation. Most will recover within 10 weeks from the time of injury. However, the prognosis is poor for axillary nerve palsies persisting beyond 10 weeks.

132. Recurrence is the most common complication following traumatic anterior dislocation of the shoulder. Age at the time of initial dislocation is probably the most important factor. Patients under the age of 20 years are thought to have a recurrence rate in the range of 80%. Athletes are at greater risk for recurrence than nonathletes. After the age of 40 the recurrence rate falls to approximately 10%. Males have a higher recurrence rate than females and the majority of recurrences occur within 2 years of the initial traumatic dislocation. Extremity dominance is unrelated to recurrence. Recurrence varies inversely with the severity of the initial trauma, such that if a minor traumatic event caused the initial dislocation, the likelihood of recurrence is relatively high.

QUESTIONS

133. How should postreduction management proceed in a patient with an uncomplicated traumatic anterior shoulder dislocation?

134. A 22-year-old college football lineman has had three episodes of traumatic anterior dislocation of the shoulder. This first occurred after trying to make an arm tackle 4 years ago. On physical examination he has evidence of anterior instability of the shoulder. Radiographs of the shoulder are negative. How should this patient be managed?

135. Limiting external rotation is the goal of most surgical procedures to treat anterior instability of the shoulder. What are the risks of this method of treatment and for which patients should this procedure generally not be recommended?

136. A 20-year-old patient demonstrates the ability to cause a "clunk" sensation in his shoulder with certain maneuvers which result in a bony prominence posteriorly in the shoulder. The patient has noted his ability to do this since a young age. This does cause intermittent pain in the shoulder and some difficulty with his job as a construction worker. How should this problem be managed?

ANSWERS

133. Postreduction management after traumatic anterior dislocation of the shoulder is controversial, especially in the younger patient in whom risk of recurrence is relatively high. However, in the younger patient (<30 years old) sling immobilization in a position of comfort of adduction and internal rotation for a period of 3 to 5 weeks is recommended. In the older patient (>30 years) in whom the risk of developing stiffness is greater and the risk of recurrence is decreased, sling immobilization for 1 to 2 weeks is recommended. During the period of immobilization, progressive isometric exercises, especially for internal and external rotation, are initiated. More vigorous strengthening exercises are initiated after the period of immobilization. Range of motion of the glenohumeral joint is rarely a problem after dislocation, but more vigorous range of motion exercises may be initiated 6 weeks after the time of injury if this is a problem. Return to overhead labor or athletic activities is not allowed until normal rotator strength and full forward elevation of the shoulder have been demonstrated.

ANSWERS

134. In the young athlete with significant trauma causing initial dislocation, the likelihood of recurrence and recurrent instability is high. Initial treatment of any anterior dislocation of the shoulder should begin with strengthening of the internal and external rotators to improve dynamic stability. If instability persists, surgical intervention is recommended. While many procedures have been described, current recommendations favor repair of the Bankart lesion (if present) with anterior capsulorrhaphy or a subscapularis tightening procedure, or both. Of importance is to ensure that instability is solely anterior with these procedures. Anterior glenoid osteotomies have, for the most part, fallen out of favor.

135. For patients who require normal or supranormal range of motion of the shoulder (swimmers, baseball pitchers) a surgical procedure resulting in limitation of external rotation is likely to cause significant limitation so that they would not be able to return to their presurgical level of activity. Aggressive strengthening of the rotator muscles is the recommended treatment for such patients. Not only is limitation of motion a problem with these procedures but if excessive tightness of anterior repair has been performed (e.g., unable to externally rotate beyond 0 degrees), these patients are at greater risk to develop osteoarthritis of the glenohumeral joint due to change in joint mechanics.

136. The patient who is able to voluntarily dislocate the shoulder frequently has multidirectional instability and a history where minimal trauma has resulted in the initial dislocation. Frequently, these patients have other emotional or psychiatric problems and they should be referred for psychiatric evaluation. Surgery for these patients is rarely recommended. Those patients without psychiatric problems who are voluntary dislocators usually respond to a rehabilitation program involving strengthening of the rotator muscles of the shoulder increasing dynamic stabilization. Only after 6 to 12 months of intensive physical therapy and after the patient has demonstrated the desire to discontinue voluntary dislocation should surgical stabilization be considered.

QUESTIONS

137. An 18-year-old swimmer complains of increasing bilateral shoulder pain with swimming activities. There has been no history of shoulder dislocation. The physical examination is remarkable for the ability to hyperextend at the knees and elbows bilaterally. Multidirectional instability of both shoulders can be demonstrated. Radiographs of the shoulders are negative. How should this patient be treated?

138. Modifications of the Bristow procedure have been previously used for treatment of anterior shoulder instability, in which the tip of the coracoid process is transferred to the anterior glenoid. What muscles are attached to the coracoid process, what nerve is at risk for injury, and why is this procedure generally no longer recommended for the treatment of anterior shoulder instability?

139. The C5 nerve root emerges superior or inferior to the C5 vertebral body?

140. After emerging from the vertebral foramina, nerve roots of the brachial plexus descend between what anatomic structures?

141. What is the function of the dorsal rami of C5–T1?

142. The phrenic nerve arises from which nerve root(s)?

143. The phrenic nerve lies in what position relative to the scalene muscles?

ANSWERS

137. In patients with atraumatic shoulder instability, this tends to occur bilaterally, with multidirectional instability and generalized ligamentous laxity as demonstrated in this case. These patients frequently respond to rehabilitation. Aggressive physical therapy with strengthening of the rotators of the shoulder frequently provides sufficient dynamic stability. If the patient does not respond to conservative treatment, an inferior capsular shift should be included as part of the surgical procedure.

138. Three muscles are attached to the coracoid process. The pectoralis minor inserts proximally and at the tip is the origin of the conjoined tendon (i.e., the short head of the biceps and the coracobrachialis). The musculocutaneous nerve runs medial to the coracoid process and obliquely through the coracobrachialis muscle, at variable distances from the coracoid process, and is at risk for injury. Because of the multiple complications of this procedure, including recurrent subluxation, coracoid nonunion, screw-related problems, injury to the musculocutaneous nerve, and shoulder weakness, this procedure is no longer the treatment of choice.

139. The brachial plexus is normally composed of the C5–T1 nerve roots. The C5–7 nerve roots emerge superior to their respective cervical vertebral bodies. C8 emerges below C7 and T1 below the T1 vertebral body.

140. The anterior primary rami of the nerve roots forming the brachial plexus descend between the anterior and middle scalene muscles.

141. The dorsal rami of C5–T1 supply innervation to the muscles and skin of the dorsal neck.

142. The phrenic nerve arises primarily from the C4 nerve root. However, there may be additional contributions form C3 or C5. Determination of the functioning of the C4 neurologic level is especially important in determining if the tetraplegic patient will be respirator-dependent.

143. The phrenic nerve lies anterior to the anterior scalene muscles. This differs from the remainder of the nerves to the brachial plexus which descend *between* the anterior and middle scalene muscles.

QUESTIONS

144. The lateral cord of the brachial plexus is composed of which nerve divisions?

145. The cords of the brachial plexus are named relative to the position of what anatomic structure?

146. What are the terminal branches of the lateral cord of the brachial plexus?

147. What are the terminal branches of the medial cord of the brachial plexus?

148. What are the terminal branches of the posterior cord of the brachial plexus?

149. What is the innervation of the pectoralis minor muscle?

150. What is the innervation of the teres major muscle?

151. What is Horner's syndrome?

152. Horner's syndrome results from injury to or interruption of which nerve fibers?

ANSWERS

144. The lateral cord is composed of the anterior divisions of the upper and middle brachial plexus trunks. The anterior division of the lower trunk becomes the medial cord and the posterior divisions of the upper, middle, and lower trunks become the posterior cord.

145. The lateral, medial, and posterior cords of the brachial plexus are named with respect to their positions surrounding the axillary artery.

ANSWERS

146. The lateral cord of the brachial plexus arises from the C5–7 nerve roots. The terminal branches of the lateral cord include the lateral pectoral nerve, the lateral root of the median nerve, and the musculocutaneous nerve.

147. The medial cord of the brachial plexus arises from the C8 and T1 nerve roots. The terminal branches of the medial cord include the medial pectoral nerve, the medial brachial cutaneous nerve, the medial antebrachial cutaneous nerve, the medial root of the median nerve, and the ulnar nerve.

148. The posterior cord of the brachial plexus arise from the C5–T1 nerve roots. The terminal branches of the posterior cord include the upper and lower subscapular nerve, the thoracodorsal nerve, the axillary nerve, and the radial nerve.

149. The medial pectoral nerve innervates the pectoralis minor muscle. The pectoralis major muscle is innervated by both the medial and lateral pectoral nerves.

150. The lower subscapular nerve innervates the teres major muscle. The upper and lower subscapular nerves innervate the subscapularis muscle.

151. Horner's syndrome results from loss of sympathetic innervation and produces the characteristic physical findings of ptosis, enophthalmus, and myosis as well as anhydrosis to the ipsilateral side of the face.

152. The sympathetic nerve fibers arise from the cervicothoracic ganglia and the C8–T1 nerve roots to accompany the trigeminal nerve to the orbit where they become the ciliary nerves. These fibers control the tarsal muscles, the orbital muscles of Müller, and the dilator muscles of the pupil. Interruption of these sympathetic nerve tracts due to injury or local anesthetic instilled at the C8–T1 nerve root level or cervicothoracic ganglia will produce Horner's syndrome.

QUESTIONS

153. After a motorcycle accident, a patient is found to have a flail and anesthetic upper extremity. Three weeks after the injury the patient's physical examination is unchanged. Nerve conduction velocity studies obtained at this time reveal absent motor conduction, but sensory conduction is intact. What is the significance of this finding?

154. When should baseline EMG studies be obtained after a brachial plexus injury? In the presence of denervated muscles, what kind of EMG findings can be demonstrated?

155. Cervical myelography is frequently used to demonstrate the presence of nerve root avulsions after brachial plexus injury. What radiographic findings suggest nerve root avulsion?

156. After brachial plexus injury, what findings suggest a preganglionic lesion?

ANSWERS

153. After brachial plexus injury, the finding of absent motor conduction with intact sensory conduction on nerve conduction velocity studies suggests a preganglionic injury to the involved nerve roots. Since the cell bodies of the afferent sensory fibers reside in the dorsal root ganglion, a lesion proximal to this site (i.e., nerve roots) will not result in wallerian degeneration of these sensory nerve axons and nerve conduction velocity of these fibers will remain normal. As there is interruption of the sensory pathways to the central nervous system, sensation cannot be perceived and the corresponding area remains anesthetic. If nerve conduction velocity studies demonstrate absence of both sensory and motor conduction, this suggests a postganglionic injury level or a combination of pre- and postganglionic injury levels.

ANSWERS

154. EMG is used to detect muscle denervation. After axonal interruption, wallerian degeneration of the axon occurs over a 3-week period. Muscle denervation potentials are not likely to be demonstrated until wallerian degeneration of the affected axons has occured. Therefore baseline EMG studies should probably be postponed until approximately 3 weeks after the time of injury. Under normal conditions muscle at rest is electromyelographically silent. After denervation small electrical potentials are generated spontaneously by the denervated muscles. Therefore, the positive finding by the EMG study of denervated muscle is one of spontaneous fibrillation potentials.

155. Avulsion injury to the nerve roots of the brachial plexus commonly damages both the nerve root and the surrounding meninges. The characteristic findings with cervical myelography in the presence of any avulsion injury include inability to visualize the nerve root as well as the presence of meningeal diverticula referred to as a traumatic meningocele at the level of the avulsed nerve root. However, these findings are not pathognomonic of a preganglionic lesion as cases have demonstrated the presence of traumatic meningocele without nerve root avulsions (false positive) as well as nerve root avulsions existing in the presence of a normal myelogram (false negative). With cervical myelography, positive findings are only suggestive and not conclusive for the presence of a preganglionic nerve root avulsion.

156. In patients with complete brachial plexus involvement, findings consistent with a preganglionic lesion on physical examination will demonstrate, in addition to a flail arm, Horner's syndrome due to involvement of the sympathetic cervicothoracic ganglia, winged scapula due to interruption of the long thoracic nerve, paralysis of the rhomboids secondary to injury proximal to the dorsal scapular nerve, and diaphragmatic paralysis if there is C4 nerve root involvement. Cervical myelogram may demonstrate traumatic meningocele. Nerve conduction studies should demonstrate sensory conduction to be intact with absent motor conduction and EMG will demonstrate denervation of cervical paraspinal as well as peripheral musculature of the affected extremity.

QUESTIONS

157. After brachial plexus injury, what findings suggest a postganglionic lesion?

158. A 22-year-old patient sustains an incomplete brachial plexus injury after a motorcycle accident. Three months after the injury there are no signs of recovery of the C5–6 neurologic deficit. How should this patient be managed?

159. How should a 68-year-old patient with C8–T1 brachial plexus lesion be managed who has no evidence of recovery 6 weeks after the time of injury?

160. A 38-year-old mail carrier experienced severe weakness of his nondominant shoulder with abduction and external rotation. He exhibits moderate tenderness over the site where his mailbag strap passes over the scapula. Impingement sign of the shoulder is negative. What diagnostic study should be done to confirm the diagnosis?

161. How should this patient be managed?

162. What anatomic structure(s) pass beneath the superior transverse scapular ligament?

163. Injury to what nerve results in winging of the scapula?

ANSWERS

157. A consistent finding is a physical examination demonstrating a flail arm. However, Horner's syndrome, winged scapula, diaphragmatic paralysis, and paralysis of the rhomboids should be absent. Cervical myelography should be normal. Nerve conduction studies should demonstrate absence of both motor and sensory conduction and EMG will demonstrate normal cervical paraspinal musculature with denervation of peripheral musculature.

ANSWERS

158. In the young patient with a brachial plexus injury without signs of recovery, it is recommended that surgical exploration of the involved portion of the brachial plexus be undertaken and where transection exists, nerve repair, nerve grafting, or neurotization be applied, depending upon the intraoperative findings. Current recommendations are that surgical exploration should be undertaken within the first 5 to 6 months after injury. In the young patient surgical exploration should be undertaken despite the fact that pseudomeningocele may be seen on myelogram owing to the possibility of a false-positive result with intact nerve roots at this level.

159. In the older patient with brachial plexus injury, the chances of nerve regeneration are relatively poor, even with surgical intervention. Therefore in this case, appropriate early tendon transfer is warranted and surgical exploration of the brachial plexus is relatively contraindicated. Additionally, one would expect poor results from surgical exploration of the brachial plexus in this case owing to the relatively long length of axonal regeneration necessary to reinnervate the C8–T1 muscle groups.

160. Weakness of the shoulder on abduction and external rotation is not always due to rotator cuff tendinitis or tear. With a negative impingement sign and evidence of local irritation over the suprascapular notch, suprascapular nerve compression neuropathy should be suspected. The diagnostic study of choice is nerve conduction study with EMG.

161. Begin with elimination of the activity which precipitated the neuropathy (i.e., removal or change of position of the mailbag). Most suprascapular nerve palsies respond to conservative measures including activity modification, local anesthetic, and cortisone injection into the region of the scapular notch as well as physical therapy to maintain shoulder range of motion. If conservative treatment measures fail or fibrillation potentials are noted on EMG studies of the spinatus muscles, then surgical decompression of the suprascapular nerve is indicated.

162. The suprascapular nerve. The suprascapular artery passes over this ligament.

163. Dynamic winging of the scapula is caused by injury to the long thoracic nerve resulting in paralysis of the serratus anterior muscle.

QUESTIONS

164. An 18-year-old man fell out of a tree and landed on his shoulder. Radiographs obtained at the time of injury were found to be negative. Three weeks after injury his right shoulder pain has resolved, but he notes delayed winging of the scapula. What is the likely cause of this scapular winging and why was this finding not apparent immediately after the injury?

165. How should traumatic winging of the scapula be treated?

166. Thoracic outlet syndrome is most frequently confused with compression neuropathy of which peripheral nerve?

167. What structure(s) is commonly compressed in thoracic outlet syndrome?

168. What is the differential diagnosis of thoracic outlet syndrome?

169. What are the provocative tests used on physical examination to diagnose thoracic outlet syndrome?

ANSWERS

164. Winging of the scapula in this case is likely due to a traction injury to the long thoracic nerve. This results in paralysis of the serratus anterior muscle. While paralysis of the serratus anterior muscle probably occurred at the time of injury, winging of the scapula will not be clinically evident until stretching of the overlying trapezius has occurred.

ANSWERS

165. Traumatic winging of the scapula is usually due to a traction neuropraxia of the long thoracic nerve. Therefore, in most cases these should be treated symptomatically. A short period of rest with sling immobilization of the involved upper extremity should be followed by range-of-motion exercises. Most resolve with time and benign neglect. If there is no resolution after approximately 2 years, appropriate stabilization procedures may be undertaken.

166. Signs and symptoms consistent with thoracic outlet syndrome are closely related to those associated with ulnar neuropathy. Features which distinguish thoracic outlet syndrome from ulnar neuropathy are sensory deficit along the ulnar aspect of the forearm or upper arm and motor involvement of the thenar muscles found in thoracic outlet syndrome and not in ulnar neuropathy.

167. Vascular symptoms are due to compression of the subclavian artery and subclavian vein. Neurologic symptoms result from compression of the lower trunk of the brachial plexus. Less commonly, there is middle trunk involvement of the brachial plexus. Therefore, most neurologic symptoms in thoracic outlet syndrome are related to C8–T1 motor and sensory symptoms.

168. Cervical radiculopathy, tumors of the apical portion of the lung (Pancoast), and peripheral nerve compression, most notably that of the ulnar nerve.

169. In the classic Adson test, the patient is seated with the neck extended and rotated toward the ipsilateral side while the breath is held in full inspiration. The disappearance of the radial pulse along with reproduction of the patient's symptoms signifies a positive result. In Wright's hyperabduction test, the patient's arm is abducted 90 degrees with the arm in full external rotation. Again, diminution of the radial pulse concurrent with reproduction of symptoms signifies a positive test. In the overhead exercise test, the fingers are rapidly and repeatedly flexed and extended, with the arms abducted. Forearm and hand pain and paresthesias occurring in less than a minute of this activity constitute a positive test. Finally, the costoclavicular maneuver places the patient's shoulders in a military brace position, with the arms drawn downward and posterior. Diminution of the radial pulse and reproduction of the symptoms constitute a positive test. False-positive results may be obtained in these tests.

QUESTIONS

170. What diagnostic study confirms the diagnosis of thoracic outlet syndrome?

171. What are the most common complaints and physical findings in a patient with suspected thoracic outlet syndrome?

172. How should the patient with suspected thoracic outlet syndrome be treated?

173. After a low velocity gunshot wound to the upper extremity with resultant nerve injury, what would be the expected percentage of spontaneous recovery?

ANSWERS

170. No specific diagnostic study can be relied on to confirm the diagnosis of thoracic outlet syndrome. This diagnosis is made strictly on a clinical basis. Special studies may, however, be beneficial. Radiographs of the cervical spine may demonstrate the presence of cervical ribs, supporting the diagnosis of thoracic outlet syndrome, or may demonstrate cervical spondylosis suggesting nerve root compression at the level of the intervertebral foramen. Electrophysiologic studies may demonstrate slowing of nerve conduction velocities in the region of the supraclavicular fossa, supporting thoracic outlet syndrome, or may demonstrate compression of other peripheral nerves mimicking thoracic outlet syndrome. In the event that there is a vascular component to the thoracic outlet syndrome, transfemoral subclavian angiography is warranted.

ANSWERS

171. Symptoms are variable. However, most patients complain of paresthesias radiating from the cervical region of the neck to the shoulder and down along the medial aspect of the limb to the ulnar two to three fingers. Pain frequently accompanies these paresthesias and is described as gnawing or burning. Nocturnal pain and paresthesias are common. Weakness of the hand as well as decreased dexterity are also frequent complaints. Symptoms are usually aggravated by placing the involved extremity in an elevated or overhead position. If there is an involved vascular element, intermittent or constant swelling, cyanosis and cold intolerance may be present. On physical examination sensory changes usually involve the ulnar aspect of the hand as well as the medial aspect of the forearm and arm. Muscle wasting and weakness may be demonstrated in the intrinsic muscles of the hand including the thenar muscles. Vascular changes may include diminished distal pulses, decreased blood pressure compared with the opposite side, color and temperature changes (with the extremity pale, blue, or cold), as well as the presence of a thrill or bruit over the subclavian artery.

172. The treatment of choice for thoracic outlet syndrome is conservative, if possible. Initially, a period of rest from activities that provoke symptoms followed by postural reeducation, muscle stretching, and strengthening exercises are indicated. Activity modification must also be undertaken in order to reduce the provocative activities which induce symptoms. In the obese patient, weight reduction may be of benefit and proper breast support may be beneficial in women. If after 4 months of conservative treatment, significant symptoms persist or if there is a significant vascular component to this disorder, surgical intervention is indicated. In order to provide adequate decompression of the thoracic outlet, most recommend first rib resection as the procedure of choice.

173. Gunshot velocities are normally divided into several categories with low velocity less than 1,200 ft/sec, medium velocity 1,200 to 2,500 ft/sec, and high velocity greater than 2,500 ft/sec. With low velocity gunshot wounds, spontaneous nerve recovery is expected between 3 and 6 months after injury in 69% of patients.

QUESTIONS

174. After a high velocity gunshot wound to the upper extremity with resultant nerve injury, what would be the expected percentage of spontaneous nerve recovery?

175. In what position should the shoulder be placed for shoulder arthrodesis?

176. Name the three types of prostheses used after upper extremity amputations.

177. The aesthetic hand prosthesis is made most commonly of what material?

178. Which prehensile terminal device for body-powered upper extremity protheses is most commonly used—the voluntary opening or voluntary closing split hook?

179. What are the advantages of a split hook for the terminal prehensile device of the body-powered prosthesis?

180. With the wrist-powered prosthesis, which motions are commonly used to produce which hand functions?

ANSWERS

174. Spontaneous nerve recovery would be expected between 4 and 7 months after the time of injury in 69% of patients. Studies have demonstrated that spontaneous recovery of nerve injuries does not depend upon the velocity of the gunshot wound. Timing of recovery, however, would be expected to be slightly longer for high velocity gunshot wounds. This is probably related to the greater concussive effect of such wounds. Most gunshot wounds result in an axonotmesis. Gunshot wounds above the elbow would be expected to have a longer period of recovery than below the elbow and injury to multiple nerves would be expected to have longer recovery than single nerve involvement.

ANSWERS

175. Abduction of 25 to 40 degrees, forward flexion of 20 to 30 degrees, and internal rotation of 25 to 30 degrees. A simple rule of thumb is 30-30-30.

176. They are classified into three types: (1) passive prosthesis, which is primarily for cosmesis with minimal functional capacity; (2) body-powered prosthesis, in which the motion of the prosthesis is controlled by movements of the remaining, naturally articulated body segments; and (3) externally powered prosthesis, in which the motivating energy is provided by some portable external energy source. In reality, most prostheses are "hybrid" prostheses, being a combination of these three types.

177. Silicone polymers are most commonly used for the aesthetic hand prosthesis rather than the previously used polyvinylchlorides. The use of silicone produces more realistic hand detail, natural hand colors, and texture. Its tear strength is relatively high and mechanical properties are not appreciably changed by temperatures within the normal climatic range (it does not become brittle in cold weather). Its chemical inertness allows for easy cleaning with soap and water.

178. The voluntary opening split hook. The advantage of voluntary opening is that grasp can be maintained without the user maintaining continuous attention and providing continuous tension on the motivating cord.

179. It is strong, lightweight, simple, reliable, and very functional. It resists wear and tear, its cost is relatively low, and maintenance and repairs are relatively simple. Its major disadvantage is that it is less cosmetically appealing.

180. Wrist dorsiflexion results in hand opening while wrist palmar flexion results in hand closing. This is the opposite of the normal tenodesis effect of the natural hand. This motion is, however, better adapted to table surface pick-up.

QUESTIONS

181. What are the disadvantages of the myoelectric prosthesis?

182. What are the advantages of the myoelectric prosthesis?

183. What is the biggest problem that limits efficient functioning of upper limb prostheses?

184. For the above-elbow amputee with a body-powered prosthesis, what motion produces elbow flexion?

185. In the above-elbow body-powered prosthesis, motion of the terminal device is dependent on elbow locking. How is this accomplished?

186. For the C4 quadriplegic patient, what is the appropriate upper extremity orthosis?

187. For the C5 quadriplegic patient what is the appropriate upper extremity orthosis?

188. For the C6 or C7 quadriplegic patient, what is the appropriate upper extremity orthosis?

189. At what age should prosthetic fitting be considered for congenital upper limb deficiency?

190. What are the advantages of early fitting of prostheses for congenital upper limb deficiency?

ANSWERS

181. It is not designed for heavy work; its weight is considerably greater, which limits its use in short amputation stumps; it is prone to breakdown and requires much greater servicing, and in most locations, repair and maintenance facilities are not readily available; its cost is usually three to four times greater than the body-powered prosthesis; a battery source must be maintained and recharged for use of this prosthesis.

ANSWERS

182. It is more cosmetically appealing; there is no body harness necessary for its operation; it tends to be more comfortable; it operates more effectively close to the body and with overhead activities than does the body-powered prosthesis.

183. Inability to replicate or reproduce sensory and proprioceptive feedback mechanisms. Visual monitoring or sound cues must be relied upon to control specific motions. This greatly impairs efficiency of the motion and limits the ability to produce finely controlled movements.

184. Motion of the prosthesis is produced by increasing tension on the motivating cable, which passes obliquely from the harness on the contralateral shoulder across the posterior aspect of the chest. Tension is increased with protraction of the shoulders combined with abduction and flexion of the amputated extremity. This results in cable shortening and subsequent elbow flexion.

185. Shoulder extension and depression locks as well as unlocks the elbow mechanism.

186. The long opponens hand splint. This does not improve function but prevents hand contractures.

187. A flexor-hinged ratchet. Since some shoulder and elbow function should be intact, the wrist and hand can be positioned for functional use with this orthosis.

188. The wrist-driven flexor-hinged orthosis. The tenodesis effect of wrist motion can be used to produce and control grasp and pinch motions with this orthosis.

189. The infant begins to execute useful gross grasping motions at the age of 3 months. Most recommend placement of at least a primitive prosthetic fitting at this time.

190. (1) Early prosthetic tolerance, (2) equalization of limb lengths (for crawling), (3) bimanual pattern of activity, and (4) acceptance of the prosthesis as an integral part of the body (becomes a part of the infant's self-image).

QUESTIONS

191. How should prostheses be prescribed for a newborn with a congenital below-elbow deficiency?

192. How should prostheses be prescribed for the newborn with congenital above-elbow deficiency?

193. In the below-elbow body-powered prosthesis, is more body motion required to operate the terminal device with the elbow flexed or extended?

194. The standard harness for the below-elbow body-powered prosthesis consists of an axillary loop connected by a stainless steel ring to an inverted Y suspension strap. Where should this ring be positioned?

195. How are displaced extraarticular fractures of the glenoid neck treated?

196. How are displaced fractures of the scapular body and spine treated?

197. How are displaced intraarticular glenoid fractures treated?

ANSWERS

191. The infant with a congenital below-elbow deficiency is fitted at age 3 months with a below-elbow prosthesis, using a figure-8 harness and passive mitten as a terminal device. At 12 to 14 months of age, the passive mitten is replaced with a functional terminal device (Plastasol-covered hook). At 18 months of age, training for use and activation of the terminal device begins. It is not until the age of 18 months that the child's attention span and mental capacity are adequate for obtaining functional use of the terminal device.

192. At 3 months of age the infant with congenital above-elbow deficiency should be fitted with a unit arm (no elbow motion) with a terminal plastic mitten. At 14 to 18 months this prosthesis is replaced with a friction elbow prosthesis and terminal device (hook) using a single control. At 3 years of age, an inside locking elbow prosthesis is prescribed.

193. The amount of motion required to operate the terminal device is the same with the elbow flexed as it is with the elbow extended. The terminal device is operated independently of elbow positioning.

194. Below the spinous process of C7 and slightly to the nonamputated side.

195. Symptomatically, with early ice and sling immobilization, followed in a few days by passive range-of-motion exercises.

196. The significance of scapular body and spine fractures is the high incidence of other significant associated injuries (35%–98%). With these fractures, nonunion is rare and normal body anatomy is not necessary for good function. Therefore they are treated symptomatically with ice, sling, and early range-of-motion exercises.

197. Treatment is controversial. However, most agree that displaced fractures involving 25% or more of the articular surface should undergo open reduction and internal fixation. Although surgery is difficult, it may reduce the chances for recurrent instability, and posttraumatic arthritis (especially in the younger patient).

QUESTIONS

198. Identify the numbered structures in this cross section of the arm at the midhumeral shaft level.

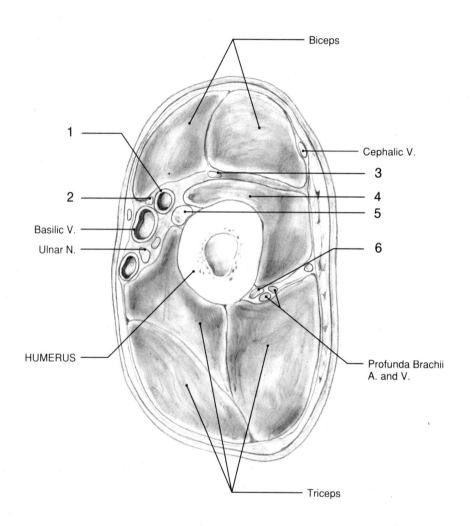

POSTERIOR

ANSWERS

198. *1*, Brachial artery; *2*, median nerve; *3*, musculocutaneous nerve; *4*, brachialis muscle; *5*, coracobrachialis tendon; *6*, radial nerve.

QUESTIONS

199. Identify *1* through *7* in the Figure.

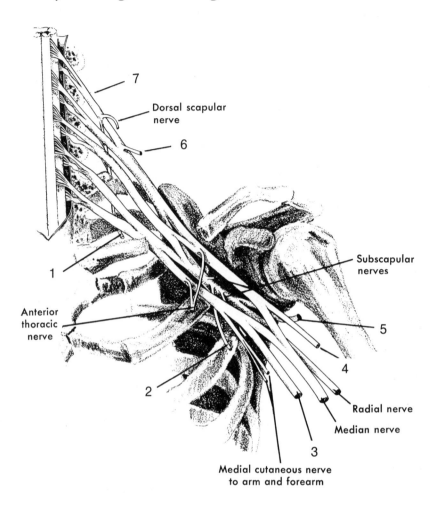

ANSWERS

199. *1*, Long thoracic nerve; *2*, thoracodorsal nerve; *3*, ulnar nerve; *4*, musculocutaneous nerve; *5*, axillary nerve; *6*, suprascapular nerve; *7*, C5 nerve root.

CHAPTER 7

Hand and Wrist

Timothy S. Loth, M.D.

QUESTIONS

1. What is the origin and insertion of the sagittal band?

2. Describe the anatomy of the extensor digitorum communis (EDC) distal to the MCP joint.

3. Describe the interosseous hood (interosseous aponeurotic expansion).

4. What is the function of the transverse portion of the interosseous hood?

5. Describe the origin, insertion, function, and pathophysiology of the oblique and transverse retinacular ligaments.

ANSWERS

1. The origin is the extensor tendon over the metacarpophalangeal (MCP) joint, passing superficial to the MCP joint capsule and the phalangeal attachment of the medial tendon of the superficial head of the interosseous tendon and deep to the lateral tendon of the deep head of the interossei. The insertion is the volar proximal phalanx and edge of the volar plate.

ANSWERS

2. It trifurcates over the proximal one half of the proximal phalanx. The central slip inserts in the base of the middle phalanx joined by the interosseous medial band. The lateral two slips join the interossei and lumbricals forming the lateral bands.

3. All dorsal and volar interossei insert into the interosseous hood, which runs from the proximal portion of the proximal phalanx to the insertion at the base of the middle phalanx. The proximal portion of the hood contains transverse fibers which run dorsally over the common extensor tendon and help flex the MCP joint. Oblique fibers of the distal interosseous hood insert into the lateral tubercles through the medial bands at the dorsal base of the middle phalanx. They assist in proximal interphalangeal (PIP) extension. Lateral slips from the common extensor tendon combine with fibers from the extensor hood to create the conjoined lateral bands distally.

4. MCP flexion.

5. The *oblique retinacular ligament* originates from the volar lateral aspect of the proximal phalanx coursing dorsally, volar to the axis of the proximal phalangeal joint to terminate in the terminal extensor tendon. It links motion of the distal (DIP) and proximal interphalangeal joints. With PIP flexion, the ligament is relaxed, allowing DIP flexion. PIP extension tightens the ligament facilitating DIP extension. Flexion contracture of the PIP joint and extension of the DIP joint occur in Dupuytren's contracture. The ligament may be reconstructed to correct a swan-neck or mallet finger deformity. The *transverse retinacular ligament* prevents dorsal shift of the lateral bands. It attaches to the edge of the flexor sheath at the level of the PIP joint and attaches dorsally to the lateral aspect of the lateral bands. Swan-neck deformity results from attenuation of the transverse retinacular ligament, allowing dorsal translation of the lateral bands. The boutonnière deformity develops as a result of tightening of the transverse retinacular ligaments in association with disruption of the central slip and triangular ligament, allowing volar displacement of the lateral bands.

QUESTIONS

6. Describe the origin, insertion, and function of the triangular ligament.

7. Describe the origin, course, insertion, and function of Cleland's ligament.

8. Describe the origin, course, insertion, and function of Grayson's ligament.

9. Describe the insertions for the interossei muscles.

10. Describe the origins and insertions of the lumbricals.

11. Describe the origin, insertion, and function of the adductor pollicis.

ANSWERS

6. The triangular ligament is a triangular-shaped part of the extensor mechanism that lies over the dorsal middle phalanx between the lateral bands, and distal to the central slip insertion and proximal to the terminal extensor. Its transversely oriented fibers prevent volar shift of lateral bands during digital flexion.

7. The major fascicles of Cleland's ligament come off around the PIP joint (volar plate, proximal and distal phalanges) and fibro-osseous sheath and pass dorsal to the neurovascular bundle to insert into the digital fascia. It holds the skin in place on the digit.

8. Grayson's ligament comes off the volar flexor tendon sheath, passes volar to the neurovascular bundle, and inserts into the skin. It prevents bowstringing of the neurovascular bundle as the digit is flexed.

9. The first, second, and fourth dorsal interossei have two muscle bellies. The superficial one courses deep to the sagittal bands through its medial tendon and inserts at the base of the proximal phalanges. The deep head courses superficial to the sagittal bands through its tendon (the lateral tendon) and inserts into the dorsal aponeurosis. The three volar and the third dorsal interossei have one tendon, which inserts into the dorsal aponeurosis.

10. The first and second lumbricals come off the radial aspect of the index and middle finger flexor digitorum profundus (FDP) tendons in the palm, pass volar to the transverse metacarpal ligament, volar to the axis of MCP motion, and insert into the radial lateral band over the midproximal phalanx. The third and fourth lumbricals arise from contiguous FDP tendons of the middle and ring and ring and small fingers, respectively. They insert into the radial lateral bands over the midproximal phalanx.

11. The adductor pollicis has two heads of origin (oblique and transverse). The transverse head is the distal two thirds of the palmar long finger metacarpal. The oblique head is the capitate, the bases of the index and long metacarpals, the palmar ligaments of the carpus, and the flexor carpi radialis (FCR) sheath. The two heads converge and insert into the ulnar sesamoid (uniting with the volar plate to the proximal phalanx). The adductor pollicis adducts the first metacarpal and extends the distal phalanx.

QUESTIONS

12. Identify the labeled structures on this representation of the dorsal apparatus of the finger.

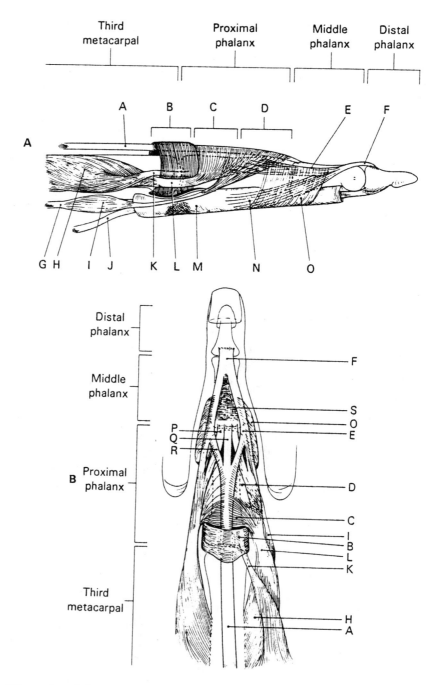

13. How should acute open or closed ruptures of the central slip be treated?

ANSWERS

12. **A**, radial side of the left middle finger. **B**, dorsum of the left middle finger. *A*, extensor digitorum communis tendon; *B*, sagittal bands; *C*, transverse fibers of intrinsic muscle apparatus; *D*, oblique fibers of intrinsic apparatus; *E*, conjoined lateral band; *F*, terminal tendon; *G*, flexor digitorum profundus tendon; *H*, second dorsal interosseous muscle; *I*, lumbrical muscle; *J*, flexor digitorum superficialis tendon; *K*, medial tendon of the superficial belly of the interosseous; *L*, lateral tendon of deep belly of interosseous; *M*, flexor pulley mechanism; *N*, oblique retinacular ligament; *O*, transverse retinacular ligament; *P*, medial band of oblique fibers of intrinsic expansion; *Q*, central slip; *R*, lateral slips; *S*, triangular ligament.

13. An open rupture is directly repaired and treated with Kirschner wire and a splint in extension for 6 to 8 weeks, leaving the DIP free. After K-wire removal, a night splint is used for 2 months. If extensor lag persists after 4 months, tendolysis of the extensor mechanism may help. A closed tear is treated with a splint to hold the PIP in extension for 8 weeks, after which the splint is gradually removed and replaced by night splinting for 2 months.

QUESTIONS

14. What are the pathologic conditions causing boutonnière deformity of the PIP joint?

15. How is a chronic boutonnière deformity prepared for surgical reconstruction?

16. What is the most disabling element of the boutonnière deformity?

17. What causes limitation of flexion of the DIP joint in boutonnière deformity?

18. How should closed acute posttraumatic tendinous boutonnière lesions be treated?

19. How should boutonnière deformities with displaced avulsion fractures of the base of the middle phalanx of significant size be treated?

20. What reconstructive options are available for chronic boutonnière deformity with full passive range of motion?

21. Describe the treatment of an extensor laceration at the level of the MCP joint?

ANSWERS

14. (1) An insufficient central slip; (2) tear or attenuation of the triangular ligament; (3) migration of the lateral bands volarly; (4) flexion contracture of the PIP joint; (5) hyperextension of the DIP from tension by the shortened lateral bands; (6) contracture of the oblique retinacular ligament.

ANSWERS

15. The preoperative goal is to obtain full passive extension of the PIP joint. A dynamic splint is applied until the PIP reaches neutral, followed by static splinting of the PIP in neutral, with the DIP flexed to stretch the contracted oblique retinacular ligament, for 4 weeks. If the PIP cannot be splinted to neutral, a persistent volar capsular contracture is present. Volar release may be necessary. This usually produces good intraoperative range of motion, which unfortunately is rarely maintained after extensor reconstruction.

16. Limitation of DIP joint flexion.

17. A tenodesis effect caused by volar displacement of the lateral bands and contracture of the oblique retinacular ligaments.

18. Closed treatment can be successful if the patient can maintain PIP joint extension actively, after passively extending the digit. (The triangular ligament is competent.) Treatment is PIP extension splinting for 6 to 8 weeks with the DIP free. A night splint is used for 4 to 8 weeks after discontinuing daytime splinting. If the patient is unable to maintain active PIP extension after passive PIP extension, surgical repair is indicated.

19. Open reduction and internal fixation with repair of the triangular ligament to correct the volar subluxation of the lateral bands.

20. (1) Oblique or stepcut tenotomy of the lateral bands distal to central slip insertion over the proximal metaphysis of the middle phalanx (Dolphin, Fowler, or Nalebuff); (2) dorsal transposition and suture of the lateral bands (Littler); (3) transposition of the lateral bands to the central slip (Matev and Littler); (4) V-Y plasty of the central slip to achieve appropriate tension.

21. Repair by direct suture. Postoperatively the wrist is held in extension of 45–60 degrees. The MCP and PIP joints are held in extension for 3 weeks. Movement of the PIP joints is begun at 3 weeks, of the MCP joints at 4 weeks, and of the wrist at 6 weeks, followed by night splinting of the wrist for 3 months. Newer postoperative protocols for dynamic splinting, which allow early mobilization of the interphalangeal joints, and protected range of motion of the MCP joints, appear promising.

QUESTIONS

22. Describe the finger pully system (Doyle and Blythe).

23. What are the flexor tendon injury zones?

24. Name these structures on the dorsum of the hand.

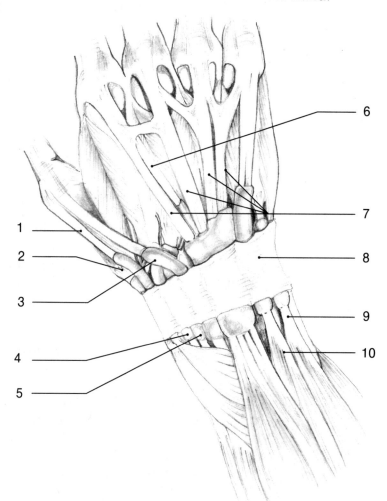

25. What is the most common finger infection?

ANSWERS

22. Odd-numbered annular (A) pulleys overlie joints: A1—MCP, A3—PIP, and A5—DIP joints. Even-numbered pulleys overlie bone: A2—proximal phalanx, A4—middle phalanx. Cruciate (C) pulleys lie between: C1—A2–3, C2—A3–4, and C3—A4–5.

23. Zone I is the area between the FDP insertion and the sublimis insertion; zone II is the area between the sublimis insertion and the proximal edge of the fibro-osseous tunnel (level of the distal palmar skin crease); zone III is the area between the proximal flexor tendon sheath and the distal edge of the carpal tunnel; zone IV is the carpal tunnel; zone V is the area between the proximal carpal tunnel and the volar forearm.

24. *1*, extensor pollicus brevis; *2*, abductor pollicus longus; *3*, extensor pollicus longus; *4*, extensor carpi radialis longus; *5*, extensor carpi radialis brevis; *6*, extensor indicis proprius; *7*, extensor digitorum; *8*, extensor retinaculum; *9*, extensor carpi ulnaris; *10*, extensor digiti minimi.

25. Paronychia.

QUESTIONS

26. Name these fingernail anatomic structures.

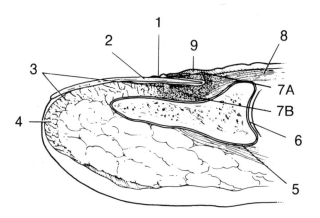

27. What are the three compartments of the forearm which may require decompression in compartment syndrome?

28. Name the labeled structures on this cross section of a supinated right hand at the level of the MCP joints.

VOLAR

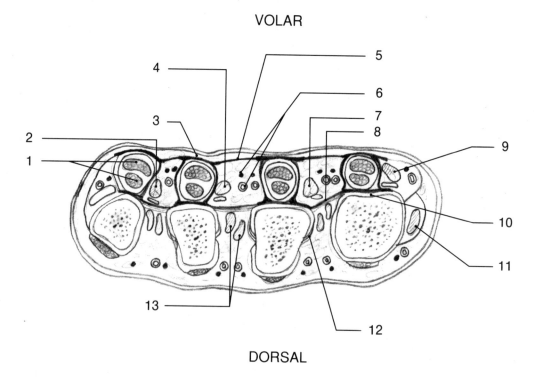

DORSAL

ANSWERS

26. *1*, eponychium; *2*, lunula; *3*, nail bed; *4*, hyponychium; *5*, periostium; *6*, distal interphalangeal joint; *7A*, dorsal roof of nail fold; *7B*, ventral floor of nail fold; *8*, insertion of extensor tendon; *9*, nail wall.

27. (1) Volar compartment (it will decompress the dorsal compartment 50% of the time and the mobile wad nearly 100% of the time); (2) dorsal compartment; (3) mobile wad.

28. *1*, superficialis and profundus tendons; *2*, fourth lumbrical; *3*, longitudinal slips of palmar aponeurosis; *4*, third lumbrical; *5*, superficial transverse metacarpal (natatory) ligament; *6*, palmar digital nerve and artery; *7*, second lumbrical; *8*, deep transverse metacarpal ligament; *9*, first lumbrical; *10*, palmar ligament (volar plate); *11*, first dorsal interosseous; *12*, MP joint radial collateral ligament; *13*, palmar and dorsal interossei.

QUESTIONS

29. What are the compartments of the hand?

30. What are recommended compartment pressure levels above which fasciotomy is performed?

31. Describe the elements of the crush syndrome.

32. What are the treatment principles for severe Volkmann's contracture?

33. Describe the surgical treatment of FCR tunnel syndrome.

34. What is a "complete" vascular arch in the hand?

35. Describe the anatomic variations of the superficial palmar arch.

ANSWERS

29. The four dorsal interosseous muscle compartments (which are not interconnected); three volar interosseous compartments; the adductor pollicis compartment; the thenar compartment; and the hypothenar compartment.

30. This is controversial. There are varying levels of pressure at which compartment decompression is recommended: (1) within 10 to 30 mm Hg of the patient's diastolic blood pressure (Whitesides); (2) compartment pressure greater than 30 mm Hg (Mubarak); (3) compartment pressure greater than 45 mm Hg (Matsen); (4) within 25 to 35 mm Hg of the patient's diastolic blood pressure (Gelberman).

ANSWERS

31. Muscle necrosis can lead to myoglobinuria, renal failure, and shock. Cardiac complications result from acidosis and hyperkalemia.

32. Release nerve compression and contractures. Transfer muscles, if available.

33. Reflect the thenar muscles. It may be necessary to partially resect the scaphoid tubercle and trapezial crest, release the entire FCR sheath to insertion, and start early motion.

34. An arch is considered "complete" when the arteries of all five digits arise from the arch.

35. *A*, the radial and ulnar arteries contribute to form a complete arch (34.5%). *B*, complete arch exclusively from the ulnar artery (37%). About 80% of hands have a complete arch. It is incomplete in 20% of hands.

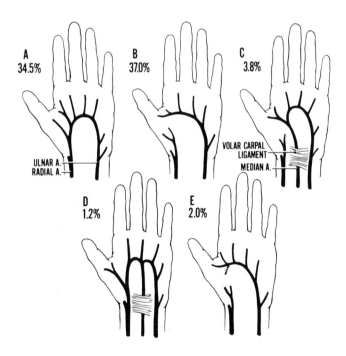

QUESTIONS

36. What are the synovial changes associated with rheumatoid arthritis?

37. What joint changes occur in rheumatoid arthritis?

38. What are the indications for surgery in rheumatoid arthritis?

39. Describe wrist deformities seen in rheumatoid arthritis.

40. What are the potential causes of trigger finger in rheumatoid patients?

41. What are the most frequent tendon ruptures seen in rheumatoid arthritis?

42. Describe ways to restore ruptured extensors in rheumatoid arthritis.

43. Describe rheumatoid arthritic MCP joint deformities.

44. What are the principles of treatment of early MCP joint disease in rheumatoid arthritis?

45. What is the most common deformity of the PIP joint in rheumatoid arthritis?

ANSWERS

36. Inflammation, hyperemia, increased synovial fluid production, proliferation of synovial lining.

37. Increased joint pressure from an increase in synovial fluid production leads to interference with nutrition, and distention of the capsule and ligaments. Periarticular osteoporosis, cysts, spurs, and joint destruction and collapse are also seen.

ANSWERS

38. The indications for surgery include severe pain and chronic synovitis not responding to good medical therapy, nerve entrapment, tendon ruptures, and deformity resulting in functional loss. Some patients with rheumatoid arthritis can have horrible-looking hands that function well without much pain. It is better not to operate until the patient meets the aforementioned criteria.

39. Ulnar translocation of the carpus, erosion of the carpus and radial metacarpal shift, supination and volar dislocation of the carpus beneath the radius, rupture or attenuation of radial wrist extensors, dorsal subluxation or dislocation of the distal ulna.

40. There are several sites for triggering in rheumatoid arthritic hands. (1) the A1 pulley (as with conventional trigger finger); (2) flexor digitorum superficialis (FDS) decussation (may require excising the slip of the sublimis or an intratendinous nodule); (3) a nodule in the FDP near A2 can cause the finger to lock into extension; this requires tenosynovectomy and nodule excision.

41. In order of occurrence: the ring and small finger extensor tendons, the extensor pollicis longus (EPL), other extensor tendons, the flexor pollicis longus (FPL), and other flexor tendons.

42. End-to-side repair to adjacent intact extensors; interposition tendon grafts (palmaris longus or plantaris); tendon transfers: extensor indicis, FDS, wrist extensor.

43. Initially there is enlargement and swelling of the knuckles; later, volar subluxation of the joint, ulnar displacement of extensor tendons, and ulnar deviation of fingers.

44. Conservative care consisting of maximal medical management, intraarticular steroid injections, and instruction in joint protection techniques. Synovectomy, soft tissue reconstructive procedures (intrinsic releases, extensor realignment, and crossed intrinsic transfer) are considered if the articular surfaces of the MCP joints are mildly involved.

45. The swan-neck (28%) and boutonnière (15%) deformities.

QUESTIONS

46. What are the early treatment options for type I swan-neck deformity in rheumatoid arthritis?

47. A 42-year-old man with rheumatoid arthritis complains of the appearance of both hands. The physical examination reveals swan-neck deformities in which there is limitation of motion of the PIP joints when the MCP joints are extended or radially deviated. The PIP joint flexion is normal when the MCP joint is allowed to flex and ulnarly deviate. What are your treatment recommendations?

48. A 50-year-old patient with swan-neck deformities also has marked reduction of PIP motion, regardless of the position of the MCP joints. Radiographs demonstrate the joint spaces to be well preserved. What is your approach to treating this type III swan-neck deformity?

49. What are the options for treatment of a patient with a rheumatoid swan-neck deformity that is stiff in all positions of the finger and whose radiographs show significant articular deterioration?

50. A 45-year-old woman with rheumatoid arthritis complains that she has lost active extension of the long finger. She has an active extension lag of 15 degrees at the PIP joint that is passively correctable. What do you recommend for treatment of this mild boutonnière deformity?

51. What is the approach to operative correction of the moderate boutonnière deformity in rheumatoid arthritis?

52. What constitutes a severe boutonnière deformity? How is it treated?

ANSWERS

46. Flexor synovectomy, intrinsic release, tenodesis (Littler or superficialis), dermadesis, or DIP arthrodesis (to correct primary mallet finger deformity).

ANSWERS

47. This patient has a classic type II swan-neck deformity in which the PIP range of motion is limited, depending upon the position of the MCP joint. In this circumstance, the joint pathomechanics have to be addressed. This combination of deformities is usually due to intrinsic muscle tightness. In mild cases, intrinsic release is satisfactory for facilitating improvement combined with procedures for correction of the swan-neck deformity listed in the previous answer. If the disease is far advanced, then both arthroplasty and intrinsic release are necessary.

48. A staged reconstruction is performed in which there is first restoration of passive range of motion of the digits through joint manipulation. Sometimes it is necessary to perform a dorsal skin release. Lateral bands may need to be mobilized to allow full flexion of the digit. Flexor tenosynovectomy has been used in conjunction with the above techniques if good active flexion is not present following restoration of passive motion intraoperatively. MCP arthroplasty is helpful in many instances.

49. PIP arthrodesis or replacement arthroplasty.

50. A mild boutonnière deformity consists of an extension lag of 30 to 40 degrees at the PIP joint that is passively correctable to neutral. Radiographs show minimal PIP articular surface involvement. Treatment consists of incision of the extensor mechanism over the dorsal middle phalanx. This allows the extensor mechanism to rebalance. Postoperatively it is desirable to put the patient into a dynamic extension splint at the PIP joint, leaving the DIP free.

51. Reconstruction of the extensor mechanism consists of the following: (1) shortening of the central extensor slip; (2) mobilization of the lateral banks with release of the transverse retinacular ligaments; (3) it is often necessary to release the extensor mechanism over the dorsum of the middle phalanx to facilitate DIP flexion.

52. Severe boutonnière deformities are those in which the PIP joint can no longer be passively extended to neutral. In this deformity, extensor mechanism reconstruction is usually unsuccessful. Recommended treatment consists of PIP fusion or possible arthroplasty.

QUESTIONS

53. Describe the pathomechanics of boutonnière deformity in rheumatoid arthritis.

54. Describe the pathomechanics of the rheumatoid arthritic boutonnière thumb.

55. What can be done for a mild thumb boutonnière deformity in rheumatoid arthritis?

56. Describe the treatment of a moderate thumb boutonnière deformity in rheumatoid arthritis.

57. Severe boutonnière deformity of the thumb in rheumatoid arthritis consists of fixed flexion of the MCP joint and hyperextension of the interphalangeal joint. How should this deformity be surgically treated?

58. Describe the pathomechanics of a thumb swan-neck deformity in rheumatoid arthritis.

59. Describe the treatment of swan-neck deformity in the rheumatoid thumb.

ANSWERS

53. Dorsal synovitis, capsular distention, and attenuation of the central slip and triangular ligament allow PIP extension lag and palmar displacement of the lateral bands. Extensor pull is transferred to the distal phalanx, causing DIP hyperextension. Joint destruction and fixed contracture gradually develop.

ANSWERS

54. Flexion of the MCP joint and hyperextension of the interphalangeal joint. Dorsal synovitis of the MCP joint causes attenuation of the capsule and extensor apparatus (brevis) with associated volar displacement of the EPL and intrinsic tendons. With attempted extension of the MCP joint there is hyperextension of the interphalangeal joint. The proximal phalanx subluxates volarly. Disease in this deformity is primarily at the MCP joint.

55. A mild boutonnière deformity of the thumb is passively correctable at both the interphalangeal and MCP joints and can be treated with MCP synovectomy and extensor revision.

56. A moderate rheumatoid arthritic boutonnière thumb has restricted MCP range of motion with or without articular destruction. The interphalangeal joint is still passively correctable. Treatment is arthroplasty or arthrodesis of the MCP joint.

57. Surgical options include MCP and interphalangeal arthrodesis; mobilization of the interphalangeal joint, dorsal synovectomy, capsulectomy, and MCP fusion; interphalangeal fusion and MCP arthroplasty with extensor reconstruction.

58. Hyperextension of the MCP and flexion of the interphalangeal joint develop as a result of dorsoradial subluxation-dislocation of the thumb metacarpal base on the trapezium. Hyperextension of the MCP joint results from stretching of the volar plate secondary to MCP synovitis and extension forces concentrated at the joint.

59. The source of the deformity, i.e., the carpometacarpal (CMC) joint subluxation, should be corrected. This can be performed through several procedures. A thumb metacarpal-trapezial arthrodesis, hemi- or complete trapezial replacement arthroplasty, or soft tissue tendinous reconstructions can be performed. With regard to the pathologic condition of the MCP and interphalangeal joints, nothing may be required since the corrective surgery on the trapezial-metacarpal joint may be enough to rebalance the thumb. Conversely, if there is significant deterioration in these joints, arthrodesis may be appropriate. In between these two extremes, one could consider extensor tendon rebalancing over the MCP joint with volar plate advancement.

QUESTIONS

60. Describe the principles in staging surgery for multiple-level involvement in rheumatoid arthritis of the hand, wrist, elbow, and shoulder.

61. Describe Dupuytren's disease.

62. Other than the palmar surface of the hand, what other areas can be affected by Dupuytren's?

63. What is the inheritance pattern of Dupuytren's?

64. What other conditions are associated with Dupuytren's?

65. What is the change noted in the type of collagen in Dupuytren's fascia compared with normal fascia?

66. What one structure is responsible for MCP joint contracture in Dupuytren's?

67. What problems result from Dupuytren's involvement of the natatory ligament?

68. What three structures are responsible for Dupuytren's contracture of the thumb?

ANSWERS

60. In general, reconstruct the proximal joints first, i.e., the wrist, then the MCP joints, and then the interphalangeal joints. Delay elbow and shoulder arthroplasties until after the hands and wrists are completed so that the components are not at risk while under anesthesia. Achieve motion at one level and stabilize others (i.e., MCP arthroplasty with wrist and PIP arthrodesis).

61. Palmar nodules and cords associated with flexion contractures of the MCP, less frequently the PIP, and occasionally the DIP joints caused by disease of the palmar aponeurosis and its digital prolongations.

62. The knuckle pads (Garrod's nodes), the dorsum of the penis (Peyronie's disease), and the plantar fascia (Ledderhose's disease).

63. Autosomal dominant.

64. Epilepsy, alcoholism, diabetes, trauma (can aggravate it, but is probably not a primary cause).

65. Normal fascia is mostly type I collagen. In Dupuytren's, there is an increase in type III collagen (similar to scar tissue).

66. The pretendinous cord. It does not alter the course of the neurovascular bundle.

67. The natatory ligament has fibers which run transversely at the level of the web space between digits. It also sends fibers distally in the digits. When the natatory ligament is involved in Dupuytren's, it will produce web space contractures of the involved fingers. The distal extensions will produce PIP flexion contractures. The natatory ligament to the thumb attaches at the level of the proximal thumb crease, and produces adduction flexion contractures of the thumb.

68. The pretendinous cord, natatory ligament, and superficial transverse ligament of the palm. All are superficial to the neurovascular bundles and do not disturb their courses.

QUESTIONS

69. Describe the four patterns of diseased cords in Dupuytren's disease that cause contracture at the PIP joint.

70. A 53-year-old car salesman presents with a painful nodule on the ulnar aspect of his dominant hand. The nodule is located over the distal palmar crease in the axis of the ring finger and is tender to palpation, firm, and appears to be subcutaneous. He has normal range of motion of the digits. The patient states that this hurts him when he grasps objects. His family history is positive for contractures of the ulnar digits in a maternal grandfather. How would you treat this tender Dupuytren's nodule?

71. What is the indication for surgery in a patient with Dupuytren's disease affecting the MCP joint?

72. What are the indications for surgery in a patient with Dupuytren's disease affecting the PIP joint?

73. Describe the classification system for congenital anomalies.

74. Describe the characteristics of radial clubhand (congenital radial-sided deficiencies).

ANSWERS

69. (1) The *central cord* is always in continuity with the pretendinous cord; it lies between neurovascular bundles and attaches distally to bone and tendon sheath over the middle phalanx. (2) The *lateral cord* adheres to skin throughout its course, and may attach to the tendon sheath through fibers of Grayson's ligament. Fibers extending distally can cause DIP contracture. (3) The *spiral cord* can manifest as an extension of the pretendinous cord through the spiral band or at the musculotendinous junction of an intrinsic muscle (abductor digiti minimi, ADM). The cord inserts distally to the bone and tendon sheath of the middle phalanx. (4) The *retrovascular cord*, dorsal to the neurovascular bundles, is densest at the PIP joint and is the most common cause of recurrence of PIP contracture following surgery.

ANSWERS

70. The tender Dupuytren's nodule should not be operated on since this may worsen the disease. The tenderness will usually subside spontaneously with time. Patients who have persistent pain in the nodule may benefit from an intranodular injection of steroid and the application of an antivibration glove. The natural history of the nodule is a gradual decrease in tenderness, but one should watch for the development of contractures.

71. A 20- to 30-degree flexion contracture at the MCP joint is an indication for surgery. This level of contracture is usually associated with the patient's inability to lay the hand flat on the table.

72. Although this is somewhat controversial, many authors believe that any degree of contracture at the PIP joint should be released. It has been demonstrated that the greater the degree of contracture at the PIP joint, the greater the likelihood of recurrence or incomplete correction with surgical intervention. This leads one to take an aggressive approach to PIP joint contractures in Dupuytren's

73. (A) Failure of formation of parts: Transverse (amelia) and longitudinal (radial clubhand, phocomelia, cleft hand); (B) failure of differentiation (syndactyly, synostosis); (C) duplication (bifid thumbs, polydactyly); (D) overgrowth (macrodactyly); (E) undergrowth or hypoplasia (hypoplastic thumb); (F) constriction band syndrome.

74. Hypoplasia, partial or complete absence of the radius, which can cause an unstable wrist with radial deviation of the hand; frequent hypoplasia or absence of the radial carpus and thumb, arteries, nerves, and muscles; frequently associated with cardiac (Holt-Oram syndrome), hematopoietic (Fanconi's syndrome) gastrointestinal (imperforate anus) anomalies; seen in association with VATER and TAR syndromes.* Treatment depends upon the degree of involvement as well as individual factors. Mild cases require no treatment. Patients with significant deformity benefit from centralization or radialization of the hand on the ulna after age 6 months. Early treatment consists of casting and splinting.

---

*VATER is an acronym for *ver*tebral defects, imperforate *a*nus, *t*rach*e*oesophageal fistula, and *r*adial and *r*enal dysplasia. TAR is an acronym for *t*hrombocytopenia–*a*bsent *r*adius.

QUESTIONS

75. Describe the characteristics of ulnar clubhand (congenital ulnar-sided deficiencies).

76. Describe splinting programs for the following **PIP** flexion contractures: passive extension lag of 50 to 90 degrees; of 35 to 50 degrees; and of 35 degrees or less.

77. Describe the Allen classification of fingertip injuries.

78. What are the three types of FDP avulsions from the distal phalanx, and how are they treated?

79. What forces produce apex volar angulation in proximal phalanx fractures?

80. What forces act on the middle phalanx shaft fractures to produce angulation?

81. Which angular deformity is produced by a fracture through the middle phalanx neck?

82. What is the direction of angular deformity seen in middle phalanx base fractures?

83. How are stable phalangeal fractures treated?

ANSWERS

75. This is an ulnar forearm hypoplasia ranging from a smaller but normally contoured ulna to partial or complete absence with radial head dislocation. The wrist is stable but the elbow demonstrates changes ranging from mild stiffness to complete rigidity. In contrast to radial clubhand, there usually are no associated systemic abnormalities, with the exception of musculoskeletal anomalies (synostosis or syndactyly).

ANSWERS

76. Splinting program for 50 to 90 degrees of extension lag is a short dorsal outrigger with a lumbrical bar; for 35 to 50 degrees of extension lag, a short dorsal outrigger with a lumbrical bar, or Capener splint, for 35 degrees or less of extension lag, a safety pin splint, cylinder cast, joint jack, or Capener splint.

77. *Type 1*—tip loss without exposed bone; *type 2*—tip loss to the level of the distal phalanx; *type 3*—distal phalanx exposed; *type 4*—amputation near the base of the distal phalanx.

78. In *type I* the tendon retracts into the palm, severing all blood supply and creating extensive scarring. Treatment is repair within 7 to 10 days. In *type II* the tendon retracts to the level of the PIP joint (sublimis chiasm) and the long vinculum remains intact. Early treatment is advised, but repair can be successful as late as 3 months. In *type III* a large bony fragment is trapped at the A4 pulley. Both vincula are usually intact and open reduction and internal fixation is recommended.

79. The proximal fragment is flexed by the insertions of the interossei into the base of the proximal phalanx. Although there are no tendons inserting into the distal fragment, it tends to be pulled into hyperextension by the central slip acting on the base of the middle phalanx.

80. The central slip inserts dorsally on the base of the middle phalanx. The sublimis tendon has a broad insertion extending from just distal to the flare of the base of the middle phalanx to a point only a few millimeters proximal to the neck.

81. Apex volar angulation is produced as the proximal fragment is pulled palmarward by the pull of the sublimis.

82. Middle phalanx base fractures have apex dorsal angulation, caused by the central slip extending the proximal fragment and the sublimis flexing the distal fragment.

83. Buddy taping. If there is any doubt, use 10 to 14 days of splinting, then buddy taping.

QUESTIONS

84. What type of immobilization is used following closed reduction of an unstable proximal phalanx fracture?

85. How should displaced condylar fractures of the middle or proximal phalanx be treated?

86. How should radial or ulnar avulsion fractures at the base of the proximal phalanx be treated?

87. What is the average time of clinical union of closed phalangeal fractures?

88. What is the most common complication of phalangeal fractures?

89. How long can it take before radiographs demonstrate union of a phalanx fracture?

90. How much angular deformity can be accepted in metacarpal neck fractures of the index and middle fingers?

91. What is a good way to preserve length in metacarpal fractures with bone loss secondary to gunshot wounds?

ANSWERS

84. External immobilization in a cast or splint extending to the tip of the finger with the MCP in 70 degrees of flexion, and varying degrees of PIP and DIP flexion to hold the fracture.

85. Open reduction and internal fixation or closed reduction with percutaneous pinning.

86. These are caused by avulsions of the collateral ligaments. Small or nondisplaced fragments can be treated with buddy taping. Larger displaced fractures result in articular incongruity if not restored by open reduction and internal fixation.

87. From 3 to 4 weeks. After immobilization for 3 weeks, phalangeal fractures can be treated with buddy taping to protect them for an additional 2 to 3 weeks.

88. Malunion.

89. From 4 to 5 months.

90. None. Because there is almost always some loss of alignment in plaster, it is recommended that closed reduction with percutaneous pinning be performed for index and long finger metacarpal neck fractures that are angulated and require reduction.

91. Transmetacarpal Kirschner wires inserted into the adjacent metacarpal, or external fixation will maintain length until bone grafting can be carried out.

QUESTIONS

92. Describe the technique of extension block splinting for dorsal fracture-dislocation of the PIP joint.

93. How are finger MCP joint ligament avulsions without major bony fragments treated?

94. What are the indications for surgery in bony ligamentous avulsion injuries at the finger MCP joints?

95. What are the two types of MCP joint dorsal dislocations?

96. How is a simple dorsal dislocation of the MCP joint reduced?

97. In complex dorsal MCP joint dislocations, what is the most important structure preventing reduction?

98. What is a consistent physical sign in complex MCP joint dorsal dislocation?

99. What are the radiographic characteristics of a complex dorsal MCP joint dislocation?

100. How should a complex dorsal MCP joint dislocation be treated?

101. What surgical approaches can be used for open reduction of a complex MCP joint dislocation?

ANSWERS

92. Closed reduction, confirmed by radiograph. The hand is placed in a splint or short arm cast with an aluminum splint outrigger with the PIP joint flexed adequately to maintain reduction (usually 60 degrees). Radiograph of the hand in the splint is obtained. If reduction is not maintained, external fixation, open reduction and internal fixation, or volar plate arthroplasty may be necessary. If satisfactory reduction is maintained, the PIP joint is allowed to flex and extend in the splint. The proximal portion of the finger must

ANSWERS

be stabilized to the splint so that extension of the finger is blocked in the splint. Flexion is reduced 15 degrees per week so that full extension may be achieved by 4 to 6 weeks. At this time the splint is removed and buddy taping is used for 2 to 3 weeks. This technique is not applicable to unstable fracture-dislocations (>40% of articular surface).

93. There is some controversy regarding the optimal position of immobilization. Some advocate splinting the MCP joint in 50 degrees of flexion for 3 weeks or near full extension to allow ligament healing as tightly as possible.

94. Fracture fragment displacement of greater than 2 to 3 mm, or if the displaced fragment involves more than 20% of the articular surface, open reduction and internal fixation are warranted.

95. Simple and complex.

96. Hyperextend the proximal phalanx to 90 degrees on the metacarpal maintaining contact at all times with the head of the metacarpal to prevent entrapment of the volar plate in the joint. The wrist and interphalangeal joints are flexed during the maneuver to relax the flexor tendons, and the proximal phalanx base is pushed along the metacarpal head into the reduced position. Buddy-tape postreduction or splint the MCP joint in 50 to 70 degrees of flexion for 7 to 10 days.

97. Interposition of the volar plate in the MCP joint.

98. Puckering of the volar skin.

99. A sesamoid within a widened MCP joint space indicates the presence of a complex dislocation with the volar plate in the joint.

100. One attempt at closed reduction. If unsuccessful, open reduction.

101. The volar approach (most favored) gives a good view of pathologic anatomy. The dorsal approach allows easy repair of metacarpal head fractures.

QUESTIONS

102. What structures trap the metacarpal head in the palm in complex dorsal MCP joint dislocations of the index and small fingers?

103. Which end of the volar plate is torn in dorsal MCP joint dislocation?

104. Describe open reduction of the volar plate in a complex dorsal MCP joint dislocation.

105. What are the pathologic features of the "locking" MCP joint?

106. How is the locking MCP joint treated?

107. How should a dorsal dislocation of the thumb MCP joint be reduced?

108. How should hyperextension volar plate injuries to the thumb MCP joint be treated?

109. What anteroposterior (AP) radiographic view best demonstrates the thumb CMC joint?

110. How is dislocation of the thumb CMC joint treated?

ANSWERS

102. Index finger—lumbrical on the radial side and the flexor tendons on the ulnar side. Small finger—the flexor tendons and lumbrical on the radial side and the abductor digiti quinti (ADQ) on the ulnar side. Incising these structures does nothing to achieve reduction. Retraction is helpful.

103. The proximal attachment to the metacarpal head.

ANSWERS

104. Before reduction is attempted, the volar plate must be removed from its position dorsal to the metacarpal head. This is accomplished through the use of a skin hook snagging the plate, delivering it from the joint. It may be necessary to release the volar plate radially and ulnarly from the deep transverse metacarpal ligament. After reduction, the volar plate is then repaired into the periosteum of the metacarpal neck with several sutures.

105. The locking MCP joint differs from the classic trigger finger, which typically locks at the A1 pulley and gives the appearance that the limitation takes place at the PIP joint. The key clinical finding in the locking MCP joint is fixed MCP flexion at 40 to 50 degrees and attempts to straighten the digit are very painful or impossible. The most common associated abnormality is the volar plate or collateral ligament catching on an osteophyte on either side of the volar aspect of the metacarpal head. Other possible causes include loose bodies, abnormal sesamoids, and an abnormal fibrous band across the volar aspect of the joint.

106. Observation for at least 1 month because spontaneous recovery can occur. If recovery does not occur, explore the joint through a volar approach, remove osteophytes from the metacarpal head, or divide abnormal fibrous bands.

107. Avoid traction reduction because pulling the phalanx back into position may interpose the volar plate in the joint, thereby creating a complex dislocation. Instead, hyperextend the proximal phalanx on the metacarpal with the thumb interphalangeal joint and wrist flexed, then push the base of the phalanx over the metacarpal head to effect reduction.

108. In a thumb spica cast for 3 to 4 weeks with the MCP joint in 15 to 20 degrees of flexion.

109. The Roberts (hyperpronated) view of the thumb taken with the forearm in maximal pronation.

110. By closed reduction. Because it is very unstable, pronation of the thumb combined with closed pinning is advocated. Then immobilize for 6 weeks.

QUESTIONS

111. Describe the principles of treatment of electrical burns involving the upper extremity.

112. What potential life-threatening complications are associated with electrical burns?

113. What are the prerequisites for tendon transfers?

114. At what muscle length on the Blix curve is the greatest contraction force generated?

115. What are the potential excursions of the forearm and hand muscles?

116. Describe donor selection for tendon transfers.

117. Describe postoperative care for tendon transfers.

118. In radial nerve palsy, which functions should be restored?

119. Describe tendon transfers for radial nerve palsy.

ANSWERS

111. (1) Evaluate entrance and exit sites, bearing in mind that there is almost always more injury than is apparent, as a result of proximal vascular damage. (2) Assure the blood supply; elevate the extremity to prevent edema; and perform escharotomy and compartment release if needed. (3) Allow demarcation; debride and cover with grafts or flaps; amputate as necessary.

112. Cardiac arrhythmias, renal insufficiency, and sepsis.

ANSWERS

113. Bony stability, no edema or inflammation, an adequate soft tissue bed, mobile joints; adequate strength, sufficient excursion, and expendable donor muscle; potential for proper direction of pull or pulley.

114. The greatest contraction force is exerted when a muscle is at resting length.

115. Interossei—3 cm; wrist flexors and extensors, extensor pollicis brevis (EPB), abductor pollicis longus (APL)—3 cm; brachioradialis, lumbricals, thenars—4 cm; finger extensors—5 cm; digital flexors—6 cm.

116. (1) List nonfunctional muscles; (2) list functions needed (i.e., thumb abduction, wrist extension, etc.); (3) list working muscles; (4) eliminate working muscles that have necessary functions that cannot be transferred; (5) match available motors to functions needed; (6) if the needs exceed the number of donor muscles, make a list of alternatives such as arthrodesis, capsulodesis, or tenodesis; (7) divide the surgical procedures into stages: (a) transfers on the flexor side of the hand; (b) transfers on the extensor side of the hand; (c) transfers that pass both volarly and dorsally to the joints of the hand.

117. Protect the transfer for 3 to 4 weeks, then begin active range-of-motion exercises. Continue protective splinting for an additional 3 to 6 weeks for sleeping or activities in which excessive force could occur.

118. Thumb extension and abduction; finger and wrist extension.

119. The muscles affected in radial nerve palsy are the EPL, APL, EDC, extensor carpi radialis longus (ECRL), extensor carpi radialis brevis (ECRB), and extensor carpi ulnaris (ECU). Basic needs are thumb, finger, and wrist extension. Tendon transfers are: thumb extension—palmaris longus to EPL, or FDS (ring or long finger) to EPL; finger extension—flexor carpi ulnaris (FCU) to EDC, or FCR to EDC; wrist extension—pronator teres to ECRB, or FDS (ring or long finger) to ERCB.

QUESTIONS

120. What function should be restored in low median nerve palsy?

121. Describe tendon transfers for low median nerve palsy.

122. What functions require restoration in high median nerve palsy?

123. Describe transfers in high median nerve palsy.

124. True or false? Ulnar clawing is worse in low ulnar nerve palsy than in high ulnar nerve palsy.

125. In low ulnar nerve palsies what hand functions should be reconstructed with tendon transfer?

126. Describe low ulnar nerve palsy tendon transfers.

127. In a high ulnar nerve palsy, which muscle functions often require replacement?

ANSWERS

120. Thumb abduction and opposition.

121. One third of patients do not need opponensplasty because they have adequate thumb abduction from other muscles. Basic needs are thumb abduction and opposition. Tendon transfers are: FDS (ring finger) to the dorsal-ulnar base of the thumb proximal phalanx, using FCU as a pulley; FDS (ring finger) to the abductor pollicis brevis (APB) and EPL, using FCU as a pulley; extensor indicis proprius (EIP) around the ulnar side of the wrist to the proximal phalanx or APB; palmaris longus with extended palmar fascia to APB (Camitz procedure); abductor digiti quinti (ADQ) across the palm to APB (Huber).

ANSWERS

122. Thumb opposition and interphalangeal flexion; DIP and PIP flexion of the index and long fingers.

123. The muscles affected in high median nerve palsy are the APB, opponens, index and long finger lumbricals, FPL, FDS, FDP (index and middle fingers), FCR, and pronator teres. Basic needs are thumb oppostion, interphalangeal flexion, and DIP flexion (index and middle fingers). Transfers are-opponensplasty as described above for low median palsy; brachioradialis to FPL; FDP of ring and small fingers to FDP of index and middle fingers using side-to-side suture.

124. True. The clawing tends to be worse with low ulnar nerve palsies because the ulnar profundus motors are intact in low ulnar nerve palsy, thereby enhancing the flexion deformity.

125. MCP flexion and interphalangeal extension of the ulnar digits, thumb adduction, and index finger abduction.

126. Deficits are thumb adduction, index finger abduction, clawing of ring and small fingers, abducted position of small finger. Basic needs are to increase thumb adduction, increase index finger abduction, MCP flexion, and interphalangeal extension of ulnar two or three digits. Tendon transfers are: thumb adduction—FDS (ring or middle finger) to adductor pollicis (palmar fascia, third metacarpal, or ECU as pulley) or ECRL with free tendon graft to ADP; index finger abduction—APL to first DI or ECRL with graft or EIP to first DI; correction of clawing—FDS to radial lateral bands of ulnar two or three digits or ECRL with graft to the radial lateral bands of the ulnar two or three digits.

127. In addition to those described above for low ulnar nerve palsy, there is weakness in the FDP of the ring and small fingers. Although there is a loss of FCU function, this does not require reconstruction.

QUESTIONS

128. Describe tendon transfers for high ulnar nerve palsy.

129. A 25-year-old woman presents with a painful long finger. The digit is exquisitely sensitive to cold. On physical examination there is a blue dot at the base of the nail and radiographs demonstrate a radiolucent lesion of the distal phalanx. What is the most likely diagnosis?

130. What is the most common primary tumor of the hand skeleton?

131. A 32-year-old farmer noted spontaneous onset of pain and swelling of his right long finger while lifting a bucket during milking. Physical examination demonstrates tenderness over the base of the proximal phalanx of the long finger with swelling and ecchymosis. Radiograph demonstrates a radiolucent lesion in the metaphyseal-diaphyseal area with thinning and expansion of the cortex. There are a few specks of calcification within this radiolucent area. A fracture line is noted with minimal displacement. What is the most likely diagnosis?

132. A 60-year-old woman receiving prednisone for rheumatoid arthritis accidently struck the back of her right hand against a hard table. Since that time she has had difficulty with the long finger locking intermittently. She was referred for trigger finger. On examination, however, this is not a typical trigger finger in that the MCP joint becomes stuck at about 60 degrees of flexion when the patient makes a fist. She is unable to fully extend the MCP joint. There are no problems with passive motion at the MCP, PIP, or DIP joints. There is palpable and visible snapping noted over the dorsal MCP joint and the digit ulnarly deviates once it is in the locked position. After passive extension of the digit, the patient can hold the MCP joint in full extension. What is the problem with this patient's finger?

133. How should this patient be treated?

ANSWERS

128. The deficits are the same as for low ulnar nerve palsy, plus loss of the FDP to the ulnar fingers and loss of the FCU. Basic needs are the same as for low ulnar palsy, plus one may want to increase DIP flexion of the ulnar two or three digits. Transfers are the same as for low ulnar palsy, except the FDS of the ring and long fingers should not be used. Flexion of the DIP joint of the ulnar two or three digits is achieved with side-to-side tenodesis to the FDP of the index or long finger, or both.

129. Glomus tumor. These tumors have characteristic cold sensitivity and occasional ridging of the nail with a blue spot at the base of the nail. Fifty percent are subungual. They are more common in women aged 30 to 50 years. Treatment is excision of the tumor.

130. Enchondroma.

131. The patient has probably sustained a pathologic fracture through an enchondroma. The most frequent site for enchondroma is in the proximal phalanges of the digits. There is no sex preference. The age range is 20 to 40 years.

132. She has sustained a tear of the radial sagittal band of the long finger extensor mechanism, resulting in ulnar subluxation of the tendon. The sagittal band functions to extend the proximal phalanx and stabilize the extensor tendons in the midline. With interruptions of the radial sagittal band, the extensor tendon shifts ulnarward into the web space. This produces ulnar deviation of the digit and the tendon locks around the metacarpal head, precluding active extension of the digit. This produces the locking-in flexion at the MCP joint.

133. This is somewhat controversial. A repair or reconstruction of the radial sagittal band is advocated by most. Closed treatment in an extension splint may be pursued if the problem is identified early.

QUESTIONS

134. Describe the prerequisites for elective surgery on the cerebral palsy (CP) upper extremity.

135. What functional tasks should be evaluated in each CP patient?

136. What procedure is effective in improving a weak grasp in a CP patient with flexed wrist posturing? What are the contraindications to surgery?

137. What procedure is recommended for hyperextensible swan-neck deformity of the PIP joints in CP?

138. How is the CP thumb-in-palm deformity treated?

139. Describe the Wassel classification of polydactyly of the thumb.

ANSWERS

134. This is controversial. Three major areas should be carefully evaluated prior to advising surgery: (1) cognition; (2) hand placement; (3) sensibility. Cognition: To benefit from upper extremity reconstructive surgery the patient should have an IQ of at least 50 to 70. Others believe that regardless of IQ, a child may be a candidate if he or she can cooperate with postoperative rehabilitation. Hand placement: If the patient cannot place the affected hand on the head and the opposite knee within a period of 5 seconds, upper extremity surgery will not produce a good functional outcome. Sensibility: Different testing techniques are employed based upon the patient's age and intellect. Recommended techniques for specific ages include: 2 to 3 years: texture discrimination; 4 to 5 years: object identification; 6 to 9 years: graphesthesia; older than 10 years; two-point discrimination. Children with 3/5 object discrimination, number perception in the palm or two-point discrimination of at least 10 mm can be considered surgical candidates for functional reconstructive procedures. Some surgeons believe that improved function can be achieved in patients with poor sensation (i.e., turning a poorly functioning hand into a satisfactory "helping hand"). In a child with an IQ of less than 50, hand placement from head to knee over 5 seconds, and poor sensibility, hygiene is the goal. Contracture releases and joint arthrode-

ANSWERS

sis to facilitate hygiene are surgical options. In a child with an **IQ** greater than 50, but with poor placement and sensibility, the goal should be to maintain hygiene. At the same time, these patients may desire improved aesthetics which can be accomplished through releases and arthrodesis. For children with an **IQ** greater than 50, with good placement and sensation, a functional upper extremity is a realistic goal. Releases, arthrodesis, and tendon transfers are considerations in these patients.

135. The patient's ability to dress, wash, eat, grip and release, pinch, bimanually manipulate objects, and general ability to cooperate (influences postoperative therapy).

136. Tendon transfers to the ECRB (usually the FCU) are effective. Contraindications to surgery are inability to extend the fingers with the wrist extended, poor cognition, and difficulty in placement in a patient who ignores the extremity.

137. Sublimis sling tenodesis with the PIP in 30 degrees of flexion.

138. Lengthening the FPL, and web release or adductor release with EPL rerouting, depending upon the deformity.

139. The Wassel classification is based upon the amount of bony duplication from distal to proximal. *Type I* represents a partial duplication of the distal phalanx; *Type II* is a complete duplication of the distal phalanx; *Type III* is a complete duplication of the distal phalanx with partial duplication of the proximal phalanx; *Type IV* is a complete duplication of the distal and proximal phalanges; *Type V* is partial duplication of the metacarpal with complete duplication of the distal and proximal phalanges; *Type VI* is a complete duplication of the thumb through the metacarpal; *Type VII* are thumb deformities which do not fit into the previous categories and include triphalangeal thumbs. See Figure.

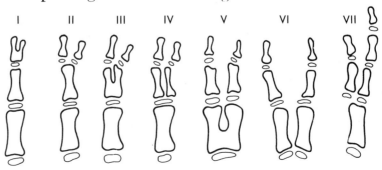

QUESTIONS

140. Describe the treatment for camptodactyly.

141. Describe the treatment for clinodactyly.

142. Describe the treatment for Kirner's deformity.

143. Which volar structures develop abnormally at the PIP joint, leading to joint contracture?

144. Which structures contribute to MCP joint extension contractures?

145. What are the principles of treatment for flexion contractures of the interphalangeal joints?

146. Describe the use of the joint jack finger splint.

147. What else can be done to mobilize resistant joint contractures?

148. What structures should be protected during checkrein ligament resection?

ANSWERS

140. Treatment early after onset includes prolonged extension splinting; release of the FDS or transfer of the FDS to the extensor apparatus through the lumbrical canal as recommended by Millesi for teenagers with flexible deformity (PIP flexion that improves with wrist flexion). In adults, osteotomy of the proximal phalanx may improve a rigid deformity.

ANSWERS

141. Surgery is usually cosmetic and can be delayed until the child is 6 years old, at which time a closing wedge osteotomy can be performed. Splinting is ineffective.

142. Progressive, painless, radiovolar curving of the distal phalanges of both small fingers. Kirner's deformity develops about age 12 years, usually in girls. There is very little functional disability but there may be difficulty in typing or playing musical instruments. Multiple opening wedge osteotomies can correct the deformity.

143. The checkrein ligaments are swallowtail extensions of the volar plate along the volar proximal phalanx which may hypertrophy, thicken, and shorten, producing marked PIP flexion contracture.

144. Thickening and shortening of the dorsal capsule and collateral ligaments. There are no checkreins at the MCP joint and the volar plate is more flexible than at the PIP joint, thus resisting development of contracture.

145. Application of nonelastic force in the direction of desired correction for long periods of time.

146. The joint jack finger splint is applied an hour before bedtime. The patient tightens the screw every 2 to 3 minutes to the point of intolerable pain. At bedtime the screw is loosened partially for comfort. The patient sleeps with the splint in place with a piece of tape around the finger and the splint. Taping prevents the splint from falling off as the finger gradually straightens. If the splint falls off, the finger resumes its contracted position. If night splinting is too painful for sleep, the joint jack is used during the day in two 1-hour sessions. Severe joint damage or trauma may require jacking 1 hour per day for up to 1 year.

147. Those not responsive to splinting may improve with serial casting.

148. The transverse communicating vessels, which supply the vincular system, and lie approximately 2 mm proximal to the volar plate, run beneath the checkreins, and merge in the midline.

QUESTIONS

149. Describe the technique of checkrein ligament release.

150. Describe the release of PIP joint extension contractures.

151. Volar plate avulsion injuries are another common cause of loss of PIP joint flexion. Describe the test for longstanding volar plate avulsion.

152. Describe the tendon, ligament, and joint capsule anatomy of the extended and flexed MCP joint.

153. What is the best initial approach to MCP extension contracture?

154. Identify the contents of the six dorsal compartments.

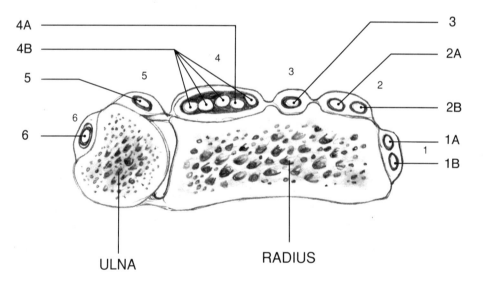

155. Describe the Frykman classification of distal radius fractures.

ANSWERS

149. Resection through either a midlateral incision or a volar V-Y plasty incision. V-Y plasty is preferred in longstanding contractures with anticipated deficiency of volar skin once the finger becomes straight. The flexor sheath distal to the A2 pulley is opened. The checkrein ligaments are cut from the proximal volar plate and are

ANSWERS

resected proximally with care to avoid injury to the transverse communicating vessels. Rarely is excision of collaterals or release of the volar plate needed to release PIP contracture. The check-rein ligaments are implicated as the major cause of contracture and their resection usually relieves the contracture.

150. These almost always involve joint contracture combined with extensor hood abnormalities and adhesions. The transverse retinacular ligament is cut, and the lateral band elevated. The dorsal capsule is excised while protecting the central slip and the joint is passively flexed. If significant adhesions of the extensor hood to the proximal phalanx are encountered, a Silastic sheet (0.005 in. or less) can be inserted between the hood and the scarred bed over the proximal phalanx after adhesiolysis.

151. Passive flexion of the joint produces significant pain. The volar plate hinges on the middle phalanx at the site of the tear. It can remain symptomatic for years, producing a voluntary loss of flexion secondary to pain which may become fixed (extension contracture). Surgical repair of the volar plate alleviates the symptoms.

152. With MCP joint extension, there are loose collateral ligaments, joint capsule, and large intrasynovial capacity. The joint abducts and adducts easily. With MCP joint flexion, collaterals are tight and intracapsular volume is decreased.

153. A knuckle-bender splint, best worn at night. If unresponsive to conservative treatment or if long standing, contractures warrant operative release. Surgery consists of capsulectomy. Collateral ligament release may be necessary. Sometimes the volar plate must be freed of adhesions.

154. *1A*, extensor pollicis brevis; *1B*, abductor pollicis longus; *2A*, extensor carpi radialis brevis; *2B*, extensor carpi radialis longus; *3*, extensor pollicis longus; *4A*, extensor indicis; *4B*, extensor digitorum communis; *5*, extensor digiti minimi; *6*, extensor carpi ulnaris.

155. *Type I:* extraarticular radius *Type III:* intraarticular radiocarpal *Type V:* intraarticular radioulnar *Type VII:* radiocarpal and radioulnar. The even-numbered Frykman categories *(Types II, IV, VI, and VIII)* consist of the preceding odd-numbered fracture pattern plus a distal ulnar fracture.

QUESTIONS

156. Describe the Lichtman classification of Kienböck's disease.

157. Describe how to measure the carpal index (carpal height ratio) and its normal range.

158. What is the natural history of scaphoid nonunions?

159. What is the humpback deformity in scaphoid nonunion?

160. What is the recommended treatment for humpback deformity in scaphoid nonunion?

161. What is the blood supply to the scaphoid?

162. What is the clinical significance of the blood supply of the scaphoid?

163. What is a DISI deformity?

164. What is a VISI deformity?

ANSWERS

156. *Stage I:* normal lunate structure; sometimes there is evidence of a compression fracture usually appearing as a radiodense or radiolucent line. *Stage II:* density change in the lunate relative to surrounding carpal bones; rarefaction along the line of previous compression fracture or increased lunate density, or both; normal size and shape of the lunate; no carpal collapse noted. *Stage III:* fragmentation or flattening of the lunate. *Stage IIIA:* lunate collapse without scaphoid collapse. *Stage IIIB:* lunate collapse with fixed scaphoid rotation. *Stage IV:* all the findings of stage III plus arthrosis of the radiocarpal and intercarpal joints.

ANSWERS

157. The carpal index is a ratio of carpal height (proximal lunate to distal capitate) to the length of the middle finger metacarpal. Normal is 0.54 ±0.03

158. Over a period of years scaphoid nonunions progress to wrist arthritis.

159. Humpback deformity is a dorsal prominence of the scaphoid. This results from a loss of volar bone, which leads to a collapse deformity of the carpus.

160. Volar inlay wedge graft with or without internal fixation.

161. The major blood supply to the scaphoid comes through a perforating artery along the dorsal ridge of the scaphoid (a branch of the radial artery). An additional smaller portion is supplied from a second radial artery branch, perforating the distal pole of the scaphoid tubercle.

162. Because of the distal-to-proximal direction of flow, fractures in the proximal portion of the scaphoid are more liable to cause interruption of the blood supply and lead to avascular necrosis of the scaphoid proximal pole and nonunion.

163. DISI deformity, or *dorsal intercalated segment instability*, refers to palmar migration of the lunate with dorsal tilt of its distal articular surface with associated palmar flexion of the distal pole of the scaphoid. It is usually associated with a scapholunate angle greater than 70 degrees and a capitate-lunate angle greater than 15 degrees. DISI deformity is associated with scapholunate instability and scaphoid nonunion.

164. In the VISI deformity, or *volar intercalated segment instability*, the lunate assumes a dorsal position in the wrist relative to the capitate and its distal articular surface faces palmarward. There is a decreased scapholunate angle. This condition is associated with ulnar-sided carpal instability such as lunotriquetral tears, as well as ligamentous laxity of the wrist.

QUESTIONS

165. A 25-year-old laborer injured his wrist 2 years ago and has had persistent radial-sided wrist pain. There are no arthritic changes noted on radiograph. The wrist arthrogram demonstrates a defect at the scapholunate joint. What are the treatment options for this patient?

166. A 35-year-old "party animal" sustained an axial blow to the right hand with dorsal dislocation of the long, ring, and small finger CMC joints. He is neurologically intact, and the skin is intact. How should these dislocations be treated?

167. A 65-year-old woman complains of persistent numbness in the index and long fingers, which is worse with driving and when doing needlepoint. She has had intermittent awakening at night from pain in the hands. What is the most likely diagnosis and what are the treatment options for this condition?

168. What factors would lead you to advocate carpal tunnel release as opposed to conservative care?

169. Describe the major variations in the motor branch of the median nerve.

170. What are the major dangers in releasing the carpal tunnel?

171. How does one differentiate carpal tunnel syndrome from pronator syndrome?

ANSWERS

165. (1) Continued conservative care with an intermittent splinting and strengthening program; (2) intercarpal arthrodesis (scaphocapitate); (3) Blatt dorsal capsulodesis; (4) Ligament reconstruction.

166. Closed reduction usually can be performed easily under intravenous (IV) sedation or local anesthesia. With multiple dislocations, however, it may be difficult to maintain the reduction and therefore closed reduction and percutaneous pinning are advisable.

167. The patient most likely has carpal tunnel syndrome. Treatment options consist of surgical release of the transverse carpal ligament (TCL), night splinting, and carpal tunnel steroid injection. Vitamin B_6 and nonsteroidal anti-inflammatory drugs have had variable success in the treatment of carpal tunnel syndrome.

168. A history of constant sensory loss, atrophy of the thenar musculature with weakness, or prolongation of two-point discrimination compared with the opposite hand are factors which indicate that conservative care is not likely to be successful. In these patients, operative release is appropriate.

169. The most common pattern of the motor branch of the median nerve is an extraligamentous takeoff from the main nerve (distal to the TCL—50%). The next most common is the subligamentous branching with the nerve exiting in a recurrent manner to innervate the thenar muscles (branches proximal to the distal edge of the TCL—30%), and the third most common course is transligamentous (through the TCL—20%).

170. Injury to the palmar cutaneous branch of the median nerve, the motor branch, the common branch to the ring and long fingers, and the superficial palmar arch. Other technical problems consist of inadequate release of the carpal tunnel which tends to occur most frequently at the distal end of the TCL.

171. A positive Tinel's sign in the forearm, reproduction of symptoms with nerve compression in the proximal forearm, frequently a negative Phalen's test, and pain with resisted pronation are present in pronator syndrome. In addition, one may see forearm pain with resisted flexion of the PIP joints of the ring and long fingers in pronator syndrome, but not in carpal tunnel syndrome.

QUESTIONS

172. What are the four potential sites of compression of the median nerve in pronator syndrome?

173. Describe the findings in anterior interosseous syndrome.

174. What are the possible sites of compression in anterior interosseous syndrome?

175. Describe the sites of compression in radial tunnel syndrome.

176. Describe the most common physical and electrodiagnostic findings in radial tunnel syndrome.

177. A 55-year-old physical education teacher complains of dorsal radial wrist pain with numbness affecting the thumb, index, and long fingers. The symptons do not waken the patient at night. They are intermittent but intense at times. On physical examination, the median nerve compression test, Phalen's test, and Tinel's sign over the median nerve from the elbow to the wrist were negative. Two-point discrimination was normal. The patient complained of shooting pains when the radial styloid was percussed. What is this patient's diagnosis and how should he be treated?

178. What are the sites and causes of compression in posterior interosseous nerve palsy?

ANSWERS

172. (1) Beneath the supracondylar process and ligament of Struthers, (2) the lacertus fibrosis, (3) the pronator teres muscle, and (4) at the arch of the FDS.

173. The patient typically describes achy forearm pain followed by weakness or loss of function affecting the FPL, and the FDP to the index and long fingers. The pronator quadratus is also affected in this syndrome. Patients frequently complain of inability to flex the thumb at the interphalangeal joint. Sensation is not affected.

ANSWERS

174. The proximal one third of the forearm, related to tendinous bands at the deep head of the pronator teres, the origin of FDS of the long finger, the origin of FCR, or secondary to accessory muscles; FDS connected to FDP, Gantzer's muscle (accessory head to the flexor pollicis FPL), palmaris profundus, and flexor carpi radialis brevis (FCRB); and enlarged bicipital bursa. Anterior interosseous nerve palsy has also been associated with fractures or thrombosis of ulnar collateral vessels.

175. Fibrous bands lying anterior to the radial head, radial recurrent vessels (leash of Henry), the tendinous margin of the ECRB, and the arcade of Frohse.

176. Pain over the radial nerve in the area of the mobile wad. The patient complains of aching in the extensor-supinator area. Maximal tenderness in radial tunnel syndrome is usually 4 to 8 cm distal to the lateral epicondyle in the supinator. Sensory changes are usually absent. The patient's pain is characteristically distal to the lateral epicondyle and should not be confused with lateral epicondylitis. Resisted long finger MCP joint extension, resisted forearm supination, or passive hyperpronation will often localize the pain in the radial tunnel and can be helpful in the diagnosis. Electrodiagnostic studies of the radial nerve are usually negative.

177. The patient most likely has Wartenburg's syndrome, also known as cheiralgia paresthetica. This is a neuritis of the superficial branch of the radial nerve. It usually occurs near the radial styloid where the nerve becomes subcutaneous. It may be posttraumatic or have no specific cause. One should ask about tight watch bands or bracelets, which might irritate the nerve. Anomalous muscles have also been described as producing neuritic symptoms. If removal of jewelry is not effective in improving the patient's symptoms, a thumb spica splint may be effective with care to mold the splint so that there is no pressure over the irritable nerve. Surgical neurolysis may be considered if conservative means are ineffective.

178. Usually the proximal edge of the supinator, although it also has been described in the middle or distal aspect of the supinator. Specific causes are ganglia, lipoma, fibroma, or rheumatoid arthritis of the radiohumeral joint.

QUESTIONS

179. A 65-year-old steelworker is referred for intermittent pain along the medial proximal forearm and numbness in the small and ring fingers. He is awakened intermittently at night with numbness in the hand and pain in the arm. Motor and sensory testing are within normal limits. Adson's test is negative. There is tenderness over the medial elbow, 3 cm distal to the medial epicondyle. There is a positive Tinel's sign in this area radiating to the ring and small fingers. The elbow flexion test is positive. Nerve conduction velocities and electromyogram (EMG) for the median and ulnar nerves are normal. What is his diagnosis? How should he be treated?

180. What are the sites of compression of the ulnar nerve in cubital tunnel syndrome?

181. What are the surgical options for treatment of cubital tunnel syndrome?

182. A 25-year-old gymnast fell from the parallel bars, landing on his dorsiflexed wrist. Since this episode he complains of intermittent numbness and tingling in the ulnar two digits. On physical examination there is pain in the ulnar palm with mild swelling. Digital range of motion and two-point discrimination are normal. The intrinsics of the hand measure 5/5 on motor testing. Allen's test demonstrates excellent flow to the hand through the radial artery. There is no filling through the ulnar artery. What is the differential diagnosis?

183. What are the borders of Guyon's canal?

184. Where does the deep motor branch of the ulnar nerve separate from the main nerve trunk?

ANSWERS

179. The patient has cubital tunnel syndrome. Although positive electrodiagnostic studies are helpful in confirming the diagnosis, mild cases frequently will have negative findings on EMG and nerve conduction velocity. The vast majority of patients present with normal two-point discrimination and motor tests. Prolongation of two-point discrimination, muscle atrophy, and weakness are usually very late signs. Initial care should be conservative, consisting of precautions in elbow posturing such as avoidance of the flexed elbow position or resting on the elbow and forearm. An elbow pad can be used depending upon how irritable the nerve is, in order to avoid direct trauma. In addition, a 45-degree elbow splint can be applied to rest the elbow either full-time or at night only, to attempt to decrease nerve irritability. If conservative care is unsuccessful, then surgical options may be considered.

180. The cubital tunnel, arcade of Struthers, anconeus epitrochlearis, medial head of triceps, aponeurosis of the FCU, and others, including osteophytes, ganglia, or lipomas, and hypermobility of the ulnar nerve.

181. Simple in situ decompression of the ulnar nerve, anterior transposition of the ulnar nerve (subcutaneous, sub- and intramuscular), and medial epicondylectomy.

182. Sensory changes may be due to irritation of the ulnar nerve and may represent a contusion of the nerve, with or without carpal fracture or CMC dislocation. What is more likely in this case, because of the abnormal vascular filling from the ulnar artery, is that the patient has sustained an ulnar artery thrombosis. This can be confirmed through Doppler evaluation or arteriogram. Radiographs of the wrist are helpful and EMG and nerve conduction studies can rule out ulnar nerve compromise in Guyon's canal.

183. Guyon's canal is a triangular-shaped area. The roof is formed by the volar carpal ligament, the lateral wall by the hook of the hamate and the insertion of the TCL, and the medial wall by the pisohamate ligament and the pisiform bone.

184. Within Guyon's canal. It then passes distally and radially around the base of the hook of the hamate to enter the deep midpalmar fat (retroflexor fat) with the deep branch of the ulnar artery. This branch continues radially to innervate the deeper intrinsics of the hand.

QUESTIONS

185. A 35-year-old factory worker noted a spontaneous inability to flex the thumb 2 weeks after a tennis elbow release. He was referred to you 6 weeks following surgery for a second opinion regarding the need for surgery. He is unable to flex the thumb interphalangeal joint, but he has good strength in the other muscle groups of the hand. EMG and nerve conduction findings are consistent with anterior interosseous nerve syndrome. What is your recommended treatment?

186. What are the indications for replantation?

187. What are the contraindications to replantation?

188. An emergency room physician in an outlying hospital wants to transfer a patient with a midforearm amputation. He wants to know how to take care of the amputated part. What is your response?

189. The patient in question 188 has arrived in your hospital and the replantation is initially successful. Circulation has been restored to the limb and he has done well postoperatively until you enter the room on a postoperative check to find that the extremity is cool with poor capillary refill. What measures should be taken to save the failing replant?

ANSWERS

185. This patient has a partial anterior interosseous nerve syndrome as evidenced by lack of involvement of the index and long finger FDP. Patients with this presentation have resolution of their syndrome nonoperatively. Conservative treatment is advised. A complete anterior interosseous nerve palsy that has not improved in 6 to 12 weeks, and which is not associated with previous trauma, is a candidate for exploration of the nerve.

ANSWERS

186. Most thumb amputations at or proximal to the interphalangeal joint would benefit from replantation, as would multiple-digit amputations, metacarpal-level amputations, and wrist and forearm amputations. Only sharp or moderately avulsed elbow and arm amputations should be considered for replantation. Almost any extremity level in a child (excluding soft tissue fingertip injuries) is an indication for replantation.

187. Concomitant life-threatening injury (head injury); multilevel injuries; extreme crush, avulsion, or contamination (farm injuries); pre-existing systemic illness (unstable angina, pneumonia, congestive heart failure); and distal fingertip amputations.

188. The goal of care of an amputated part is to decrease the warm ischemic time. One should wrap it in sterile saline or lactated Ringer's–soaked sterile gauze and place it in a plastic cup or bag, which is then placed on ice. Do not use dry ice since this will freeze the part and make it unsuitable for replantation. Partial amputations, which are dysvascular, should be treated similarly. Align the partially amputated segment, then dress and splint to prevent additional trauma. Pack ice around the dysvascular parts.

189. Replants may fail referable to arterial or venous problems or both. If a venous outflow problem is identified, then elevating the extremity may help. If it appears to be an arterial problem, lowering the limb may help. Loosening the dressing may improve blood flow to the extremity as well, particularly if there has been swelling. Patient agitation can lead to vasospasm. Sedation will help reverse this. In addition, the patient may be hypovolemic resulting in vasospasm, and hydrating the patient and assuring that his blood count is satisfactory may save the replant. If the patient has become cool, this too may lead to peripheral vasoconstriction. Keeping the patient in a warm room with a K-pad over the replanted extremity may improve perfusion. A heparin bolus of 5,000 units IV may be successful in patients who have had crushing injuries and subsequent clot formation. Axillary block anesthesia or sympathetic block may also reverse vasospasm. Leach therapy has been successful in saving replants that have had venous outflow problems. If these measures are unsuccessful, return the patient to the operating room for inspection of the arterial and venous anastomoses (The last may be the best initial maneuver if the replant is obviously compromised.)

QUESTIONS

190. What are the usual results from replantation of digits?

191. What is the maximal warm ischemic time which will not produce deleterious effects in a digital replantation?

192. What is the maximal cold ischemic time that will not deleteriously effect digital performance following replantation?

193. A 29-year-old hairdresser has been transferred to the emergency room following a motor vehicle accident, which partially amputated the left arm at the level of the shoulder. There is a transverse comminuted fracture at the humeral neck, with evidence of an avulsion injury of the extremity. Ragged skin edges are heavily contaminated and the only structures intact are the radial nerve and a severely stretched ulnar nerve. The patient was initially evaluated at an outlying hospital and subsequently transferred to the replantation center. The accident occurred 8 hours ago. The emergency room physician has asked whether this is a replantable extremity. What is your response?

194. A 23-year-old medical student has just amputated the long, ring, and small fingers in a table saw. The level of amputation is through the midproximal phalanges. Describe the sequence of repair of the severed structures and your rationale for this sequence.

195. In the previous case, how many arteries and how many veins should be repaired for each digit?

ANSWERS

190. Viability is achieved in 70% to 90% of patients. Cold intolerance develops in all patients and supposedly disappears in 2 to 3 years. Good range of motion is difficult to achieve (usually only 50% of normal). Sensibility is 10 mm or less in 50% of adults, 5 mm or less in children.

191. Six hours.

192. Twenty-four to 30 hours of cold ischemic time is tolerated in digital replantation.

193. A number of factors militate against replantation in this case. The long ischemic time is the major factor. With major upper extremity replantations there is a significant mass of muscle which can undergo necrosis if it is not reperfused rapidly. The warm ischemic time should be under 6 hours and the cold ischemic time under 12 hours in making the decision to replant an amputation such as this. The risk of toxic products being liberated into the general circulation after revascularization of a nonviable extremity is significant and would contraindicate replantation if this extremity had not been kept cooled. Another contraindication is the mechanism of injury. Avulsion injuries have extensive zones of injury. The anticipated recovery of nerve function in this extremity is poor. The degree of contamination is also troublesome.

194. With any amputation, a primary goal of replantation is to reestablish blood flow both into and out of the extremity. This goal, however, must be deferred until other more gross surgical procedures are performed. In order to protect the arterial and venous repairs, it is recommended that the bony and tendinous repairs be performed prior to the vascular repairs. My recommended sequence is as follows: (1) bony fixation, (2) flexor and extensor tendon repairs, (3) nerve repairs, (4) arterial repairs, (5) venous repairs, (6) skin coverage. (*Note:* Nerve repairs can be deferred until after the vascular repairs depending upon the individual circumstances of the replantation.)

195. Two veins for each artery repaired, and a minimum of one artery for each digit.

QUESTIONS

196. A 60-year-old farmer amputated his index finger at the level of the MCP joint with a hatchet while chopping wood. The digit was immediately placed on ice. He is otherwise healthy. It was a clean amputation with comminution of the articular surface of the base of the proximal phalanx and metacarpal head. The injury was 1 hour ago. What is your recommendation regarding treatment?

197. A 65-year-old retired minister has a long history of bilateral hand pain. His major complaints, however concern the index and long finger PIP joints. He has been treated with splinting and nonsteroidal anti-inflammatory drugs without significant relief. On physical examination he has Heberden's and Bouchard's nodes on all fingers. There appears to be more swelling and greater loss of motion in the index and long finger PIP joints. The range of motion in each of these joints is from 40 to 60 degrees of flexion. The remainder of his hand has satisfactory pain-free motion. Radiographs demonstrate narrowing of the long and index finger PIP joints with large osteophytes noted dorsally and palmarly as well as 10 degrees of ulnar subluxation. There is involvement to a lesser degree in the other interphalangeal joints of the hand. The MCP joints have been spared. What do you recommend for treatment of the index and long fingers?

198. What is the recommended position for arthrodesis of the wrist?

199. What is the optimal position for a shoulder arthrodesis?

200. What is the recommended position for arthrodesis of the elbow?

201. What are the components of a nerve fiber?

202. What are the connective tissue elements supporting the fasciculi?

203. What is the difference between myelinated and unmyelinated fibers?

ANSWERS

196. Although somewhat controversial, in general, replantation of single finger amputations proximal to the sublimis insertion in elderly laborers produces poor results with regard to function, and revision of the amputation would be indicated. If this same patient had presented with an amputation of the thumb at the MCP joint level, replantation would be performed.

197. This patient has characteristic osteoarthritis of the hand. Treatment options include arthrodesis or arthroplasty. The index finger, because of the need for stability in pinch, is best served by arthrodesis. The long finger could function with a PIP arthroplasty, although an arthrodesis would be more reliable. Both options have a high likelihood of relieving pain. PIP arthroplasty, however, is at risk for breakage and bony resorption, which could necessitate revision in the future.

198. Neutral to 15 degrees of dorsiflexion.

199. This is controversial. Paralytic shoulders requiring fusion should be fused in 50 degrees of abduction, 15 to 25 degrees of flexion, and 25 degrees of internal rotation. Older patients with degenerative shoulder disease requiring an arthrodesis should be fused in 20 degrees of abduction, 30 degrees of flexion, and 40 degrees of internal rotation.

200. Ninety degrees of flexion if the elbow fusion is unilateral. With bilateral fusions, 50 degrees of extension in one elbow and 110 degrees of flexion in the other.

201. Axons surrounded by the Schwann cell sheath.

202. The epineurium, perineurium, and endoneurium. The epineurium is the superficial layer. Blood and lymphatic vessels run in the epineurium. Each funiculus is surrounded by perineurium. Endoneurium is the extracellular space surrounding the Schwann cells and axons.

203. Unmyelinated fibers are those in which axons lie in furrows on the surface of the Schwann cell. The myelinated fibers are encased in concentrically arranged lamellae which are the wrappings of the Schwann cell plasma membrane around the axon.

QUESTIONS

204. What is the node of Ranvier?

205. Describe wallerian degeneration.

206. When does proximal axonal budding occur?

207. What is the usual sequence of healing following laceration of a peripheral nerve?

208. What effect does nerve degeneration have on the skeletal muscle it supplies?

209. Is electrical stimulation of denervated muscle effective in delaying deterioration of the motor end plates?

210. What are the three periods of regeneration delay seen after peripheral nerve injury as the nerve begins to grow?

211. List suture and needle sizes for microsurgical repairs at the wrist, palm, proximal digits, and distal digits.

ANSWERS

204. An axonal segment which lacks myelin sheath.

205. Schwann cells digest fragmented myelin in endoneurial tubules distal to axonal interruption and in the proximal axonal zone of injury. The debris is removed by 2 to 8 weeks and then there is progressive shrinkage in the fascicular cross-sectional area. Shrinkage may reach a maximum as early as 3 months after injury. The fascicular cross-sectional area may be only 17% of normal by 2 years.

206. About 4 days after injury; it may be delayed 14 to 21 days in severe crush or avulsion injuries.

ANSWERS

207. The perikaryon (cell body) responds to injury by increasing its metabolic activity by the fourth day. Anywhere from 15% to 80% of the cell bodies die following section of the nerve trunk. Another factor which may prevent full recovery following nerve injury is that the injured axon segment, which must be regenerated, may be too long. It may, in a sense, exceed the cell body's capacity for repair. The axon distal to severance undergoes wallerian degeneration. While the axon and myelin sheath degenerate, the Schwann cells and macrophages remove the necrotic debris. Unmyelinated axons degenerate within 1 week. The fascicular cross-sectional area also decreases with time. Wallerian degeneration also occurs over a shorter distance in the proximal stump in the zone of injury. Ninety-six hours after a sharp traumatic injury, axonal sprouting begins. In extreme trauma, axonal sprouting may be delayed as long as 3 weeks. Schwann cells form tubules for the regenerating axons. The new nerve fibers pass down new endoneurial tubules. This results in a loss of specificity of the nerve fibers as some of the sensory and motor fibers pass into tubules for end organs for which they were not intended.

208. Muscle atrophy develops with progressive destruction of motor end plates. The motor end plates begin to deteriorate by the third month after denervation.

209. Measurements of capacity for work of muscle after denervation, as well as histologic evaluation of denervated human muscle with and without electrical stimulation, have not shown significant differences.

210. (1) Neuronal survival (4–20 days); (2) axonal traversing of the suture line or area of injury (3–50 days); (3) end-organ connection (the axon grows down the distal end of the neural tube at approximately 1 mm/day).

211.

Location	Needle Size (μm)	Suture Size
Wrist	150	9–0
Palm	100	10–0
Proximal digit	50–75	10–0
Distal digit	50	11–0

QUESTIONS

212. Describe methods to facilitate group fascicular alignment of the proximal and distal stumps of a severed nerve.

213. What is Panner's Disease?

214. Describe the treatment for osteochondritis dissecans of the radial head.

215. Describe the Martin-Gruber anastomosis.

216. Describe the Riche-Cannieu anastomosis.

217. What provisions should be made in the fabrication of a standard socket for a wrist disarticulation patient to preserve maximal motion of the extremity?

218. Describe the characteristics of a long below-elbow amputation socket with regard to design features to preserve function.

ANSWERS

212. (1) Observe blood vessel patterns on epineural sheaths; (2) match the pattern of fascicular groups within the two nerve stumps; (3) electrical stimulation (within 72 hours) for identification of ''motor'' groups in the distal stump; (4) electrical stimulation for identification of ''sensory'' groups in the proximal stump; (5) histologic staining to differentiate motor and sensory fascicles.

213. This is an osteochondrosis of the capitellum. This usually occurs in boys from 5 to 10 years of age and affects the right elbow. This should be distinguished from osteochondritis dissecans of the radial head. In Panners's disease one sees fragmentation and deformity of the entire ossific nucleus of the capitellum. The lesion heals with reconstitution of the capitellum and no surgery is necessary.

ANSWERS

214. Although somewhat controversial, treatment is for the most part nonoperative. Activity modification and rest are usually prescribed. In patients who are older, arthroscopy may be helpful in evaluating the lesion. Drilling and pinning the lesion may be possible in this manner. Arthroscopy may be helpful also in removal or replacement of loose bodies.

215. The Martin-Gruber anastomosis is a connection between the median and ulnar nerves in the forearm in which the median nerve carries ulnar motor fibers to the adductor pollicis and first dorsal interosseous until the midforearm where they branch to join the ulnar nerve. Thus, in high ulnar nerve lesions, there may be some ulnar intrinsic motor function preserved.

216. The Riche-Cannieu anastomosis is a variation in neural supply to the thenar muscles, which are usually supplied by the median nerve. These muscles can be innervated to varying degrees by anastomosis of the ulnar motor branch to the recurrent motor branch of the median nerve in the hand.

217. To facilitate transmission of stump rotation to the socket, it is flattened to produce an elliptic cross section in the mediolateral plane. The socket covers only about 50% of the radial surface of the forearm to ensure that there is no restriction of elbow flexion. The opposite socket border runs along the ulnar aspect of the forearm to the olecranon which aids in prosthesis stability and in resisting bending moments when lifting.

218. Since a long below-elbow stump maintains pronation and supination of the forearm, it is desirable to accommodate this motion through prosthetic fitting. The techniques used for long below-elbow stump fitting are the same for a wrist disarticulation, mainly flattening of the distal end of the prosthesis into an elliptic configuration which conforms with the contour of the distal forearm—a low trim line over the radius, and a high trim line over the ulna.

CHAPTER 8

Lower Extremity

Timothy S. Loth, M.D.

QUESTIONS

1. What is the function of the popliteus muscle?

2. What is the function of the semimembranosus muscle?

3. Which meniscus is more mobile?

4. How should acute complete ruptures of the quadriceps tendon be treated?

5. How should a partial quadriceps tendon rupture be treated?

6. How should chronic complete quadriceps tendon ruptures be treated?

7. What is the conventional way of designating the direction of a dislocation of the knee?

8. What is the mechanism of injury in anterior knee dislocation?

ANSWERS

1. Internal rotation of the tibia on the femur.

2. Flexion and internal rotation of the tibia.

3. The lateral meniscus.

4. Operative repair, sometimes using a reinforcing Scuderi flap.

5. In a cylinder cast in extension for 5 to 6 weeks, or cast brace.

6. Quadricepsplasty and repair with protection of the repair using a pull-out wire and a McLaughlin tibial bolt.

7. The direction of tibial displacement.

8. Knee hyperextension leads to tear of the posterior capsule and rupture of the posterior (PCL) and anterior (ACL) cruciate ligaments.

QUESTIONS

9. Describe the Hohl and Moore classifications of proximal tibial plateau fractures and fracture-dislocations.

ANSWERS

9. **A,** proximal tibial plateau fractures are classified as: type 1—minimally displaced; type 2—local compression; type 3—split compression; type 4—total condyle; type 5—bicondylar. **B,** proximal tibial fracture-dislocations are classified as: type I—split; type II—entire condyle; type III—rim avulsion, type IV—rim compression; type V—four-part fracture.

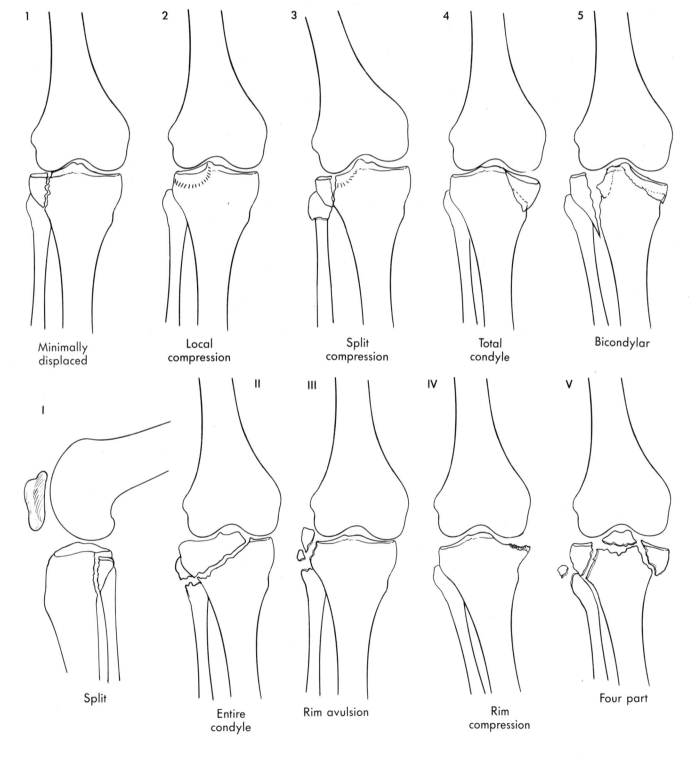

1	2	3	4	5
Minimally displaced	Local compression	Split compression	Total condyle	Bicondylar

I	II	III	IV	V
Split	Entire condyle	Rim avulsion	Rim compression	Four part

QUESTIONS

10. How are plateau rim avulsion fractures treated?

11. What is the mechanism of injury in tibial plateau rim compression fractures?

12. How should rim compression fractures be evaluated and managed?

13. What are the treatment options for four-part tibial plateau fracture-dislocations?

14. What are the types of tibial spine avulsion fractures?

15. How are tibial spine avulsion fractures treated?

16. How should peroneal nerve injury in association with fibular head fracture be treated?

17. When treating nondisplaced plateau fractures, what else should one evaluate?

18. How should medial and lateral total condyle fractures of the tibial plateau be treated?

ANSWERS

10. Plateau rim avulsion fractures are often seen on the lateral knee associated with avulsion fractures of the fibular head or with Gerdy's tubercle and cruciate injuries. They cannot be reduced by closed means because of the capsular attachments. Open reduction and internal fixation with capsular and ligament repair, augmentation, or both, are carried out, and a long leg cast or cast brace is applied postoperatively.

11. The impact of the femoral condyle after the contralateral collateral ligament ruptures. Assessment of the ligament injury and its repair are vital to successful management. Cruciate disruption occurs in three fourths of cases.

ANSWERS

12. (1) Rule out ligament instability with intraoperative stress radiographs; (2) repair the ligaments; (3) correct the rim compression; (4) apply a cast for 4 to 6 weeks; (5) watch for stretch of the peroneal nerve and for vascular injuries.

13. Open reduction and internal fixation if traction does not align the fragments satisfactorily, or use an Ilizarov-type external fixator, casting, or cast brace.

14. Type I is tilted up at the anterior margin only. In type II the anterior portion is lifted completely from its bed with some posterior opposition remaining. Type IIIA is completely displaced. Type IIIB is completely displaced and rotated.

15. Types I and II may be reduced with closed manipulation under anesthesia with the knee in full extension. Then apply a long leg cast for 5 to 6 weeks. Type III is treated with open reduction and internal fixation with the reduction held with sutures or screws, followed by a long leg cast in extension for 5 to 6 weeks.

16. If the lateral knee is unstable, repair the ligament, and explore the nerve. If the knee is stable, then follow the patient clinically for 3 months. Explore if no return occurs. Repair requiring ligament healing to bone should be protected for at least 3 to 4 weeks and repair of ligament to ligament requires protection for a minimum of 4 weeks.

17. Knee stability. If ligaments are torn, most advocate repair, although some believe that cast immobilization may be satisfactory. If the cause of instability is from fracture displacement or depression, open reduction and internal fixation is usually indicated.

18. Medial condyle fractures although displaced or depressed only a few millimeters, need open reduction and internal fixation (ORIF) to prevent fracture migration. Lateral condyle fractures of less than 5-mm displacement are treated with traction for a few days, then a cast brace until healed. If displaced more than 5 mm, ORIF is indicated. Traction with early motion for fractures of either condyle for the nonambulatory patient is a satisfactory option.

QUESTIONS

19. What is the most frequent complication in tibial plateau total condyle depression fractures?

20. How should bicondylar tibial plateau fractures be treated?

21. In the assessment of a tibial plateau fracture, an examination under anesthesia is performed to determine stability. If 15 degrees of valgus deflection is noted with stress application, how should this patient be managed?

22. Describe the treatment of nondisplaced tibial plateau fractures.

23. What is the blood supply to the patella and what segment of the patella can undergo avascular necrosis (AVN) after transverse fracture?

24. What are the indications for surgery in patellar fracture?

25. How are undisplaced patella fractures treated?

26. How are displaced patella fractures treated?

ANSWERS

19. Loss of reduction.

20. First try distal tibial traction and observe the degree of restoration of the tibial condyles. If reduced, use 4 to 6 weeks of traction with range-of-motion exercises as the fracture pain subsides. Traction is contraindicated when the medial condyle is unstable. A varus knee deformity is a frequent problem. Open reduction and internal fixation with buttress plate(s) is reserved for fractures that will not reduce in traction.

ANSWERS

21. If there is more than 10 degrees of varus or valgus instability to stress testing through an arc of 0 to 90 degrees of flexion, this is considered unstable. The instability may result from fracture displacement or depression, or ligamentous injury. Open repair of the cause of the instability is indicated.

22. For the best results, these patients should be treated with early motion and protected weightbearing to prevent displacement. Traction, a knee immobilizer with intermittent motion, or a fracture brace with protected weightbearing may be appropriate for various fracture patterns and patient personalities.

23. A patella plexus which enters in the central portion and at its distal pole supplies the patella. In transverse fractures the proximal pole may undergo AVN.

24. This is controversial with regard to the ranges of acceptable limits of fragment separation (>3–4 mm), and joint surface incongruity (>1–3 mm). Comminuted fractures with displacement of the articular surface, osteochondral fractures with displacement into the joint, marginal or longitudinal fractures with displacement, or any fracture in which there is disruption of the extensor mechanism should be explored.

25. Displacements of no more than 1 to 2 mm with smooth articular surfaces and with the quadriceps mechanism intact are treated with a cylinder straight-leg cast for 3 to 6 weeks.

26. Open reduction and internal fixation, or, if the fracture is through the distal pole, excision of the smaller fragment with suturing of the patellar tendon to the remaining fragment and repair of the quadriceps mechanism.

QUESTIONS

27. How are comminuted patellar fractures treated?

28. How is an anterior dislocation of the knee reduced?

29. How is a posterior knee dislocation reduced?

30. What can prevent reduction of a posterolateral knee dislocation?

31. How are knees treated after closed reduction for dislocation?

32. What are the rates of vascular and nerve injuries in knee dislocations?

33. Dislocation of the proximal tibiofibular joint is a rare injury. What is the most frequent activity causing this injury?

34. What are the three types of acute proximal tibiofibular dislocations?

ANSWERS

27. This depends upon whether the fragments are displaced or not. Minimally displaced fragments with intact quadriceps can be treated by placing the patient in a long leg cast. Excision of the multiple displaced fragments by shelling them out of the quadriceps and patellar tendons and reestablishing the quadriceps mechanism by suturing the expansions is best for displaced comminuted fractures. Partial patellectomy or a fragmented displaced distal pole with preservation of the intact proximal fragment is also acceptable.

ANSWERS

28. By longitudinal traction, with care to avoid hyperextension of the knee, and then lifting the distal femur into the reduced position. Try to avoid pressure in the popliteal area. Pushing the proximal tibia posteriorly also produces reduction, but care must be taken not to hyperextend the knee in doing so.

29. Longitudinal traction. Extend the knee and lift upward on the proximal tibia. Lateral and medial dislocations are reduced by longitudinal traction and force is applied to correct the deformity of the tibia and femur.

30. The medial capsule and collateral ligament can be trapped in the joint or a buttonhole tear in the medial capsule may trap the medial femoral condyle.

31. Arteriography or Doppler pulse pressure evaluation, splints with the knee in 15 degrees of flexion for 1 to 2 weeks, then a long leg cast for 6 to 8 weeks; others advocate aggressive open repair of all torn structures.

32. The rate of vascular injuries is 20% to 50%; of nerve injuries, 25% to 35%.

33. Parachute jumping. It is also called horseback rider's knee. The fibular head may be bumped against a gate post as the rider rides through, dislocating the fibular head posteriorly.

34. (1) Anterolateral (most common); (2) posteromedial (most serious; it leads to peroneal injury and recurrent subluxation); (3) superior (associated with severe interosseus membrane disruption).

QUESTIONS

35. How are acute proximal tibiofibular dislocations treated?

36. What is the recommended salvage procedure for patients who have persistent pain at the proximal tibiofibular joint following a successful reduction of a proximal tibiofibular dislocation?

37. What are the surgical options for treatment of displaced supracondylar fractures of the femur?

38. Describe the AO classification system for supracondylar fractures (Muller).

39. How are anterior dislocations of the hip reduced?

40. How are anterior hip dislocations treated post reduction?

41. How should anterior hip dislocations with associated femoral head fractures be treated?

ANSWERS

35. In treating anterolateral dislocation the knee is flexed 70 to 90 degrees, the foot is dorsiflexed, and direct pressure is applied to the fibular head to produce reduction. Posteromedial and superior dislocations are more likely to be unstable and recur but can be reduced by using a similar technique except that the direction of manual pressure on the fibular head varies and is opposite the direction of its displacement. The type of postreduction immobilization does not affect the recurrence rate. Soft dressing and crutches are used for 1 to 2 weeks with return to activities after 5 to 6 weeks. If reduction is unobtainable or unstable, perform open reduction and internal fixation.

36. Persistent symptoms should be addressed with a proximal fibula resection. Proximal tibiofibular arthrodesis is not recommended because of development of subsequent ankle problems.

ANSWERS

37. Condylar compression screws, condylar buttress plates, interlocking intermedullary reamed nails, Ender's nails, Rush pins, and the Zickle supracondylar system.

38. There are three major groups in this classification: type A—extraarticular; type B—unicondylar; and type C—bicondylar. Type A fractures are subdivided into simple, two-part, and comminuted fractures. Type B fractures are subdivided based upon the location of the condylar fracture. Type BI fractures are lateral condyle, sagittal plane; type BII are medial condyle, sagittal; and type BIII are coronal fractures of the condyles. Type C fractures are subdivided based upon the presence or absence of comminution and its location. Type CI fractures are noncomminuted bicondylar fractures. Type CII are bicondylar fractures which have supracondylar comminution. Type CIII are bicondylar fractures that have supracondylar or intracondylar comminution.

39. In the *Stimson method*, the patient is prone, the hip flexed 90 degrees. The operator holds the ankle and knee at 90 degrees and applies gentle downward pressure just distal to the knee. Gentle rotation of the hip may facilitate reduction. Using the *Allis technique*, the patient is supine, with the knee slightly flexed to relax the hamstrings. While an assistant stabilizes the pelvis and applies lateral traction to the affected thigh, longitudinal traction is applied with continued hip flexion to 60 to 70 degrees. The femur is adducted and internally rotated to achieve reduction.

40. The hip is managed in skin traction until painless range of motion is attained, usually in 2 to 3 weeks, then weightbearing is allowed as tolerated. Avoid extremes of abduction and external rotation to avoid redislocation.

41. If pre- and postreduction films demonstrate a displaced transchondral fracture of the femoral head, excision is recommended. Open reduction and internal fixation (ORIF) may be indicated for fractures greater than one third of the head diameter. Indentation fractures of the head were thought not to be amenable to ORIF, and had a poor prognosis, but recently there have been attempts to elevate and graft bone in the depressed fragments, which may improve the long-term outcome.

QUESTIONS

42. How are posterior dislocations of the hip reduced?

43. How are posterior hip dislocations treated after reduction?

44. Describe the classification for traumatic hip dislocations.

45. What are frequent complications following hip dislocation?

46. What is the Pipkin classification of femoral head fractures?

47. How are Pipkin fractures treated?

ANSWERS

42. (1) Open reduction as described by Epstein. (2) The Stimson method: The patient is prone with the hip flexed over the table edge. An assistant stabilizes the pelvis by applying pressure over the sacrum. The hip and knee are flexed to 90 degrees. Downward pressure is applied behind the flexed knee with gentle rotation of the femur. (3) The Allis maneuver: The patient is supine. The pelvis is stabilized by an assistant. Traction is applied in direct line of the deformity, followed by gentle flexion of the hip to 90 degrees, then gentle internal and external rotation with continued traction to produce reduction.

43. After radiographic evaluation, postreduction stability is assessed. Provided there are no large displaced posterior or posterosuperior acetabular wall fractures or displaced acetabular column fractures, the hip is flexed to 90 degrees in neutral abduction-adduction and a strong posteriorly directed force is applied to the femur. If subluxation or dislocation occurs with this test, additional studies and surgery may be necessary. A computed tomography (CT) scan is obtained to evaluate the articular surfaces of the hip and detect entrapped osteochondral fractures. Apply Buck's traction with the hip in abduction to prevent flexion and internal rotation and adduction, which can cause dislocation. Traction is continued until the patient is pain-free (several days to 2 weeks). Weightbearing is allowed after 4 to 12 weeks.

ANSWERS

44. Type I: dislocation without fracture; type II: irreducible dislocation secondary to soft tissue interposition (i.e., capsule, tendon, or muscle); type III: unstable hip following reduction, or incarcerated fragments of bone, cartilage, or labrum; type IV: dislocation with fracture of the acetabulum which requires operative reconstruction; type V: dislocation with fracture of the femoral head (Pipkin fractures and head impaction fractures) or neck.

45. *Avascular necrosis* of the femoral head is seen in from 1% to 17% of dislocations. *Posttraumatic arthritis* is another problem following hip dislocations and can be seen in varying degrees in from 20% to 90% of all injuries. The uncomplicated hip dislocations without associated fractures have the lowest rate of arthritis which has been reported to be as high as 24%. Posttraumatic arthritis associated with fracture-dislocations tends to occur more frequently and has been reported in as many as 88% of injuries. *Recurrent dislocation* of the hip is fairly rare. *Sciatic nerve* injuries occur in 8% to 19% of dislocations. *Heterotopic bone formation* tends to occur more frequently in head-injured patients and those with acetabular fractures. Prophylaxis with indomethacin is appropriate for these.

46. Type I: posterior dislocation of the hip with fracture of the femoral head caudad to the fovea centralis; Type II: hip dislocated with fracture line extending cephalad to the fovea centralis. (usually including the fovea); Type III: type I or II with fracture of femoral neck; Type IV: type I or II with acetabular rim fracture.

47. This is controversial. Type I: If closed reduction produces congruence of the fragment, treatment is 4 to 6 weeks in traction followed by protected weightbearing for 4 weeks. If a step-off of 1 mm or greater is present, open reduction and internal fixation (ORIF) is recommended through an anterior approach using Herbert or small cancellous screws. Others believe that primary open reduction of the hip with displaced fragment excision is best. Type II fractures are treated by closed reduction. If congruent, traction is used. If incongruent, ORIF is carried out. Type III: ORIF of the femoral neck fracture followed by treatment of the head fracture as in type I and II, or ORIF of the femoral head fracture followed by screw fixation of the femoral neck fractures. Type IV: After selecting treatment for the acetabular fracture, the femoral head fracture is treated as in types I and II.

QUESTIONS

48. What are the indications for surgery after closed reduction of a posterior fracture dislocation of the hip?

49. How should you treat a hip fracture-dislocation with ipsilateral femoral shaft fracture?

50. How much angular deformity is acceptable in femoral shaft fractures?

51. What is the major cause of disruption of vascular repairs in associated femur fractures?

52. What is the most common angular deformity associated with femur fractures?

53. How much shortening is acceptable in femur fractures in adults?

54. How should fractures of the femur that have become infected after operative fixation be treated?

55. What are the major prerequisites in achieving bony union in infected fractures?

56. Which muscles contribute to the fracture displacement and angulation seen in femoral supracondylar fractures?

57. What complication should be watched for in supracondylar fractures?

ANSWERS

48. Instability at 70 to 90 degrees of flexion, trapped intraarticular fragments, or loss of 40% or greater of the posterior wall.

ANSWERS

49. First reduce the hip dislocation (the Stimson maneuver is useful). If this cannot be done, perform open reduction if the patient is stable enough for surgery. Then treat the femoral fracture with open reduction and internal fixation, or traction.

50. Varus—8 degrees; valgus—15 degrees; malrotation—internal 15, external 20 degrees; anterior bow—less than 15 degrees.

51. Infection.

52. Varus secondary to overpull of adductors.

53. 0.5 in.

54. (1) Thorough debridement of the infected area and thorough wound irrigation; (2) with stable internal fixation of the fractured femur, keeping the implant in place; if loose, the fixation device should be removed and replaced with one that achieves stability without devascularizing of bony fragments; (3) as soon as the infection begins to resolve, bone grafting should be considered to fill the defects; (4) intravenous (IV) antibiotics 3 to 6 weeks; (5) removal of all implants after bony union is achieved; thorough debridement of local soft tissue; sometimes overreaming an infected medullary canal is necessary to remove infected granulation tissue.

55. Bony stabilization, control of infection, adequate blood supply, and soft tissue coverage.

56. Posterior angulation and displacement secondary to pull of the quadriceps, hamstrings, and gastrocnemius.

57. Vascular injury. An unusual and tense swelling in the popliteal area as well as signs of ischemia in the lower leg suggest rupture of a major vessel.

QUESTIONS

58. How should impacted supracondylar fractures be treated?

59. How are displaced supracondylar fractures treated nonoperatively?

60. How are displaced supracondylar femur fractures treated operatively?

61. How are condylar fractures of the femur treated?

62. What are the normal limits of symphyseal separation in males and females?

63. What is the treatment for a postpartum patient with symphysis separation?

64. Describe the treatment of isolated, nondisplaced sacroiliac joint injury.

65. How are isolated pelvic straddle fractures treated?

66. How should unstable pelvic fractures be treated?

67. How should displaced sacral fractures be treated?

ANSWERS

58. Because the powerful thigh muscles may cause angular deformity, a short period of traction may be advisable. Once pain and swelling have subsided, a cast or fracture brace can be applied. Careful monitoring should continue because angulation and displacement may occur in the cast brace.

ANSWERS

59. With closed reduction with 15 to 20 lbs of tibial traction with the knee, thigh, and leg supported in balanced suspension traction with some knee flexion. Traction is used for 8 to 12 weeks or until the fracture stabilizes, at which time a cast or brace can be applied.

60. (1) Reduction of displaced articular fragments; (2) reduction of the shaft to the condyles indirectly or assisted by traction; (3) fixation with a locking IM nail or blade plate or screw plate device. A bone graft is done for severely comminuted fractures.

61. Open reduction and internal fixation or percutaneous fixation to avoid further fracture displacement, planning for early motion.

62. Males: 0.5 mm; females: 1.5 mm. Diastasis of the symphysis greater than 2.5 cm requires fixation.

63. A 3-in.-wide circumferential strap is placed that runs below the iliac crest and above the trochanters. Place on bed rest in the lateral position.

64. Symptomatic treatment with bed rest and a pelvic sling or belt followed by a slow gradual return to activities over 10 to 16 weeks.

65. Bed rest is recommended. The length of the extremities and the weightbearing arch are unaffected. Symptomatic care is appropriate. (*Note*: Look for urinary tract or abdominal visceral injury in these fractures, which have a 20% mortality rate).

66. Most authors advocate open reduction and internal fixation or external fixation. Traction with external fixation may be an option if the patient is hemodynamically unstable.

67. Reduction in traction or open reduction with or without fixation. Some transverse sacral fractures may require decompression but may not be amenable to fixation.

QUESTIONS

68. Which two intertrochanteric fractures require special treatment?

69. How are pathologic intertrochanteric fractures treated?

70. How are fractures of the greater trochanter treated?

71. How are isolated fractures of the lesser trochanter treated?

72. What are the three main clinical problems seen in subtrochanteric fractures of the femur?

73. What two factors are responsible for malunion and nonunion seen in subtrochanteric fractures?

74. Describe the criteria for recognizing unstable intertrochanteric fracture patterns.

75. What are the key factors in stable reduction of intertrochanteric fractures?

76. How are intertrochanteric fractures reduced?

77. How are fractures of the femoral neck treated when metastatic lesions are present?

ANSWERS

68. (1) An irreducible fracture secondary to iliopsoas obstruction. The long spike on the head-neck fragment is caught between the iliopsoas and the lesser trochanter. The varus position remains, even with the application of strong traction. Release of the iliopsoas insertion from the lesser trochanter allows reduction. (2) A reversed oblique fracture line often necessitates notching of the distal shaft to allow impaction of the neck fragment, preventing medial migration of the shaft. Other approaches include anatomic reduction with a 95-degree blade plate or condylar compression screw device fixation, a Zickle supracondylar, gamma nail, or reconstruction nail.

ANSWERS

69. Open reduction and internal fixation with screw and side plate, possibly with PMMA and radiotherapy.

70. Fractures with greater than 1 cm of displacement are treated by open reduction and internal fixation if not comminuted. If the displacement is less than 1 cm, treatment is bed rest for several days, then protected weightbearing for 3 to 4 weeks.

71. These usually occur in adolescents. If displaced more than 2 cm, treatment is bed rest for 3 weeks, then mobilization. With displacement greater than 2 cm in a young athletic patient, consider open reduction and internal fixation. Surgery is not necessary in elderly patients.

72. Malunion, delayed union, and nonunion.

73. (1) The subtrochanteric area is cortical bone which has a decreased blood supply and is prone to comminution. (2) Large biomechanical stresses in the subtrochanteric area can lead to failure of fixation devices.

74. (1) Fractures with reversed obliquity which have a tendency toward medial displacement of the shaft secondary to adductor muscle pull, (2) medial and posterior comminution or displacement of fracture fragments which may preclude bone-to-bone contact. (3) fractures that cannot be reduced adequately (i.e., four-part fractures, displaced greater and lesser trochanteric intertrochanteric fractures).

75. Restoration of medial and posterior cortical contact between the major fracture fragments.

76. By traction, slight abduction, and slight external rotation. Sometimes posterior displacement at the fracture site requires lifting of the femur to complete the reduction. "Overreduction" may be desirable in unstable fractures through a valgus overcorrection and internal rotation.

77. By cemented hemiarthroplasty or total joint replacement.

QUESTIONS

78. What are the indications for surgery of pathologic lesions of the femoral neck?

79. What is the Singh index?

80. What is the function of the meniscus?

81. Describe the contents of the compartments of the leg.

82. What constitutes a satisfactory reduction in closed diaphyseal tibia fractures?

83. What are the options for closed treatment of tibia fractures?

84. What are the operative fixation options for tibial fractures?

85. Describe the clinical findings in a patellar ligament rupture.

86. Describe repair of an acute patellar ligament rupture.

ANSWERS

78. (1) A painful lytic lesion of 50% or greater of the cross-sectional diameter of the bone; (2) a painful lytic lesion involving a length of cortex greater than the cross-sectional diameter of the bone or more than 2.5 cm in axial length; (3) bone pain unrelieved by radiotherapy. Impending fractures across the neck of the femur have stresses too high for simple prophylactic pinning to be successful.

79. This method for grading osteopenia ranges from 1 to 6 and is based upon trabeculae patterns in the proximal femur. Grade *6* is normal (well-defined primary and secondary tension and compression trabeculae); and *1* is severe loss of trabeculae consistent with extreme osteopenia.

ANSWERS

80. Menisci function in shock absorption, knee stability, and articular cartilage nutrition.

81. The *anterior compartment* consists of the extensor digitorum longus, extensor hallucis longus, peroneus tertius tibialis anterior, tibial artery, and deep peroneal nerve. The *lateral compartment* encloses the peroneus longus and brevis and the superficial peroneal nerve. The *superficial posterior compartment* consists of the gastrocnemius and soleus. The *deep posterior compartment* encompasses the tibialis posterior, flexor hallucis longus, flexor digitorum longus, tibial nerve, posterior tibial artery, and peroneal artery.

82. No more than 5 degrees of varus or valgus or 10 degrees of anterior or posterior angulation are acceptable. The rotational alignment should be comparable to the opposite uninjured extremity. Less than 50% of displacement and no more than 5 to 10 mm of shortening are acceptable.

83. The types of external mobilization consist of long and short leg casts or fracture braces, splints, pins and plaster, external fixators, and traction.

84. Compression plating, intermedullary nailing (Enders', Küntscher, or, Lottes nails, and locked nail devices).

85. The patient complains of pain about the knee with inability to extend the knee. There may be a palpable defect in the patellar ligament and the patella will be in an abnormally proximal position.

86. Bony avulsions from the tibial tuberosity are best treated by fixation of the bony fragments. Intrasubstance tears of the patella ligament should be treated with debridement of frayed ends with suture approximation of the tendon. McLaughlin wire over the superior pole of the patella attached through the tibial tuberosity is effective in reducing tension on the repair. Postoperatively, a long leg cast is worn for approximately 6 weeks. A cast-brace may also be employed with passive extension assist to reduce tension on the repair.

QUESTIONS

87. A 16-year-old girl was playing soccer and had severe pain in her knee as she fell to the ground. She has been able to ambulate on the leg and there is pain throughout her knee. Physical examination demonstrates the knee to be in a slightly flexed position with the patella laterally dislocated. What factors predispose to dislocation of the patella?

88. How should this patient be treated?

89. What are the complications associated with dislocation of the patella?

90. What is the main reason for obtaining radiographs following reduction of the patella dislocation?

91. What is the most sensitive test for anterior knee instability?

92. What is the danger of arthroscopy in an acutely injured knee?

93. What is the best approach to PCL repair?

94. A 35-year-old office worker had been on a 3-week exercise binge to lose weight. After losing 20 lbs, he presents complaining of severe shin pain. He states that he had "shin splints" in high school and this pain feels similar. He has increased his mileage to 3 miles per day over the course of his first 2 weeks of exercise. On physical examination he is tender over the proximal third of the tibia with minimal swelling noted. There is no crepitation noted. Radiographs are normal. There is no swelling in the compartments. What is your diagnosis and how can you confirm it?

ANSWERS

87. Predisposing factors include hypermobility of the patella due to poor muscle tone, genu valgum, attenuation of the medial support structures, weakened vastus medialis, patella alta, shallow patellofemoral groove, increased femoral neck anteversion, excessive external tibial torsion, laterally inserted patellar tendon, and genu recurvatum, which causes laxity in the extensor mechanism.

ANSWERS

88. Reduction of the dislocated patella through knee extension and medial-directed pressure on the patella. For first-time dislocators, if no articular fractures are present, a cylinder cast or knee immobilizer may be used for 4 to 6 weeks. Quadriceps exercises should be performed after the acute tenderness of the dislocation subsides.

89. (1) Recurrent dislocation, (2) osteochondral fractures, (3) chondromalacia patella, (4) degenerative joint disease.

90. To look for osteochondral fracture fragments.

91. The Lachman test. With the patient in a supine position and the knee in approximately 15 degrees of flexion, the distal femoral condyle is gripped in one hand, thereby stabilizing the femur. The proximal tibia is drawn anteriorly with the other hand. Abnormal tests demonstrate anterior displacement of the tibia without a firm end point compared with the uninjured knee.

92. There is a risk of extravasation of arthroscopic fluid through tears in the capsule which can lead to acute compartment syndrome. It is recommended that knee arthroscopy after acute injury be performed with attention to extravasation of fluid, not using infusion pump techniques, but rather a gravity irrigation system, and limiting the arthroscopy to 30 to 45 minutes.

93. If there is an isolated injury to the PCL, a posterior approach offers the best visualization of the ligament. One does not see the joint well, however. Preceding the repair with knee arthroscopy allows excellent visualization of the joint to rule out other abnormalities.

94. This patient likely has a stress fracture of the tibia. These occur most frequently in the posterior or medial aspect of the tibia. Radiographs may be negative for the first 2 to 4 weeks. Serial radiographs after this may show some periosteal reaction or sclerosis. One of the best ways to diagnose stress fracture before radiographic changes are evident is by bone scan.

QUESTIONS

95. How should this patient be treated?

96. Describe the treatment of a fracture of the lateral margin of the patella.

97. What is the usual mechanism of injury associated with medial margin fractures of the patella?

98. An 18-year-old man has had recurrent locking of the knee. He has a history of previous patellar dislocations. What is the most likely diagnosis and what should the treatment consist of?

99. List three negative prognostic factors in the healing of a tibia fracture.

100. What is the recommended position for arthrodesis of the hip?

101. What is the most common cause of an iliac hernia?

102. What are some common problems that can develop in patients with hip arthrodesis?

103. What is the optimal position for a knee fusion?

104. What is the major problem with arthrodesis of a Charcot knee?

105. What is the recommended position for arthrodesis of the ankle?

ANSWERS

95. Non–weight-bearing crutch ambulation until the patient is asymptomatic, then partial weight-bearing on crutches without a cast for about 2 to 3 months. Cessation of athletic activity is advised during this period.

ANSWERS

96. Treatment typically consists of excision of the osseous fragment with repair of the lateral retinaculum and capsule. The joint should be evaluated for loose bodies.

97. These are associated with lateral dislocations of the patella and represent avulsion fractures.

98. This patient most likely has loose bodies, which are causing the knee to lock. These are the result of shearing of osteochondral fragments with the previous knee dislocations. Treatment is knee arthroscopy. A less likely diagnosis is meniscal tear. Arthroscopy helps to clarify the diagnosis.

99. Increasing amounts of displacement, open injuries, and comminuted fractures.

100. Thirty degrees of flexion, 0 degrees of abduction, and 0 to 30 degrees of external rotation.

101. Iliac hernias occur following harvest of a full-thickness iliac crest bone graft. They tend to occur more frequently in the middle of the ileum as opposed to the anterior or posterior portion.

102. Lumbar spine pain, osteoarthritis in the ipsilateral knee, and osteoarthritis in the contralateral hip.

103. Zero to 20 degrees of flexion, slight valgus, and 10 degrees of external rotation.

104. Pseudarthrosis. This can be minimized through meticulous excision of the capsule, meticulous bone carpentry, and rigid internal fixation. (Charcot ankle joints also have a higher pseudarthrosis rate than ankle arthrodeses done for other causes.)

105. Neutral flexion-extension, neutral heel to 5 degrees of valgus, and rotation equivalent to the opposite unaffected extremity.

QUESTIONS

106. What problems result from common peroneal palsy?

107. What deformities develop with palsy of the tibial nerve?

108. What is the only isolated muscle with sufficient strength to produce active plantar flexion in the presence of a paralyzed triceps surae?

109. What functional difficulties do patients have with femoral nerve palsy?

110. What is the recommended muscle transfer for a femoral nerve palsy?

111. A 10-year-old boy has had right knee pain for about 3 months without any previous history of trauma. He has a mild effusion and moderate quadriceps atrophy. Radiographs demonstrate a 2- × 1-cm subarticular lucent area in the medial aspect of the lateral femoral condyle. What is the diagnosis and treatment?

112. An 18-year-old man has the same symptoms and radiographic findings as the patient described above. How does this patient's treatment differ?

113. Describe a grading system for chondromalacia.

ANSWERS

106. Loss of dorsiflexion and eversion of the foot.

107. Cavus foot from plantar fascia contracture; the Achilles tendon becomes elongated and the calcaneus is rotated into dorsiflexion.

108. The tibialis anterior muscle. This muscle can be transferred through the interosseous membrane.

ANSWERS

109. These patients do well ambulating on level surfaces. They are unable, however, to effectively climb stairs or inclined surfaces.

110. Biceps femoris transfer to the extensor mechanism.

111. The patient has osteochondritis dissecans. It occurs more frequently in males than in females. Treatment depends upon the age of the patient. For a patient up to the age of 13, rest or immobilization typically allow for resolution of symptoms. Activity modification is recommended for a brief period as well. This lesion in children through early adolescence rarely evolves into loose bodies. Drilling the lesion is usually not indicated. If the child has persistent symptoms that do not respond to cast immobilization, then arthroscopic drilling of the lesion may be helpful.

112. Arthroscopy to evaluate the fragments is a good idea in this instance. If the cartilage is not separated, the patient may heal with rest and immobilization. Drilling under arthroscopic control is an alternative which may be considered. Separated, undisplaced fragments should be drilled, curetted, and pinned or stabilized with bone pegs arthroscopically. In non–weight-bearing surfaces where the cartilage has become completely separated, removal of subchondral bone to cancellous bone in the crater should be carried out. Loose bodies should be removed. In weight-bearing areas large loose bodies consisting of cartilage and bone should be replaced and pinned. In patients with loose bodies, treatment is determined by whether the resultant defect is located in weight bearing or non–weight-bearing portions of the femoral condyle. With defects in the non–weight-bearing area, excision of the fragment, curettage of the defect, and drilling are appropriate treatments. For defects in the weight-bearing area, treatment depends upon the presence or absence of bone in the loose body. Treatment is also influenced by the shape of the loose body. If it fits the defect, it is replaced following curettage of the defect and drilling. If the loose body has no bone or does not fit at the crater, it should be discarded and the crater curetted and drilled.

113. Grade 0: normal cartilage; grade 1: soft swollen cartilage; grade 2: extensive fibrillation with localized fissuring or fragmentation; grade 3: erosion to subchondral bone with fissuring or fragmentation.

QUESTIONS

114. A 13-year-old female basketball player collided with an opposing player, sustaining forced flexion to the right knee. She had immediate pain and was unable to bear weight on the extremity. On examination she had a high-riding patella with marked tenderness over the tibial tubercle. Radiographs demonstrated an avulsion of the tibial tubercle. Describe the treatments for the various types of tibial tubercle avulsion fractures.

115. True or false? A transverse or short oblique fracture at the tip of the femoral stem is the most common fracture pattern seen about a prosthesis.

116. What is the treatment of choice for a transverse fracture at the tip of the femoral prosthesis?

117. Why is open reduction and internal fixation selected in short oblique or transverse fractures at the tip of a femoral prosthetic stem?

118. In fractures of the proximal femur that extend around the proximal femoral component stem, is revision of the prosthesis necessary?

119. Describe the Gustillo and Anderson classification of open fractures.

ANSWERS

114. The Watson Jones classification of tibial tubercle avulsion fractures is *type I*—fracture through the secondary ossification center; *type II*—tonguelike projection of the epiphysis lifted anteriorly and upward, involving the secondary center of ossification and the proximal tibial epiphysis without articular involvement; and *type III*—the line of fracture passes upward and backward into the joint across the primary ossification center. Open reduction and internal fixation (ORIF) is the treatment of choice for displaced type III fractures. Type I and II fractures can usually be reduced closed in an extension cast or splint. Lateral radiograph of the knee in full extension will allow determinination of the adequacy of reduction. If there is any residual displacement (≥ 0.5 cm), ORIF should be performed.

115. True. A stress riser at the transition point between the prosthesis segment and the adjacent less stiff bone leads to fractures in this area.

ANSWERS

116. These fractures should be internally stabilized. The options include replacement with a long-stem prosthesis, with wiring or plate and screws (using unicortical or tangential screws in the proximal segment to avoid the stem of the prosthesis). Other options are the use of a plate with bicortical screws in the distal fragment, and unicortical screws and cerclage wires in the proximal fragment. One final option for a stable prosthesis includes the use of intramedullary rods such as Ender's pins.

117. These fractures are at high risk for displacement, shortening, and nonunion, and are not amenable to closed treatment. Minimally displaced spiral or long oblique fractures at the tip of the prosthesis are more amenable to treatment in traction with subsequent cast-brace or fracture bracing.

118. This fracture usually cannot occur unless there is loss of fixation of the proximal femoral component. The fracture may have produced disruption of the bone-cement prosthesis interface or there may have been preexisting loosening which predisposed the proximal femur to fracture. Management here consists of open reduction and internal fixation with revision of the femoral component.

119. This is a descriptive classification of the severity of injury for open fractures that is helpful in determining prognosis and in describing the types of soft tissue injury associated with fracture. *Type I* is a low-energy injury in which the length of the skin defect is less than 1 cm. Type I injuries are usually associated with injuries in which the skin is punctured by fracture fragments piercing the skin rather than by an external penetration. *Type II* open fractures have sustained an increased degree of injury with moderate muscle damage and usually a wound which is larger than 1 cm in length. *Type III* open fractures have extensive muscle damage and significant skin interruption measuring more than 10 cm. These high-energy injuries are also associated with displaced segmental fractures, fractures with diaphyseal segmental loss, concomitant vascular injuries requiring repair, farmyard injuries, other injuries in which significant contamination has occurred, and shotgun or high-velocity gunshot wounds. Type III fractures are further subdivided into types A, B, and C. Type IIIA has a limited periosteal stripping, type IIIB involves extensive periosteal soft tissue stripping from bone, and type IIIC involves a major vascular injury requiring repair.

QUESTIONS

120. A 25-year-old patient is admitted with a grade IIIB open fracture in the proximal one third of the tibia. Following fracture stabilization and debridement, a 4-cm open area of exposed tibia remains. What are the options for coverage of this defect?

121. What are the options for soft tissue coverage for a grade IIIB open fracture in the middle one third of the tibia?

122. What options are available for soft tissue coverage of a grade IIIC open fracture in the distal one third of the tibia following successful revascularization?

123. A 32-year-old accountant was playing racquetball and felt severe infrapatellar pain when he abruptly changed direction to make a shot. Since that episode he has been unable to walk on the leg. On physical examination, there is swelling in the area of the patellar ligament with tenderness. There is a palpable defect in the patellar ligament. He is unable to actively extend the knee. What is the diagnosis and how should this problem be treated?

124. What is the most common complication associated with hip fractures in geriatric patients?

ANSWERS

120. Provided there is no extensive trauma to the posterior aspect of the leg, consideration can be given to a gastrocnemius muscle flap and skin graft. An alternative muscle flap would be a soleus flap. If the defect is extremely large with a significant cavity to be filled, a free tissue transfer should be considered, such as a latissimus dorsi transfer. If free tissue transfer is not feasible, a cross-leg flap may be considered.

121. The best local flap is the soleus muscle flap with skin graft. In the distal segment of this zone, the flexor digitorum longus muscle may be taken with the soleus to cover an extensive defect. An extensively injured leg may require a free tissue transfer.

ANSWERS

122. Local muscle flaps are usually not successful at this level. Small shallow defects may be treated with fasciocutaneous rotation flaps. Vascularized free tissue transfer is the treatment of choice for most of these defects. Flap choice varies from latissimus dorsi for larger defects to gracilis and serratus for smaller ones. A simplified approach to soft tissue defects in the tibia requiring soft tissue coverage is as follows: upper one third of the tibia—gastrocnemius and skin graft; middle one third of the tibia—soleus muscle and skin graft; lower one third of the tibia—free tissue transfer.

123. This patient has ruptured his patellar ligament. These injuries usually occur in patients under the age of 40. Surgical repair should be performed if the patient is unable to extend the knee against gravity. It is possible to treat these injuries nonoperatively if the retinacular attachments of the vastus medialis and lateralis are intact, thus allowing some extension of the knee. However, a surgical repair should be performed if there is any evidence of proximal migration of the patella. Knee flexion will frequently demonstrate a high-riding patella, whereas if the knee is held in extension, this may not be obvious. An end-to-end suture repair should be performed. If the patellar ligament has been avulsed from the tibial tuberosity, repair through drill holes is helpful. The semitendinosus tendon can be looped through viable tissue in late-presenting cases. A number of techniques have been described to relieve tension on the repair. These consist of wires or pins in the patella and in the proximal tibia to prevent excessive stress on the repair site.

124. Venous thrombosis is seen in 40% to 90% of patients in whom no prophylaxis has been given.

QUESTIONS

125. Describe the Russell-Taylor classification for subtrochanteric fractures.

126. What is the clinical significance of the Russell-Taylor classification of subtrochanteric fractures of the femur?

127. What constitutes the anterior column of the pelvis?

128. What is the posterior column of the pelvis?

ANSWERS

125. The Russell-Taylor classification has two major groups. *Group I fractures* do not extend into the piriformis fossa; therefore IM nailing is possible. *In type IA* fractures (A), comminution of the fracture lines extend from below the lesser trochanter to the femoral isthmus. *In type IB* fracture (B), lines extend from the lesser trochanteric area to the isthmus. *Group II fractures* extend proximally into the greater trochanter involving the piriformis fossa. *Type IIA* fractures (C) extend from the lesser trochanter into the piriformis fossa, maintaining medial cortical stability with lack of comminution or major fracture of the lesser trochanter. *Type IIB* fractures (D) have extension of the fracture line from the piriformis fossa into the greater trochanter as well as loss of continuity with the lesser trochanter. Significant medial cortical comminution may be present.

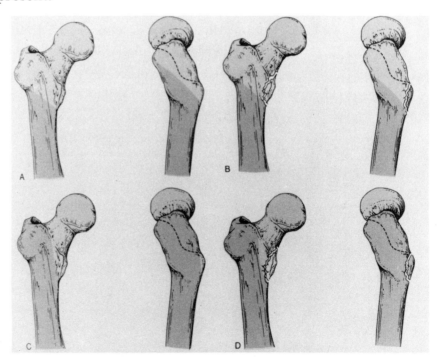

ANSWERS

126. Because the fracture line does not extend into the piriformis fossa in group I fractures, intramedullary nailing is a reasonable option. Group II fractures have extension of the fracture line into the greater trochanter and the piriformis fossa which makes intramedullary nailing much more difficult. Type IIA and IIB fractures can be surgically approached with hip compression screws supplemented with lag screws and iliac crest bone grafting.

127. The anterior column includes the anterior ilium, pelvic brim, superior pubic ramus, and anterior wall of the acetabulum.

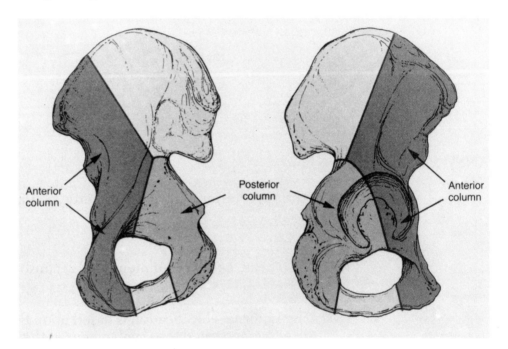

128. The posterior column is the ischial portion of the pelvis which consists of the ischial tuberosity and posterior wall of the acetabulum, extending superiorly to the greater sciatic notch. The anterior and posterior columns bisect the acetabulum in the coronal plane.

QUESTIONS

129. What radiographic views are recommended for the evaluation of acetabular fractures?

130. Following routine radiographic evaluation, what additional imaging studies may be obtained to help delineate acetabular fractures?

131. Describe the Letornel classification of acetabular fractures.

ANSWERS

129. Anteroposterior (AP) and 45-degree oblique views (Judet) of the pelvis.

130. A CT scan, and three-dimensional reconstruction CT scan.

131. The Letornel classification is based upon the location of the fracture fragments and the involvement of the anterior or posterior columns. There are five basic fracture types which can be combined to form five additional categories of acetabular fractures. The five simple fractures consist of: (A) posterior wall, (B) posterior column, (C) anterior wall, (D) anterior column, and (E) transverse fractures (p. 433, *top*). The more complex, combined categories include: (F) posterior column and posterior wall fractures, (G) transverse fractures with posterior wall fracture, (H) T-shaped fracture, (I) anterior column and posterior hemitransverse fractures, and (J) fractures of both columns (p. 433, *bottom*).

ANSWERS

131.

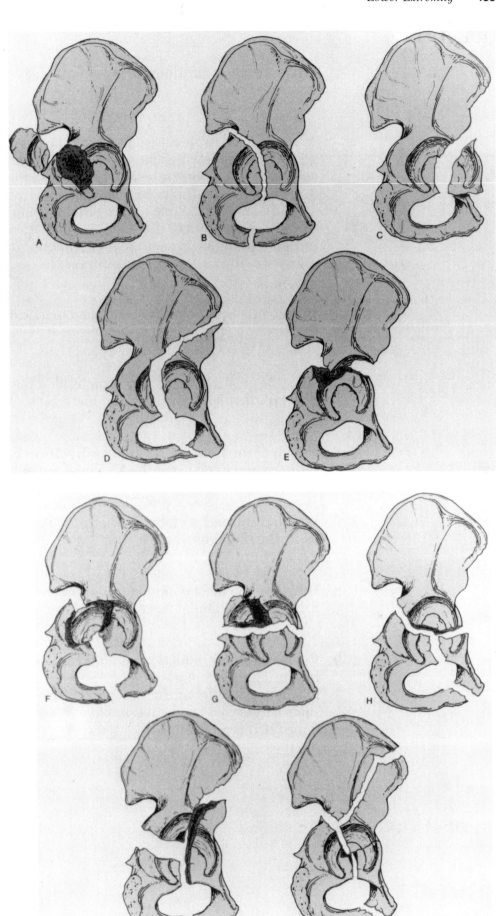

QUESTIONS

132. What are the indications for surgery in displaced acetabular fractures?

133. A 25-year-old professional baseball player is brought to the emergency room following a motor vehicle accident. Pelvic radiographs and CT scan demonstrate a displaced transverse acetabular fracture with a large displaced posterior wall fracture. The patient is hemodynamically stable and is without other injuries. Assume that surgical restoration of the pelvis is mandatory to attempt to return this patient to his previous level of functioning. How long after the injury would you schedule his surgery?

134. What is the best operative approach to a posterior acetabular wall fracture?

135. What surgical approach is recommended for posterior column fractures involving the acetabulum?

136. Which of the Letornel acetabular fractures can be satisfactorily reduced and fixed using the Kocher-Langenbeck approach?

137. Which displaced acetabular fractures are amenable to treatment using the ilioinguinal approach?

138. What are the most common perioperative complications seen after fixation of acetabular fractures?

139. Following open reduction and internal fixation of a acetabular fracture the patient awakens with footdrop. The patient had a normal neurovascular evaluation preoperatively. It has been 6 months since surgery and there has been no recovery. What should be done for this problem?

ANSWERS

132. Most of these fractures require open reduction and internal fixation to obtain suitable alignment and early patient mobilization. Closed reduction and skeletal traction generally do not achieve satisfactory alignment. Unless there are specific individual contraindications to surgery (osteoporosis, systemic infection, etc.) operative intervention should be strongly considered.

133. The ideal time to perform surgery is between 2 and 10 days after injury. A delay of 2 to 3 days is desirable to help decrease local intraoperative hemorrhage. Beyond 10 days, the fracture fragments are not as easily manipulated. After a 3-week delay callus can complicate fracture reduction.

134. A Kocher-Langenbeck approach with the patient in lateral decubitus allows excellent visualization of the fracture.

135. A Kocher-Langenbeck approach with the patient prone.

136. Posterior wall and posterior column, transverse, associated transverse and posterior wall, and T-shaped fractures. If an associated anterior column fracture is irreducible through the Kocher-Langenbeck approach, the posterior column fractures are fixed and the patient is then turned supine for an ilioinguinal approach. Other options for T-shaped fractures include the extended iliofemoral and triradiate approaches.

137. Anterior wall and anterior column fractures, and fractures of both columns. The last-named, with displaced fracture lines into the sacroiliac joint and complex posterior column involvement, may be better approached through an iliofemoral approach.

138. Infection, nerve palsy, ectopic bone formation, and thromboembolic complications.

139. This complication is the result of excessive retraction of the sciatic nerve. It can be prevented by careful intraoperative monitoring of the amount of tension applied by assistants retracting the nerve. Early treatment consists of ankle-foot orthosis. Sciatic nerve recovery may occur over a 3-year period. Tendon transfer to correct the footdrop should not be performed until this 3-year period has elapsed.

QUESTIONS

140. Which approaches to the acetabulum are most frequently associated with ectopic bone formation?

141. Which radiographs are necessary to complete the evaluation of an unstable pelvic fracture?

142. Describe the pathologic changes associated with osteochondritis dissecans in the adolescent.

143. Describe the most common location of osteochondritis dissecans in the knee.

144. Which radiographic view most often identifies osteochondritis dissecans?

145. What is the best management for the nondisplaced osteochondritis dissecans of the medial femoral condyle identified in a skeletally immature boy?

146. What is the appropriate management of the loose fragments of osteochondritis dissecans in the skeletally mature adolescent?

147. Describe the pathologic changes in Osgood-Schlatter disease.

148. At what age is Osgood-Schlatter disease most common?

149. What is the natural history of Osgood-Schlatter disease?

150. In the presentation of Osgood-Schlatter disease, what study is mandatory to rule out other possible pathologic conditions such as tumors?

151. Which of the following treatment modalities is contraindicated in Osgood-Schlatter disease—rest and immobilization, isometric knee exercises, knee pads, or steroid injections?

ANSWERS

140. The iliofemoral approach, followed by the Kocher-Langenbeck approach. The ilioinguinal approach rarely is associated with ectopic bone formation.

141. AP, inlet and outlet views, and CT scanning. Oblique radiographs may be used if a CT scan is not available.

142. Periarticular osseous necrosis with overlying cartilage softening, occasionally associated with fragment displacement.

143. The lateral aspect of the medial femoral condyle.

144. The tunnel view of the knee.

145. Activity modification and a short period of immobilization supplemented with isometric strengthening exercises of the knee.

146. If the fragment is less than 5 mm, simple excision. If the fragment is larger, placement into the recipient bed and internal fixation is suggested.

147. Apophysitis secondary to repetitive microtrauma results in inflammation and new bone formation at the tendon-bone junction.

148. Age 13 to 14 years in boys, 10 to 11 in girls.

149. In the majority of cases, complete resolution within 1 to 2 years of onset.

150. AP and lateral radiographs of the knee.

151. Steroid injections, because they can induce weakening of the patellar tendon and subcutaneous fat necrosis.

QUESTIONS

152. Describe the most common cause and location of Baker's cyst in childhood.

153. What is the natural history of Baker's cyst in childhood?

154. Describe the two phases of a normal gait cycle and approximate time percentage attributed to each.

155. Describe the subdivisions of stance phase.

156. Toe-off signals which phase?

157. Provide the average percentage of time spent in each phase of gait.

158. Describe the function of efficient gait.

159. In normal gait cycle, when is hip flexion maximized?

160. Describe the postion of the knee at heel strike.

161. Describe the position of the knee at mid single limb stance.

162. Describe the relationship of shoulder girdle rotation to pelvic rotation.

163. Describe the characteristics of gait in a 1-year-old child.

164. At what age is the adult gait pattern achieved?

165. What are the characteristics of antalgic gait?

ANSWERS

152. Synovial popliteal cysts which arise between the semimembranosus and gastrocnemius tendons.

153. Spontaneous resolution within 2 to 5 years.

154. Stance phase, 60%; swing phase, 40%.

155. (1) Weight acceptance, (2) single limb stance, (3) weight release.

156. Swing phase.

157. Weight acceptance, 11%; single limb stance, 39%; weight release, 11%; swing phase, 39%

158. Forward body progression allowing only small oscillations in the center of gravity in three planes.

159. At foot strike hip flexion approximates 40 degrees.

160. Ten degrees of flexion.

161. Zero degrees of flexion.

162. A reciprocal transverse rotation occurs through the vertebral column.

163. Slower velocity, shorter step length, and increased cadence are accompanied by lack of reciprocal swing of the upper and lower limbs and a wider step length.

164. Gait characteristics are similar to those of an adult by age 7.

165. Decreased stance phase time on the affected limb, with a shorter swing phase in the contralateral limb.

QUESTIONS

166. Name the labeled structures on the posterior thigh.

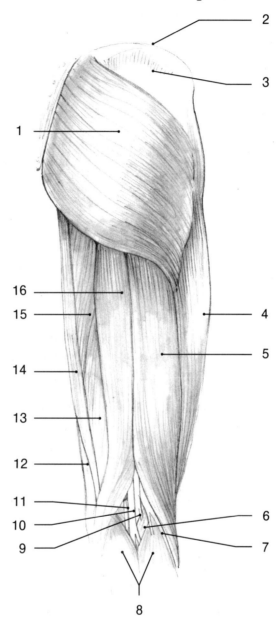

ANSWERS

166. *1*, gluteus maximus; *2*, iliac crest; *3*, fascia over gluteus medius; *4*, iliotibial tract; *5*, biceps femoris, long head; *6*, plantaris; *7*, common peroneal nerve; *8*, gastrocnemius, medial and lateral heads; *9*, tibial nerve; *10*, popliteal vein; *11*, popliteal artery; *12*, sartorius; *13*, semimembranosus; *14*, gracilis; *15*, adductor magnus; *16*, semitendinosus.

QUESTIONS

167. Name the structures in the deep aspect of the buttock.

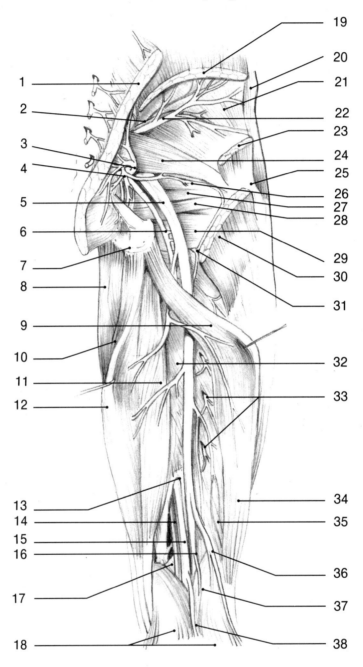

ANSWERS

167. *1*, gluteus maximus (cut); *2*, superior gluteal artery; *3*, inferior gluteal nerve; *4*, inferior gluteal artery; *5*, sciatic nerve; *6*, posterior femoral cutaneous nerve; *7*, ischial tuberosity; *8*, gracilis; *9*, biceps femoris, long head; *10*, adductor magnus; *11*, semimembranosus; *12*, semitendinosus; *13*, adductor hiatus; *14*, popliteal artery; *15*, popliteal vein; *16*, tibial nerve; *17*, adductor tubercle of femur; *18*, gastrocnemius, medial and lateral heads; *19*, gluteus medius (cut); *20*, tensor fasciae latae; *21*, gluteus minimus; *22*, superior gluteal nerve; *23*, gluteus medius (cut); *24*, piriformis; *25*, greater trochanter; *26*, superior gemellus; *27*, obturator internus; *28*, inferior gemellus; *29*, quadratus femoris; *30*, gluteus maximus (cut); *31*, medial femoral circumflex artery; *32*, adductor magnus; *33*, perforating arteries; *34*, biceps, long head (retracted); *35*, biceps, short head; *36*, common peroneal nerve; *37*, medial sural cutaneous nerve; *38*, lesser saphenous vein.

QUESTIONS

168. Name these structures from the posterior hip and thigh.

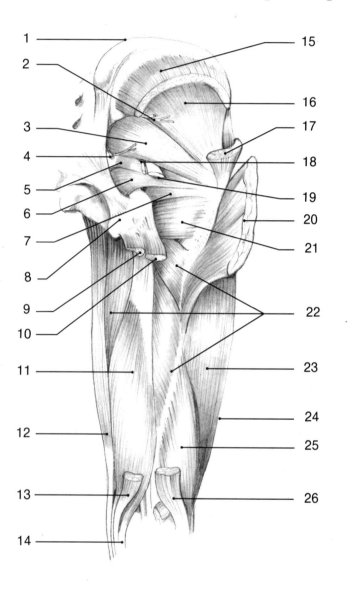

ANSWERS

168. *1*, iliac crest; *2*, superior gluteal vessels and nerve; *3*, piriformis; *4*, inferior gluteal vessels and nerve; *5*, superior gemellus; *6*, obturator internus; *7*, inferior gemellus; *8*, ischial tuberosity; *9*, semitendinosus (cut); *10*, biceps femoris, long head (cut); *11*, semimembranosus; *12*, gracilis; *13*, semitendinosus (cut) *14*, semimembranosus; *15*, gluteus medius (cut); *16*, gluteus minimus; *17*, gluteus medius (cut); *18*, posterior femoral cutaneous nerve; *19*, sciatic nerve; *20*, gluteus maximus; *21*, quadratus femoris; *22*, adductor magnus; *23*, vastus lateralis; *24*, iliotibial tract; *25*, biceps femoris, short head; *26*, biceps femoris, long head (cut).

QUESTIONS

169. Name these medial thigh structures.

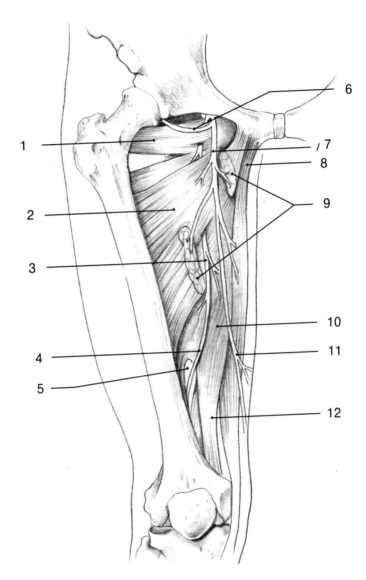

ANSWERS

169. *1*, obturator externus; *2*, adductor brevis; *3*, posterior branch of obturator nerve; *4*, articular branch of (knee) obturator nerve; *5*, hiatus of adductor canal; *6*, articular branch of (hip) obturator nerve; *7*, anterior branch of obturator nerve; *8*, gracilis; *9*, adductor longus (cut); *10*, adductor magnus; *11*, cutaneous branch of obturator nerve; *12*, adductor magnus tendon.

QUESTIONS

170. Name the labeled structures from this cross section of the thigh.

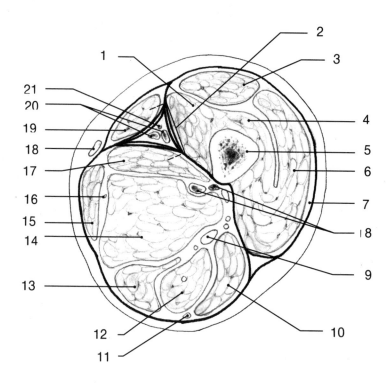

ANSWERS

170. 1, vastus medialis; 2, adductor canal; 3, rectus femoris; 4, vastus intermedius; 5, femur; 6, vastus lateralis; 7, iliotibial tract; 8, deep (profunda) femoral artery and vein; 9, sciatic nerve; 10, biceps femoris, long head; 11, posterior femoral cutaneous nerve; 12, semitendinosus; 13, semimembranosus; 14, adductor magnus; 15, gracilis; 16, anterior division of obturator nerve; 17, adductor longus; 18, saphenous vein; 19, sartorius; 20, femoral artery and vein; 21, saphenous nerve.

QUESTIONS

171. Identify each labeled structure on this anterior leg.

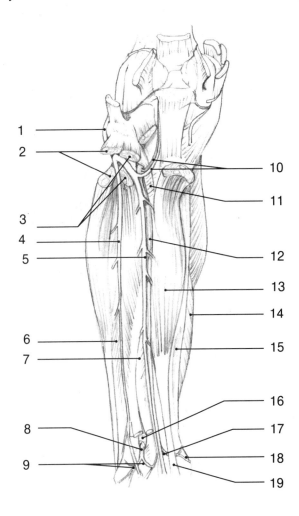

ANSWERS

171. *1*, common peroneal nerve; *2*, peroneus longus (cut); *3*, extensor digitorum longus (cut); *4*, superficial peroneal nerve; *5*, deep peroneal nerve; *6*, peroneus brevis; *7*, extensor hallucis longus; *8*, perforating branch of peroneal artery; *9*, anterior lateral malleolar arteries; *10*, anterior tibial recurrent artery and recurrent articular artery; *11*, interosseous membrane; *12*, anterior tibial artery; *13*, tibialis anterior; *14*, soleus; *15*, tibia; *16*, interosseous membrane; *17*, anterior medial malleolar artery; *18*, medial malleolus; *19*, tibialis anterior tendon.

QUESTIONS

172. Identify the structures from this cross section of the midleg.

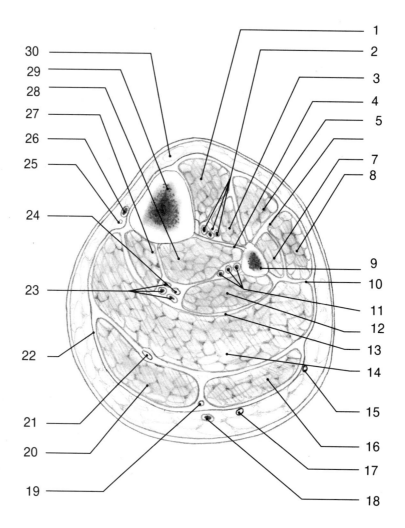

ANSWERS

172. *1,* tibialis anterior; *2,* anterior tibial artery and veins and deep peroneal nerve; *3,* extensor hallucis longus; *4,* interosseous membrane; *5,* extensor digitorum longus; *6,* anterior intermuscular septum; *7,* peroneus brevis; *8,* peroneus longus; *9,* fibula; *10,* posterior intermuscular septum; *11,* peroneal artery and veins; *12,* flexor hallucis longus; *13,* transverse intermuscular septum; *14,* soleus; *15,* lateral sural cutaneous nerve; *16,* gastrocnemius (lateral head); *17,* communicating branch of lateral sural cutaneous nerve; *18,* lesser saphenous vein; *19,* medial sural cutaneous nerve (sural nerve); *20,* gastrocnemius (medial head); *21,* plantaris tendon; *22,* crural fascia; *23,* posterior tibial artery and veins; *24,* tibial nerve; *25,* saphenous nerve; *26,* greater saphenous vein; *27,* flexor digitorum longus; *28,* tibialis posterior; *29,* tibia; *30,* subcutaneous tissue.

QUESTIONS

173. Name the labeled arteries in this lower extremity arteriogram.

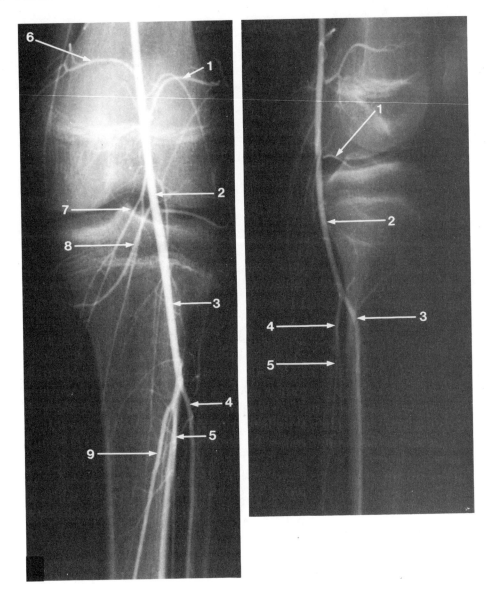

ANSWERS

173. Arteriogram of left leg, frontal view. *1,* lateral superior genicular artery; *2* and *3,* popliteal artery; *4,* anterior tibial artery; *5,* peroneal artery; *6,* medial superior genicular artery; *7,* middle genicular artery; *8,* medial inferior genicular artery; *9,* posterior tibial artery. Arteriogram of left leg, sagittal view *1,* middle genicular artery; *2,* popliteal artery; *3,* anterior tibial artery; *4,* posterior tibial artery; *5,* peroneal artery.

CHAPTER 9

Total Joint Reconstruction

Douglas McDonald, M.D.

Timothy S. Loth, M. D.

Robert E. Burdge, M. D.

David Strege, M. D.

QUESTIONS

1. What were two of Sir John Charnley's greatest contributions to total hip arthroplasty?

2. How does methylmethacrylate provide fixation of hip components?

3. What intraoperative principles and techniques will maximize the interference fit achieved with bone cement?

4. What are some other methods used to fix prosthetic components to bone?

5. What theoretical parameters are important in deciding what head size to use in total hip arthroplasty?

6. Does a larger or smaller head size result in a greater theoretical range of motion?

7. From a theoretical standpoint, which is more stable—a large head diameter or a small head diameter?

ANSWERS

1. Although he made many contributions to orthopedic surgery, the use of methylmethacrylate for fixation of the prosthetic components, as well as the use of high-density polyethylene plastic to articulate with the metal, were two of his greatest contributions.

2. Methylmethacrylate is not an adhesive as such, but rather provides a strong mechanical interference fit between the prosthesis and the bone.

3. The cement itself should be mixed uniformly and allowed to reach a doughy state before the components are inserted. Surgical fields should be as dry as possible to allow the cement to interdigitate the bony trabeculae and not be mixed with blood. The use of cement restrictors in the femoral canal will allow for increased pressurization of the cement during component insertion. Finally, efforts to achieve a relatively uniform and complete cement mantle a few millimeters thick is considered the optimum.

4. In principle, there are primarily two other methods to achieve prosthetic fixation. One method relies purely on mechanical press fitting of components with a so-called macrofit. Examples of this type of fixation include the Austin-Moore–type press fit stem or threaded acetabular cups. The other prosthetic fixation technique relies on porous surfaces on components which attempt to achieve biologic tissue ingrowth on a microscopic level.

5. From a theoretical standpoint different head sizes may make a difference in range of motion, stability, force transmission, and surface wear.

6. Assuming the neck size is the same, a larger head size will result in a greater arc of motion. From a clinical standpoint, however, the patient's preoperative range of motion and soft tissue constraints have a much greater effect on the ultimate postoperative range of motion.

7. Purely from a theoretical standpoint, a larger head size is more stable since it would require a greater degree of displacement to dislocate it from the acetabulum.

QUESTIONS

8. In clinical experience, does a larger head size lead to a lower incidence of hip dislocation?

9. How does head size affect the transmission of force to the acetabulum after total hip arthroplasty?

10. Since force transmission across the acetabulum, particularly frictional torque, has been implicated in acetabular loosening, is there any clinical experience that suggests that head size makes a difference?

11. What are the surface wear characteristics associated with different head sizes?

12. What is the clinical implication of surface wear in hip arthroplasty?

ANSWERS

8. No. Dislocation after total hip arthroplasty is truly a multifactorial problem. Factors such as previous surgery, surgical approach, component position, soft tissue reconstruction, and patient compliance are factors that have a much greater influence on clinical dislocation rates.

ANSWERS

9. Stress transmission to the acetabulum can be either direct force transmission, as compression or tension, or indirect force as a result of frictional torque. Femoral head size, acetabular size, and acetabular component thickness are all variables that determine the amount of the stresses. Theoretically, frictional torque is lessened if the acetabular component is large, but is increased if the femoral head is large. With all polyethylene cups, a thicker cup is also associated with lower frictional torque. Lower frictional torque is also believed to be associated with metal-backed components using a thinner polyethylene wall. From a theoretical standpoint, using finite element models, a greater direct surface stress is seen with a smaller head size than with a larger head size, as the former tends to concentrate the stress. But actual stress transmission to the acetabular bone is also influenced by the size and thickness of the acetabular component. A larger acetabular size and thickness results in less compressive stresses. Therefore a small (22 mm) head results in a higher surface stress of the polyethylene. Stress to the bone may be compensated by allowing for a greater acetabular polyethylene thickening.

10. Yes, there is some evidence that suggests that a large head size (32 mm) is associated with an increased incidence of radiolucent lines, as well as acetabular revision, compared with 28-mm or 22-mm heads. The use of a 32-mm head is also associated with a thinner acetabular component.

11. The coefficient of sliding friction when polyethylene moves against the polished metal surface is approximately $0.1 \, \mu_s$ to $0.2 \, \mu_s$. Within a given system, the actual wear is proportional to the load and the sliding distance. Therefore, on a theoretical basis, a larger femoral head size has a greater sliding distance, which should result in a greater amount of wear particles. Yet a small (22 mm) head produces greater local stresses and, in some experimental studies, shows higher wear rates than an intermediate size (28 mm) implant.

12. Surface wear generates wear debris. The biologic response to particulate foreign debris has been associated with an increased risk of loosening.

QUESTIONS

13. In summary, is there an optimal head size for total hip arthroplasty?

14. What are the important prerequisites for biologic ingrowth into a porous surface?

15. What are the common surgical approaches to the hip for arthroplasty?

16. Is one approach to the hip any better than another?

17. What are some of the risk factors associated with a dislocated total hip arthroplasty?

18. What is the optimal acetabular component orientation?

19. What is an optimal femoral component position?

20. Does trochanteric osteotomy affect the incidence of dislocation?

ANSWERS

13. Probably an intermediate size, such as 26 or 28 mm, is optimal. Most experimental and clinical evidence suggests that a 32-mm head should probably be avoided. A 22-mm head should probably be used with small acetabular components (44 or 46 mm) to allow for optimal acetabular thickness.

14. Ingrowth requires a biologically compatible material with optimal pore size, intimate aposition with viable tissue, implant stability, and the absence of infection.

ANSWERS

15. The most commonly used approaches are the standard posterior approach with a posterior dislocation of the hip and an anterolateral approach with an anterior dislocation of the hip. In addition, there are combined approaches designed for greater exposure for revision arthroplasty. These approaches involve either a trochanteric osteotomy or a partial skeletonization of the proximal femur, leaving an intact soft tissue sleeve in which the abductors are still attached to the thigh musculature.

16. For primary arthroplasty the personal preference of the surgeon is probably most important. There is some evidence to suggest a posterior approach is associated with a higher incidence of dislocation, although this is somewhat controversial and dislocation in general is a multifactorial problem. For revision arthroplasty one of the more extensile approaches is often warranted.

17. The risk factors associated with dislocation can be divided into preoperative, perioperative, and postoperative factors. Of the potential preoperative factors, only prior surgery has been recognized as a significant factor. The incidence of dislocation after primary arthroplasty ranges from 1% to 3%, whereas after a revision arthroplasty the incidence varies between 4% and 20%. Perioperative factors include the previously mentioned surgical approach and component head size. But probably most important is component orientation.

18. Although somewhat difficult to measure, the cup should be positioned in a so-called safe zone of abduction of 40 ± 10 degrees, and anteverted 15 ± 10 degrees. It is also important that the cup be placed inferiorly near the anatomic inferior margin of the acetabulum.

19. Again, this is almost impossible to measure adequately from a plain radiograph. An intraoperative position of 0 to physiologic 15 degrees of anteversion is probably appropriate.

20. If done correctly and if the osteotomy heals, there is probably no association with dislocation. Trochanteric nonunion and migration, however, has been associated with a higher dislocation rate.

QUESTIONS

21. What are two important factors which influence the incidence of infection after total joint arthroplasty?

22. What organisms are the most common pathogens in an infected hip arthroplasty?

23. In evaluating a patient with a painful hip arthroplasty, what radiographic features are suggestive of component loosening?

24. In evaluating a patient with a loose component, how does one decide whether it is infected?

25. What principles should be adhered to in managing an infected implant?

ANSWERS

21. Prior surgery, particularly prior arthroplasty, and the use of prophylactic antibiotics.

22. *Staphylococcus aureus* and *Staphylococcus epidermidis.*

23. The development of a complete radiolucent line between the bone-cement interface, particularly if it is 1 mm and progressive, is generally a sign of loosening. In addition, fractures in a cement mantle are also a sign of loosening. Certainly any change in a component's position in a linear direction or a rotational position is indicative of loosening (see Figure). (AP radiograph in a 72-year-old man, 10 years status post total hip arthroplasty. This figure shows many of the radiographic signs of loosening noted at the *arrows.* Proximally and laterally there is a separation between the prosthesis and cement mantle and proximally and medially there is a crack in the cement mantle. Distally there is lucency at the bone-cement interface.)

ANSWERS

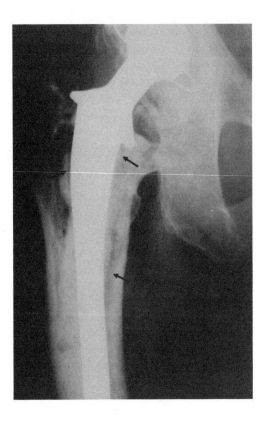

24. If a patient has obvious clinical signs, such as a draining wound, marked erythema or swelling, or systemic evidence of infection, such as an elevated white blood cell count or markedly elevated sedimentation rate, one would have to be suspicious. In the absence of obvious clinical signs, however, infection may be difficult to determine, particularly from plain films alone. Bone scans will show increased activity around a loose implant whether it is infected or not. The indium white cell–labeled scan is probably the most specific test. Hip aspiration and culture, even in a hip that later proves to be infected, will only identify an organism preoperatively two thirds of the time.

25. Complete removal of all foreign material including cement, and identification of the causal organism(s) with appropriate parenteral antibiotic therapy. Reconstruction can be done in one stage for less virulent organisms with minimal tissue involvement as delayed primary exchanges, usually after two or three operative debridements, or as secondary reconstructions in the case of more virulent organisms with more extensive tissue involvement. A final option is to leave the patient with a resection arthroplasty.

QUESTIONS

26. In principle, how does revision arthroplasty of the hip differ from primary arthroplasty?

27. When a patient with congenital hip dysplasia comes to arthroplasty, what problems should be anticipated on both the acetabular and the femoral side?

28. When doing a total knee replacement, how should fixed deformities, either varus or valgus, be corrected?

29. What is the relative incidence of deep infection in revision arthroplasty, compared with primary arthroplasty of the hip?

30. Is treatment of a deep wound infection for total joint arthroplasty with debridement, suction irrigation drainage, and without component removal likely to be successful?

ANSWERS

26. Revision arthroplasty may require different surgical exposures, techniques, and instruments for component removal, and different component selection for reconstruction and techniques and material to manage bony deficits.

27. On the acetabular side the most common problem is loss of superior and lateral bone stock. On the femoral side one must be prepared to deal with a small-sized femoral canal, as well as excessive femoral anteversion. Additionally, many patients will have had previous surgery, either on the acetabular or femoral side.

ANSWERS

28. In principle, fixed deformities should be corrected by correcting the soft tissue and not by modifying standard bony resections (see Figure). (AP radiograph of the knee in a 63-year-old woman. Marked medial joint space narrowing in varus deformity is present, typical for degenerative arthritis. Medial soft tissue release may be needed at the time of arthroplasty.)

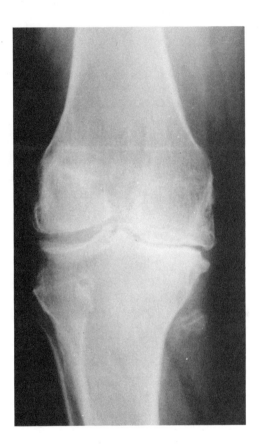

29. Deep infection occurs almost twice as often if the patient has had previous hip surgery.

30. No. Debridement without component removal may be effective for an acute deep wound infection (within a few weeks from surgery), but once the bone-cement interface becomes infected, successful treatment usually requires complete removal of all foreign bodies.

QUESTIONS

31. In the management of a fixed valgus deformity during total knee arthroplasty, what soft tissue structures may need to be released?

32. In patients who undergo total joint replacement of both the hip and the knee on the same side, how much total combined hip and knee flexion is required for them to easily climb stairs and get out of a chair?

33. What specific problems should be anticipated in performing a total hip replacement in patients with Paget disease of the involved femur or acetabulum?

34. In patients with a hip arthrodesis who complain both of low back pain and knee pain, will conversion to a total hip arthroplasty relieve their discomfort?

35. What is the optimal position for arthrodesis of the hip?

36. What gait abnormalities are observed in a patient with degenerative disease of the hip joint?

37. In a patient with fixed flexion deformities of the hip, what compensatory posture does the lumbar spine assume?

38. In viewing a radiograph of the pelvis, if one notices significant protrusio acetabuli associated with hip disease, what pathologic condition should be considered?

ANSWERS

31. Generally, lateral capsular structures are initially released from the femoral side. If more release is needed, the following structures should be released, in sequence: (1) the iliotibial band, usually at a point 10 cm proximal to the joint; (2) the popliteal tendon; (3) the fibular collateral ligament. On rare occasions, one can even release the lateral head of the gastrocnemius and release or lengthen the biceps femoris tendon. It must also be remembered that a lateral retinacular release may be required for patellar instability, particularly in patients with a longstanding fixed valgus deformity.

ANSWERS

32. It generally requires a combined hip and knee flexion of 190 degrees or more.

33. There is a potential for increased blood loss during surgery and one may have to manage bony deformity of the proximal femur, which can tend to lead to a varus position of the femoral component. Additionally, in patients with Paget disease of the pelvis there may be a significant amount of protrusio acetabuli present. Postoperatively, the incidence of heterotopic bone formation is higher, as well.

34. It will generally relieve the low back pain, but is less predictable in relieving the knee pain.

35. Although somewhat controversial, most authors recommend arthrodesis in approximately 30 degrees of flexion, neutral abduction-adduction, and slight external rotation.

36. There will often be shortening of the stance phase of the affected limb, secondary to pain, and a displacement of the body over the affected hip (Trendelenburg gait) in an attempt to decrease the muscle contraction forces across the joint.

37. The patient will generally develop a hyperlordotic posture of the lumbar spine with a prominence of the buttocks with ambulation.

38. Significant protrusio acetabuli is most commonly seen in rheumatoid arthritis, but is also seen in Paget disease, Marfan syndrome, and ankylosing spondylitis. Significant protrusio is unusual in osteoarthritis.

QUESTIONS

39. In a patient with avascular necrosis of the femoral head, at what stage of the disease would you expect to see joint space narrowing?

40. What is the advantage of the bipolar prosthesis over a standard unipolar femoral endoprosthesis?

41. What are some of the options available to prevent postoperative heterotopic bone formation following total hip arthroplasty?

42. How long will patients continue to improve their range of motion after total hip arthroplasty?

43. In a patient with suspected avascular necrosis but normal-appearing plain radiographs, which imaging technique is the most sensitive in identifying early changes?

ANSWERS

39. Joint space narrowing is generally seen as a late-stage event. In the staging system of Ficat and Arlet, it would be stage IV (see Figure). (AP radiograph of the hip in a 42-year-old renal transplant patient. Subchondral sclerosis and collapse is noted in the femoral head and is consistent with Ficat stage III avascular necrosis.)

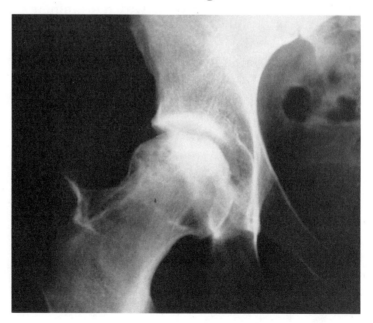

ANSWERS

40. The rationale behind the bipolar prosthesis is that the frictional forces to the acetabular cartilage will be lessened. Direct impact loading forces may also be decreased, due to the added polyethylene liner.

41. There are both intraoperative and postoperative methods that can help in the prevention of ectopic bone. Although perhaps controversial, careful surgical technique with minimal trauma to the abductor muscles, minimal periosteal stripping of the ilium, and thorough removal of bone dust and debris can be of benefit. Postoperatively there are three primary methods that have been advocated: (1) low-dose radiation, (2) anti-inflammatory medication, and (3) diphosphonates. Low-dose radiation (700–1,000 cGy) is the most effective method and is indicated for high-risk patients. Diphosphonates, most commonly etidronate disodium, prevent the mineralization of osteoid matrix, but they do not inhibit the formation of osteoid. Therefore, when the medicines are discontinued the mineralization can then occur. Although initially thought to be effective in preventing heterotopic bone formation, most authors now consider it ineffective and, in fact, long-term use can produce osteomalacia.

42. Most patients will acquire most of their motion within the first year post operation with a little improvement after that.

43. Magnetic resonance imaging (MRI) (see Figure). (Coronal T1-weighted MRI of the hip in a 32-year-old man with a normal plain film. The subchondral low signal is consistent with early avascular necrosis.)

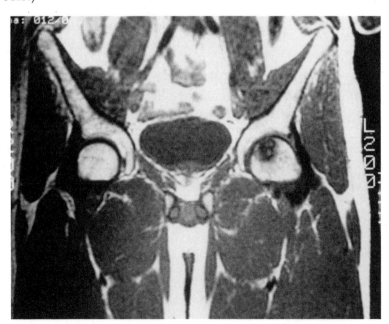

QUESTIONS

44. What are some radiographic signs of potential loosening in an uncemented femoral component?

45. What are some basic contraindications to total knee arthroplasty?

46. Does bilateral total knee arthroplasty done at a single session have a complication rate similar to staged and unilateral arthroplasty?

47. How much of the tibial plateau should the tibial implant cover?

48. How does an intramedullary stem on a tibial prosthesis affect the force distribution to the tibia?

49. What is one of the most common complications of total hip arthroplasty using an uncemented femoral stem?

50. What is the rationale for overreaming the distal canal when doing a total hip arthroplasty with an uncemented femoral component?

51. What is the most common indication for total hip arthroplasty in the adolescent?

ANSWERS

44. The development of a radiolucent interval around the prosthesis suggests a fibrous interface between the metal and bone. If this lucent area is seen over the ingrowth portion of the prosthesis, it would suggest a lack of bony ingrowth. Another sign is a shedding of beads or wires. Finally, hypertrophy of bone near the distal tip of a component, although not directly indicative of a loose component, certainly suggests an abnormal stress concentration and may represent a stress shielding of the proximal portion of the femur. Finally, as with any cemented component, migration or change in position suggests loosening.

ANSWERS

45. Probably the foremost contraindication is an active or recent septic arthritis of the knee. A second contraindication is a completely nonfunctioning extensor mechanism or severe neurologic dysfunction that prevents extension or control of the knee. Total knee arthroplasty is also generally contraindicated in a neuropathic joint. Finally, the conversion of a solid surgical arthrodesis of the knee to a total knee arthroplasty is probably not warranted.

46. Yes. There does not appear to be an adverse incidence of complications when doing simultaneous bilateral total knee arthroplasties. The initial physical therapy and rehabilitation is harder and the hospital stay may be slightly longer, but the patients are only subjected to one anesthesia and the overall rehabilitation time, compared with staged arthroplasties, is less.

47. It is important to try to maximize the area of the tibial plateau that is covered by the implant. This tends to distribute the stress to the tibia more appropriately.

48. Primarily the stem allows the implant to resist greater bending forces. In primary arthroplasty, however, a longer stem is not necessarily better since some degree of stress shielding of the tibial cortex along the length of the stem will occur.

49. Persistent thigh pain and associated limp. Many patients will have some thigh pain after uncemented femoral arthroplasty, but it can be persistent, even at 1 or 2 years, in approximately 20% of patients.

50. To avoid a tight fit distally, in deference to a tight fit proximally, although theoretically a perfectly uniform fit may be ideal. Perfection is difficult to achieve in practice. Some authors believe that rigid distal fixation, particularly if proximal fixation is less rigid, will lead to stress concentration at the distal stem tip and that this is the cause of thigh pain.

51. Juvenile rheumatoid arthritis (JRA).

QUESTIONS

52. What are some of the special problems encountered when doing a hip arthroplasty in patients with JRA?

53. If one is considering core decompression as a treatment for avascular necrosis of the femoral head, at what stage of the disease should it be performed?

54. Is bipolar hemiarthroplasty preferred over total hip arthroplasty in the treatment of avascular necrosis if the acetabular cartilage is normal?

55. What is the role of the technetium 99m bone scan evaluation of a patient with a painful hip arthroplasty?

56. Have there been any attempts to classify the bony deficiencies that arise after loosening of an acetabular component?

57. Are there any groups of patients that are particularly prone to develop heterotopic bone after total hip arthroplasty?

58. What is the mechanism of action of warfarin (Coumadin) used in the prevention of deep venous thrombosis following total hip arthroplasty?

59. When using warfarin to anticoagulate, what elevation of the prothrombin time is considered adequate?

60. How does heparin work as an anticoagulant?

ANSWERS

52. Small patient size may require the use of small components. Osteoporosis, often severe, leads to difficulty in component fixation. Joint contractures, both of the hip and the knee, are also prevalent and may require surgical correction through soft tissue releases, before or during the arthroplasty. Protrusio acetabuli may require medial bone grafting as well. Postoperatively the infection rate is generally higher.

ANSWERS

53. The best results from core decompression have been achieved prior to subchondral fracture and collapse (stage I or II).

54. Although theoretically attractive, hemiarthroplasty is not as predictable as total hip arthroplasty in relieving pain. The early clinical experience also suggests a higher revision rate or conversion to total hip arthroplasty in patients that have undergone bipolar replacement.

55. By itself, the ^{99m}Tc bone scan may only be helpful if it is normal. In this circumstance, it may rule out the arthroplasty as the source of the pain. A positive scan, however, can occur with aseptic loosening, an infected implant, fractures around an implant, or even metastatic disease. Although very sensitive, it is not very specific.

56. Yes. A few classification schemes have been proposed that try to describe the quantity and degree of host bone missing. In principle, there are two main types of deficiencies. These are either structural, noncontained defects of either the peripheral rim or medial wall, or they are cavitary, contained defects.

57. It is difficult to predict in an individual patient whether he or she will develop significant heterotopic bone. However, patients with ankylosing spondylitis and a history of ectopic bone after previous hip surgery are considered at high risk. Patients with Paget disease are also at an increased risk.

58. Warfarin inhibits the hepatic synthesis of vitamin K–dependent clotting factors II, VII, IX, and X.

59. The dosage should be adjusted to prolong the prothrombin time approximately 1.25 to 1.50 times normal.

60. Heparin acts by accelerating the antithrombin III inhibition of activated coagulation factors IX, X, XI, XII, and thrombin. Heparin will also inhibit platelet function.

QUESTIONS

61. What are relative contraindications to knee replacement arthroplasty?

62. What affect does continuous passive motion (CPM) in the immediate postoperative period have on wound healing and the incidence of thromboembolism after a total knee replacement?

63. The force across the patellofemoral joint during walking on a level surface is _____ times body weight.

64. When going up and down stairs the force across the patellofemoral joint increases to _____ times body weight.

65. What affect does squatting have on the force experienced through the patellofemoral joint?

66. What are the indications for operative treatment of patellar fracture following patellofemoral arthroplasty in a total knee replacement?

67. Describe the nonoperative treatment for a nondisplaced patellar fracture following patellofemoral arthroplasty.

68. What are the operative options for treating a comminuted displaced patellar fracture after a total knee arthroplasty?

69. What is the orientation of the tibial plateau in the coronal plane in a normal knee relative to the tibial mechanical axis?

70. Postoperative radiographs of a total knee replacement demonstrate a tibial component orientation of 0 degrees of varus-valgus angulation. What is your prediction regarding the development of radiolucencies in this patient referable to the alignment of the tibial component?

71. With regard to sagittal orientation of knee arthroplasty components, what is the normal tibial plateau posterior slope?

ANSWERS

61. Charcot joint; previous osteomyelitis of the proximal tibia or distal femur; severe vascular insufficiency; and a young patient with unrealistic and excessive physical demands for the knee.

62. There appears to be no significant effect compared to patients not receiving postoperative CPM.

63. 1.0 to 1.5.

64. Three to four.

65. It may markedly increase the force across the patellofemoral joint up to seven times body weight.

66. Surgery is indicated for disruption of the extensor mechanism, a loose implant, more than 2 mm of displacement, and comminuted patella fractures.

67. Immobilization in a cylinder cast or a knee immobilizer with protected weightbearing for 4 to 6 weeks.

68. Surgical options include open reduction and internal fixation or partial or total patellectomy. Comminuted fractures are best treated with resection of the fragments, performing either a partial or total patellectomy. Major fragments may be internally fixed. In general the operative salvage of patellar fractures is problematic, with the complication rate exceeding 40%, and satisfactory results obtainable in only about 46% of patients.

69. The tibial plateau has a 3-degree varus angulation relative to the tibial mechanical axis.

70. Adverse effects are unlikely with this tibial component alignment. A tibia cut of more than 3 or 4 degrees of varus, however, correlates with development of radiolucencies.

71. The normal tibial plateau has a posterior slope of 4 to 7 degrees.

QUESTIONS

72. What effect does anterior rotation of the femoral component have on total knee performance?

73. What effect does femoral component posterior rotation have on total knee components?

74. With regard to sagittal orientation of the femoral component, what is the orientation of the femoral cut to the shaft of the femur?

75. When comparing uncemented and cemented total knee arthroplasties, which has a higher reoperation rate?

76. What two complications are seen more frequently in uncemented total knee arthroplasties compared with cemented total knee arthroplasties?

77. What are the indications for bone graft in total knee arthroplasty?

78. As the depth of the resection increases for the tibial component, what changes occur in tibial bone strength?

79. When performing a patellar resurfacing, what patellar thickness should be retained to optimize extensor mechanics and maintain extensor strength?

80. Why is the tibial stem length kept to a minimum to achieve fixation in an uncomplicated cemented total knee replacement?

81. During a total knee arthroplasty there is inadvertent underresection of the distal femoral bone which was compensated for by increased proximal tibial resection. What clinical problem can be anticipated?

82. To compensate for overresection of the distal femur, underresection of the proximal tibia is considered. Why should this "correction" maneuver be avoided?

ANSWERS

72. The femoral cortex may be notched and the trochlear phalanx may impinge.

73. There will be increased component wear because of altered contact areas. In addition, the trochlear phalanx and patella may impinge.

74. The femoral cut is made perpendicular to the femoral shaft in the sagittal plane.

75. Based on the Mayo Clinic experience, uncemented total knee arthroplasties seem to have a higher reoperation rate.

76. Total implant loosening is more frequent in the uncemented group, as is implant subsidence into the tibia.

77. Tibial deficiency or tibial and femoral combined deficiencies exceeding 10 mm, or a defect size more than 25%–50% of the tibia, or projected cement column exceeding 5 mm in height.

78. Tibial bone strength decreases.

79. The original patellar thickness should be retained to optimize extensor mechanics and maintain strength.

80. Because a long cemented stem will stress-shield the tibia over the entire length of the cemented tibial stem.

81. The knee will be unstable at 45 to 90 degrees of flexion.

82. Because the knee will be tight in flexion, thereby limiting motion.

QUESTIONS

83. What problems can result from inadvertent posterior placement of the femoral component in a total knee replacement?

84. What is the most common organism isolated from infected knee replacements?

85. What options should be considered in treatment of a septic total knee arthroplasty?

86. Reduction in the porosity of polymethylmethacrylate (PMMA) significantly improves mechanical compression and tensile strength as well as fatigue life. What mixing technique can significantly decrease the porosity of PMMA in total joint replacement?

87. What factors are associated with supracondylar fractures of the femur following total knee arthroplasty?

88. How are supracondylar femur fractures in patients with total knee arthroplasties treated?

89. What is the major mode of failure seen in total knee arthroplasty?

90. Following total knee arthroplasties, the patient develops a clinical syndrome consistent with fat embolism syndrome. What intraoperative techniques are associated with the development of fat embolism syndrome in total knee arthroplasty?

91. Excessive internal rotation of the tibial component produces lateral displacement of the tibial tuberosity. What clinical problems can be seen in this clinical situation?

92. The sartorius muscle is innervated by the _____ nerve?

93. The gluteus medius and minimis muscles are primary abductors of the hip. They are innervated by _____ ?

ANSWERS

83. Loss of motion can occur with the knee being tight in flexion, and notching of the anterior femoral cortex can lead to supracondylar fractures.

84. *Staphylococcus aureus.*

85. Appropriate antibiotic therapy is required in conjunction with one of five options: (1) debridement with retention of components, (2) removal of implants, leaving a resection arthroplasty, (3) arthrodesis, (4) reimplantation of the prosthesis, (5) amputation.

86. Mixing and preparation of PMMA under a vacuum with centrifugation can significantly reduce cement porosity.

87. Osteoporosis, notching of the anterior femoral cortex, and trauma.

88. If satisfactory alignment can be achieved through closed techniques, nonoperative management is pursued. Open reduction and internal fixation is reserved for patients with adequate bone stock and inability to maintain adequate alignment.

89. Implant loosening. This can result from improper implant positioning, poor surgical technique, and the use of constrained implants which increase stresses at the bone-implant interfaces.

90. The use of intramedullary instrumentation for limb alignment or long-stemmed implants has been associated with fat embolism syndrome.

91. Patellar subluxation or dislocation.

92. Femoral.

93. The superior gluteal nerve.

QUESTIONS

94. What is the leading cause of death following total hip replacement?

95. What is the most common cause of sciatic nerve palsy following total hip replacement?

96. What technical errors predispose to dislocation following total hip replacement?

97. In the rheumatoid patient with both wrist and metacarpophalangeal (MCP) joint deformities that require surgical reconstruction, why would you prefer to perform the wrist reconstruction first?

98. A patient with longstanding rheumatoid arthritis presents with significant ulnar deviation and volar subluxation of the proximal phalanges of the MCP joints. Evaluation of the wrist demonstrates significant disease with palmar and ulnar subluxation of the carpus. The patient has minimal wrist pain, but the appearance and function of her hand are significant problems. Wrist range of motion is 40 degrees dorsiflexion to 40 degrees of palmar flexion with 10 degrees of radial and ulnar deviation. Radiographs of the wrist demonstrate minimal articular changes in the carpus. The MCP radiographs show the metacarpal heads to be destroyed. How would you reconstruct this hand and wrist?

99. Why have most hand surgeons stopped using silicone rubber replacements for carpal bone arthroplasties?

100. What long-term problems have been identified with the use of Silastic MCP arthroplasties?

101. Describe the Eaton classification of trapezial-metacarpal arthritis.

102. In a patient with Eaton stage IV trapezial-metacarpal arthritis, why would a hemitrapezial arthroplasty be inappropriate?

ANSWERS

94. Thromboembolic disease.

95. Postoperative hemorrhage secondary to anticoagulation.

96. Malposition of the femoral or acetabular component, use of a short femoral neck which can produce impingement that levers the head out of the acetabulum, and nonunion of trochanteric osteotomies.

97. Because uncorrected ulnar shift of the carpus will contribute to recurrence of the ulnar drift of the fingers after MCP joint surgery.

98. Before approaching the MCP joints, one should correct the wrist deformity. Otherwise one is likely to have recurrence of the ulnar deformity of the digits. In a patient with significant ulnar-palmar subluxation of the carpus without significant degenerative changes, I prefer a radiolunate arthrodesis (Chamay fusion). With the wrist corrected one could proceed to MCP arthroplasties.

99. Recent reports of silicone synovitis. Other associated problems have been implant failure through fracture or subluxation and dislocation.

100. Implant fracture and dislocation (although these may be asymtomatic), bony resorption around the implant, silicone synovitis, and recurrent deformity at the MCP joints.

101. There are four stages of progressively severe arthritis in the pantrapezial area. In stage I the trapezial-metacarpal joint is normal. There may be effusion or ligament laxity. In stage II there is slight narrowing of the trapezial-metacarpal joint with sclerotic changes of the subchondral bone. In stage III there is significant joint space narrowing, associated cystic changes, sclerotic bone, and loose bodies. Stage IV is the same as stage III, including arthritis of the scaphotrapezial joint.

102. Hemiarthroplasty would not address the scaphotrapezial arthritis. A complete trapezial arthroplasty is preferred.

QUESTIONS

103. What is the average range of motion for Swanson MCP arthroplasties in long-term follow-up?

104. What problem is present when hinging of the prosthesis is noted in testing flexion with a trial proximal interphalangeal joint (PIP) Silastic implant?

105. What should be done to correct for pistoning of the stem through a flexion-extension range of motion in PIP Silastic arthroplasty?

106. When performing a Silastic PIP arthroplasty for a chronic boutonnière deformity, extensor system rebalancing is required. What can be done surgically to accomplish this?

107. Describe the techniques for soft tissue rebalancing used in MCP arthroplasties in rheumatoid arthritis patients.

108. True or false? Silastic replacement of the trapezium has not been associated with silicone synovitis as have other carpal bone replacements.

109. What is the average range of motion anticipated in Swanson silicone wrist arthroplasty?

110. Describe three options for salvage of a failed total wrist arthroplasty.

111. When deciding on total wrist arthroplasty for treatment of a particular patient, what other treatment options should be given consideration?

ANSWERS

103. Published series report an average arc of motion of 34 to 57 degrees for Swanson MCP arthroplasties in long-term follow-up.

104. The implant fit is too tight, indicative of a need for additional soft tissue release or bony resection. This can lead to early implant failure because of excessive stress transmission to the implant.

105. Some degree of pistoning of the stem is normal and no effort should be made to correct it.

106. Central slip shortening, sometimes with lengthening of the terminal tendon to improve distal interphalangeal (DIP) flexion.

107. Soft tissue rebalancing is facilitated through intrinsic releases, bone shortening, centralization of the extensor mechanism, at times volar plate mobilization or release, radial collateral ligament reconstruction (particularly for the index finger), and crossed intrinsic transfer.

108. False. Although less frequently seen (approximately 20% of cases) silicone synovitis has been associated with Silastic trapezial replacements.

109. On average, 25 degrees of dorsiflexion to 25 degrees of palmar flexion with 5 degrees of radial deviation, and 15 degrees of ulnar deviation.

110. (1) Removal of the implant with casting in the hopes of establishing a resection arthroplasty; (2) wrist fusion; (3) revision with another prosthesis.

111. In the patient with inflammatory arthropathy of the wrist with minimal joint destruction, synovectomy may provide pain relief and improved function. Wrist denervation may also be considered in the patient with minimal joint destruction. If articular destruction is localized, limited wrist arthrodesis or resection arthroplasty (proximal row carpectomy) may be suitable alternatives. Complete wrist arthrodesis should be considered in the patient with total wrist involvement and who will be placing relatively heavy demands on the wrist joint.

QUESTIONS

112. One of the alternatives to total wrist arthroplasty in the rheumatoid patient is wrist synovectomy. What are the indications for this procedure?

113. What are the advantages of wrist arthrodesis over other procedures for wrist arthroses?

114. From a biomechanical standpoint, does wrist arthrodesis increase or decrease grip strength?

115. What are some of the problems associated with silicone interposition wrist arthroplasty?

116. What are the indications for total wrist arthroplasty?

117. What are the contraindications for total wrist arthroplasty?

118. A 34-year-old woman with rheumatoid arthritis is 10 years status post bilateral wrist arthrodesis. However, because of increasing loss of motion of the elbow and shoulders, she is having significant difficulty with daily activities owing to limitation of motion. At this point the patient desires to have wrist motion. How should this situation be managed?

ANSWERS

112. Pain with limited articular destruction and minimal wrist deformity. Distal radioulnar joint disease that threatens to rupture extensor tendons of the hand and wrist.

ANSWERS

113. Successful arthrodesis provides complete and long-term pain relief. Wrist fusion is a dependable procedure that is durable and is stable with time. No future surgery will be necessary. Excellent function of the hand is maintained.

114. Since wrist motion is eliminated after wrist arthrodesis, the mechanical advantage and excursion available to the finger flexors becomes limited without the benefit of wrist extension. This will *decrease* the strength of power grip. Clinically, wrist arthrodesis increases power by stabilizing the wrist and relieving pain.

115. Silicone interposition wrist arthroplasty is a true wrist joint replacement in that midcarpal and radiocarpal joint functions are preserved. However, as this prosthesis provides no true mechanical articulation, it functions as a spacer. This prosthesis has demonstrated poor durability and limited longevity. Fracture of the prosthesis occurs relatively frequently with conservative estimates placed at 20% after 5 years, while others have demonstrated 65% prosthesis fractures within 6 years. Subsidence of the prosthesis is common. This causes shortening of the wrist which may have an adverse effect on the extrinsic musculotendinous finger motors. Surprisingly, there has been no significant association with silicone synovitis.

116. Indications are relatively limited. The most common indication is for the rheumatoid arthritis patient who has multiple upper extremity joint involvement. There should be a distinct need for wrist motion. The patient should have significant wrist pain or significant deformity of the wrist.

117. Implantation in the very active or very young patient who places heavy demands on the wrist. There is a high likelihood that loosening of the implant will occur in such patients. Other contraindications are marked osteopenia, in which fixation of the implant is difficult and fracture is likely to occur, a past history of joint sepsis, and absence of the radial wrist extensors. Absence of the extensor carpi ulnaris is not a contraindication as this tendon is primarily an ulnar deviator of the wrist as opposed to a pure wrist extensor.

118. If the wrist extensors are intact, previous wrist arthrodesis is not a contraindication to total wrist arthroplasty. After considering options to improve shoulder or elbow motion, or both, total wrist arthroplasty may be considered as a viable option.

QUESTIONS

119. In total wrist arthroplasty, what are the indications for resection of the distal ulna?

120. At the time of surgery, a biaxial (semiconstrained) total wrist arthroplasty implant is noted to have a loose fit. How is this resolved?

121. What is the desired postoperative range of motion after total wrist arthroplasty?

122. After implantation using current total wrist arthroplasty designs, what is the likelihood that future revision will be necessary?

123. The success of resection arthroplasty of the wrist (proximal row carpectomy) is dependent on what anatomic features of the carpus?

124. Wrist arthrodesis is commonly performed as a salvage procedure for total wrist arthroplasty. What is the position of choice for wrist arthrodesis?

125. A 42-year-old rheumatoid patient with multiple joint involvement has bilateral painful wrists without appreciable sparing of the articular cartilage. How should this patient be managed?

126. A 48-year-old trucker has significant painful posttraumatic arthritis with nearly complete involvement of both wrists 10 years after his injury. What recommendations should be made?

127. What arc of motion at the elbow is necessary to carry out most daily activities?

ANSWERS

119. After radial resection and implantation of the prosthesis, a relative ulnar positive variance occurs. This can lead to ulnar abutment and therefore the distal ulna should always be resected in total wrist arthroplasty.

120. With joint capsular reconstruction and an increased period of postoperative cast immobilization (6 weeks vs. the normal 4 weeks).

121. A flexion-extension arc of 60 degrees. Excess motion leads to prosthetic imbalance, subluxation, and loosening.

122. Although limited, current information suggests that after total wrist arthroplasty there is a 33% chance of need for revision in 5 years.

123. Healthy articular cartilage of the capitate and lunate fossa as well as a nearly equal radius of curvature of the convex dome of the capitate and the concave lunate fossa of the radius.

124. Between 0 and 15 degrees of wrist dorsiflexion.

125. Maintaining motion is of utmost importance. Current recommendations favor total wrist arthroplasty of the nondominant wrist and arthrodesis of the dominant wrist.

126. If limited wrist arthrodesis is not possible due to extensive involvement of arthritis, bilateral total wrist fusion should be recommended. Because of the significant physical demands on the wrists of a laborer, total wrist arthroplasty would be at considerable risk for loosening and is therefore not recommended.

127. The normal arc of motion at the elbow is 0 to 150 degrees of flexion-extension with 75 degrees of pronation and 85 degrees of supination. As a full arc of motion is not necessary for most activities, the functional arc of motion is one of 30 to 130 degrees of extension-flexion with 50 degrees of pronation and 50 degrees of supination.

QUESTIONS

128. Describe the currently used types of implants for total elbow arthroplasty.

129. What are the surgical indications for total elbow arthroplasty?

130. What are the contraindications to total elbow arthroplasty?

131. The Coonrad-Morrey semiconstrained total elbow replacement prosthesis is designed with 7 to 10 degrees of varus-valgus laxity at the hinge joint. What is the advantage of this construction?

132. The Coonrad II total elbow arthroplasty design was modified in 1981 to the Coonrad-Morrey total elbow arthroplasty with addition of an anterior flange to the lower humeral stem. What is the purpose of this additional anterior flange?

ANSWERS

128. The evolution of total elbow arthroplasty has brought two types to the forefront. (1) Unconstrained or resurfacing implants (capitello-condylar or Pritchard) require that the surrounding soft tissue elements maintain stability. (2) In the semiconstrained implant (Coonrad-Morrey total elbow prosthesis) the humeral and ulnar components are connected by a hinge pin where ultrahigh-molecular-weight polyethylene bushings prevent metal-on-metal contact. Total constraint at the hinge is eliminated by design with 7 to 10 degrees of varus-valgus laxity which conforms to the average laxity of the normal elbow joint. Both types of implants relieve pain (in approximately 90% of implants). The resurfacing implants are more likely to subluxate or dislocate but are thought to be less likely to loosen. The semiconstrained elbow provides for elbow stability regardless of the condition of the surrounding soft tissue structures.

ANSWERS

129. Pain relief is the major indication. Both the semiconstrained and resurfacing prostheses provide pain relief in the range of 90% of implants. Additionally, total elbow arthroplasty is used to improve function. Unlike the knee or hip, loss of motion at the elbow may significantly impair function of the involved extremity, and total elbow arthroplasty may be used primarily to improve motion. The semiconstrained implant can be used to provide stability to the elbow to improve elbow function. Elbow function can also be improved by increasing strength. Because of the likelihood of loosening with placing of increased demands on the extremity after total elbow arthroplasty, this is not encouraged as one of the goals for joint replacement. However, strength is increased through pain relief.

130. Previous infection of the joint is a relative contraindication to elbow replacement. Severe soft tissue contractures at the elbow cannot be overcome with total elbow arthroplasty, leading to unsatisfactory results. Paralysis of the flexor musculature of the elbow will also significantly compromise the result. Loss of extension power can, however, be compensated for by gravity. Patients with previous elbow arthrodesis or painless ankylosis in a satisfactory position should not be considered for total elbow arthroplasty. Also, uncooperative patients and those who are unable to understand the full implications of this procedure should not undergo total elbow arthroplasty.

131. The semiconstrained total elbow replacement prosthesis conforms to normal joint laxity. Laxity at the hinged joint also decreases stresses on the bone-cement interface which allows the surrounding soft tissue envelope to absorb some of the transmitted forces. This decreases the likelihood of implant loosening which was a major complication of earlier totally constrained designs.

132. Maximal stress after semiconstrained total elbow arthroplasty is found to occur anteriorly at the site of insertion of the humeral components. Bone graft, when placed between the flange and the anterior cortex, can enhance thickening of bone stock at this site to resist these stresses. The flange and bone graft are designed to resist torsional and posteriorly directed forces occurring at this site. This will also aid in preventing loosening.

QUESTIONS

133. The infection rate after total elbow arthroplasty is higher than that seen after other total joint replacement procedures (approximately 7%). What factors contribute to this complication?

134. In the case of deep infection after total elbow arthroplasty, what treatment recommendations should be made?

135. Six months after total elbow arthroplasty a patient is found to have a septic elbow. Intraoperatively at the time of implant removal, the ulnar component is loose and is easily removed. However, the humeral component is quite stable and difficulty with removal has caused the humerus to fracture 5 cm from its distal end. How should this be treated?

136. What is the expected arc of motion after total elbow arthroplasty?

137. Instability after total elbow arthroplasty is a complication unique to resurfacing implants with an approximate 10% incidence of postoperative subluxation or dislocation. What steps can be taken to minimize this complication?

138. Four months after total elbow arthroplasty a 25-year-old patient with rheumatoid arthritis dislocates her elbow. How should this be treated?

ANSWERS

133. Several factors peculiar to the elbow place the patient with total elbow arthroplasty at risk for infection. Anatomically, the elbow is a subcutaneous joint with minimal soft tissue coverage. Also, candidates for total elbow arthroplasty are usually at risk for infection. A vast majority of these patients have rheumatoid arthritis and may be immunocompromised by chronic use of steroids. Also, frequently (especially in the patient with posttraumatic arthritis) these patients have had at least one previous surgical procedure on the joint. The type of implant used appears to have no bearing on the infection rate, as the rate is the same for both semiconstrained and unconstrained prostheses. Antibiotic-impregnated cement has been used successfully to decrease the incidence of infection in total elbow arthroplasty.

134. Implant removal is the treatment of choice, regardless of whether the prosthesis is stable or unstable. Removal of a stable infected implant, however, is an especially demanding procedure. After implant removal, total elbow arthroplasty, now converted to resection arthroplasty, is associated with a relatively good (80%) long-term patient satisfaction. Rarely is consideration given for reimplantation.

135. These fractures usually heal after casting for approximately 6 weeks.

136. Between 30 and 130 degrees of flexion-extension with 60 degrees of pronation and 60 degrees of supination. Slightly less extension (36–40 degrees) is usually noted with resurfacing implants owing to postoperative immobilization.

137. Patient selection is important because stability is dependent upon the surrounding soft tissues. The patient must have competent medial and lateral collateral ligaments. Soft tissue structures must be carefully repaired at the time of closure. As most dislocations occur early in the postoperative period, positioning the elbow in full extension is to be avoided. Postoperatively the elbow should be placed in a cast for 3 to 4 weeks.

138. After closed reduction, the elbow should be immobilized at 90 degrees for 3 to 6 weeks.

QUESTIONS

139. After total elbow arthroplasty, the patient falls and fractures the humerus at the proximal tip of the humeral component. How should this patient be managed?

140. Is radial head replacement recommended at the time of total elbow replacement?

141. A 26-year-old man sustained a gunshot wound to his elbow 2 years earlier. This resulted in nearly complete destruction of the distal humeral articular surface. While his motion is fairly well preserved, he complains of nearly constant pain in this elbow. How should this be managed?

142. In the patient with rheumatoid arthritis, what is the appropriate timing for total elbow arthroplasty?

143. Why is elbow arthrodesis generally considered a poor choice as an alternative in elbow reconstructive procedures?

144. What are the indications for total shoulder arthroplasty?

ANSWERS

139. Fractures occur more commonly with loose prostheses because a loose prosthesis can cause cortical bone resorption. Also, abnormal bone-cement interface stresses may compromise the quality of bone. If the prosthesis is loose, revision surgery should be undertaken exchanging the present implant for a long-stemmed component in order to bypass the fracture. If there is no evidence of loosening, cast immobilization is the treatment of choice.

140. Although theoretically the addition of a radiohumeral component to total elbow arthroplasty may improve stability and prevent loosening, clinically the benefits of the radiohumeral component have been outweighed by complications. The use of a radial head implant has therefore been abandoned in the capitellocondylar and Coonrad-Morrey implants. While a radiohumeral component is still available with the Pritchard prosthesis, data are not yet available to demonstrate if this component is beneficial.

ANSWERS

141. In this young male patient, relatively high demand would make total elbow arthroplasty at risk for loosening and a less desirable choice. While arthrodesis would provide good stability if strength is a necessity, in most situations loss of elbow motion is poorly tolerated and the complication rate is high. Interposition arthroplasty is the procedure of choice. Should instability become a problem, it can easily be converted to a semiconstrained total elbow arthroplasty.

142. Elbow pain unresolved with conservative treatment is the usual complaint of patients with rheumatoid arthritis. In these patients, radiographs of the elbow will assist in determining the appropriate treatment. In the presence of minimal or no joint narrowing and maintenance of joint contour, synovectomy alone is appropriate. With complete obliteration of the joint space and mild alteration of the joint contour, resurfacing arthroplasty should be considered. With severe alteration of joint contour and gross joint destruction, a semiconstrained total elbow arthroplasty is the procedure of choice. As a rheumatoid patient usually does not place great demands on the upper extremity, age is a relatively minor consideration for total elbow arthroplasty. However, it is generally recommended that for those under the age of 40 years, a resurfacing implant be used, and for those older than 40 the semiconstrained total elbow arthroplasty be done.

143. While a successful elbow arthrodesis will provide considerable strength for the extremity, other factors make this a less desirable alternative. The functional impairment of loss of elbow motion is significant. This includes being unable to extend the hand to the mouth. The loss of motion of the elbow is poorly compensated by shoulder and wrist motion. Also, solid fusion is difficult to obtain, especially if there is significant bone loss. Once fusion is attained the risk of fracture of the humerus or ulna is estimated at greater than 10%.

144. Indications for total shoulder arthroplasty are unresolved pain after conservative treatment measures due to destruction of glenohumeral cartilage. This most commonly results from osteoarthritis, rheumatoid arthritis, traumatic arthritis, osteonecrosis, cuff tear arthropathy, and previous failed reconstructive surgery. Because of excellent results and relative scarcity of complications after total shoulder arthroplasty, this procedure is by far the treatment of choice for reconstruction of the glenohumeral joint.

QUESTIONS

145. What are the contraindications to total shoulder arthroplasty?

146. In total shoulder arthroplasty what design change considerations could be made in the prosthesis to increase stability?

147. What is cuff tear arthropathy of the shoulder?

148. In making the proximal humeral osteotomy for placement of the humeral component of total shoulder arthroplasty, at what angle should the osteotomy be made?

149. What is the most common complication requiring revision surgery following nonconstrained total shoulder arthroplasty?

150. What options are available other than total shoulder arthroplasty for glenohumeral joint reconstruction?

151. Shoulder arthrodesis may be considered as an alternative to total shoulder arthroplasty in glenohumeral joint reconstruction. What are the primary indications for shoulder arthrodesis?

152. A patient is referred for total shoulder arthroplasty. Radiographs of the shoulder demonstrate nearly complete destruction of the glenohumeral joint. However, the patient has minimal discomfort. He is otherwise in good health. How should this patient be managed?

ANSWERS

145. Extreme osteoporosis rendering the glenoid quite flexible and also medial resorption of the glenoid subchondral bone, leaving only a small scapular neck to articulate with the humerus. These occur more commonly in the rheumatoid patient, making placement of the glenoid component difficult and also resulting in a high likelihood of glenoid component loosening. Other contraindications are deltoid and rotator cuff paralysis, neuropathic arthritis, and active or recent shoulder joint infection.

ANSWERS

146. Stability can be increased by decreasing the radius of curvature of the articulation, increasing the depth of the socket component, making it more cuplike, or by securing the components to each other as in the ball-in-socket designs.

147. Cuff tear arthropathy of the shoulder, also known as "Milwaukee shoulder," is a term coined by Neer to denote collapse of the humeral articular surface with glenoid instability in association with a massive and longstanding rotator cuff tear. It is usually treated with total shoulder arthroplasty and repair of the rotator cuff.

148. It should begin just medial to the supraspinatous attachment to the greater tuberosity extending distally and medially at 45 degrees with 30 degrees of retroversion.

149. Glenoid loosening. This most commonly occurs at approximately 3 to 5 years postoperatively. Humeral component loosening is quite rare.

150. Total shoulder arthroplasty is by far the procedure of choice for reconstruction of the glenohumeral joint. After failure of nonoperative treatment, including use of nonsteroidal anti-inflammatory agents, activity modification, and physical therapy modalities, consideration should be given to synovectomy if joint destruction is minimal. Resection arthroplasty and arthrodesis are other alternatives.

151. The indications are relatively limited. They include loss of motor control about the shoulder due to paralysis of the deltoid and rotator cuff muscles, previous glenohumeral joint septic arthritis, and previous failed reconstructive surgery with muscle or bone deficiencies.

152. In the patient in whom joint destruction is out of proportion to the patient's symptoms, a Charcot joint is suspected. This is a contraindication to total joint arthroplasty. In an otherwise healthy patient a cervical syringomyelia should be suspected and an MRI of the cervical spine is indicated.

QUESTIONS

153. In most total shoulder prostheses currently in use, the glenoid implant is a metal-backed component. Earlier implants used a non-metal-backed polyethylene glenoid component. What are the advantages of a metal-backed glenoid component?

154. A patient is brought to the operating room with cuff tear arthropathy of the shoulder. Intraoperatively, the patient is noted to have massive rotator cuff tear, which cannot be adequately repaired. What type of shoulder prosthesis should be implanted (unconstrained vs. constrained)?

155. What surgical approach is most commonly used for total shoulder arthroplasty?

156. What kind of results may be expected after unconstrained total shoulder arthroplasty with regard to pain relief and range of motion?

157. What are the indications for proximal humerus resection arthroplasty?

158. After failed total elbow arthroplasty, what surgical options are available for revision? What are the advantages of these options?

ANSWERS

153. The advantage of the metal-backed component is that it decreases polyethylene deformation and cold flow. It also improves fixation and distributes the interface stresses evenly to prevent loosening.

154. Regardless of whether the rotator cuff tear can be completely repaired, an unconstrained total shoulder prosthesis should be implanted. Because of the high complication and glenoid loosening rate associated with a constrained implant, the latter is currently not recommended with inability to repair the rotator cuff. There will need to be limited goals concerning the postoperative rehabilitation program.

ANSWERS

155. The deltopectoral approach.

156. Relatively good results. Pain relief occurs in greater than 90% of patients. In the osteoarthritic patient the final range of motion is approximately 75% to 80% of normal. Range of motion of the posttraumatic and the rheumatoid patient is somewhat less, at 65% to 70% of normal.

157. The indications for proximal humerus resection arthroplasty are relatively limited. It should be considered for salvage of infected total shoulder arthroplasty or for failed total shoulder arthroplasty with unreconstructable bone or soft tissue loss.

158. Arthrodesis of the elbow is, in most cases, a poor choice for revision, and should only be considered if there is adequate bone stock available for the patient who places heavy demands on the upper extremity. This is a relatively poor choice owing to the significant functional disability and relatively high complication rate. Resection arthroplasty is the recommended salvage procedure after an infected total elbow arthroplasty. Although strength and stability are a problem with resection arthroplasty, it can provide pain relief and allow elbow motion. Interposition resection arthroplasty has a somewhat unpredictable outcome. If bone loss is extensive, and in the absence of sepsis, allograft elbow replacement may be considered. However, there is a relatively high associated complication rate (approximately 30%) due to sepsis and nonunion after this procedure. The most viable option for revision in the absence of sepsis is total elbow replacement. Use of a semiconstrained prosthesis provides good pain relief and elbow stability if there is adequate bone stock available. Without adequate bone stock, special custom-designed prostheses or composite prostheses with allograft are other options.

QUESTIONS

159. A 57-year-old patient complains of significant elbow pain 15 years after open reduction and internal fixation of a comminuted T-condylar distal humerus fracture. Radiographs demonstrate extensive traumatic arthritis of the elbow joint. How should this patient be managed?

160. A 60-year-old man is seen 10 years after a gunshot wound to the elbow. He complains of significant discomfort at the elbow. There was no nerve injury to the involved extremity, but radiographs of the elbow demonstrate 2 cm of bone loss of the distal humerus. How should this patient be managed?

ANSWERS

159. In the older patient with posttraumatic arthritis who is not going to place excessive demands on the upper extremity, a semiconstrained total elbow arthroplasty is the treatment of choice. However, preoperative discussion with the patient regarding the patient's expectations of activity level after surgery are necessary. Because of the risk of loosening, the patient should be advised that lifting should be limited to 10 lb on a one-time basis and 5 lb on a repetitive basis. If the patient's activity level is greater, interposition resection arthroplasty should be recommended.

160. This patient is a candidate for semiconstrained total elbow arthroplasty. Bone loss of the distal humerus of 2 cm or less does not require special prosthesis for joint replacement. If bone loss is greater than 2 cm, consideration should be given to a custom implant or composite implant and allograft reconstruction.

CHAPTER 10

Foot and Ankle

Timothy S. Loth, M. D.

QUESTIONS

1. Identify the labeled structures on this cross section through the ankle.

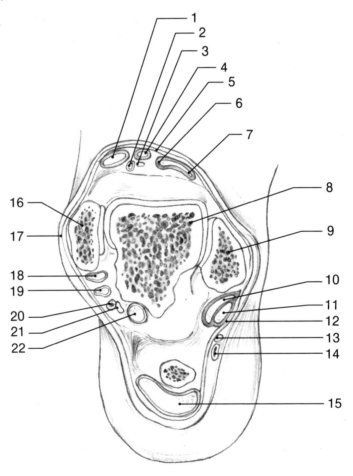

2. Describe the treatment of fractures of the lateral process of the talus—nondisplaced fractures, large displaced fractures, and comminuted fragments.

ANSWERS

1. *1*, tibialis anterior; *2*, anterior tibial artery; *3*, deep peroneal nerve; *4*, extensor hallucis longus; *5*, superior extensor retinaculum; *6*, extensor digitorum longus; *7*, peroneus tertius; *8*, talus; *9*, lateral malleolus; *10*, peroneus brevis; *11*, peroneus longus; *12*, superior peroneal retinaculum; *13*, sural nerve; *14*, lesser saphenous vein; *15*, tendo Achillis; *16*, medial malleolus; *17*, flexor retinaculum; *18*, tibialis posterior; *19*, flexor digitorum longus; *20*, posterior tibial artery; *21*, tibial nerve; *22*, flexor hallucis longus.

2. Nondisplaced fractures are treated in a cast for 6 weeks (nonweightbearing for 4 weeks). Large displaced fractures are treated by open reduction and internal fixation. Comminuted fragments are treated by primary surgical excision to avoid development of arthritic changes of the subtalar joint. A sinus tarsi incision exposes the fragments.

QUESTIONS

3. What can obstruct closed reduction of medial subtalar dislocations?

4. What is the most common obstruction to closed reduction of lateral subtalar dislocations?

5. What is the treatment for unreducible medial and lateral subtalar dislocations?

6. What is the Hawkin's classification for talar neck fractures?

7. Which fracture is associated with talar neck fractures?

8. Which radiographic views are critical in evaluating reduction of talar neck fractures?

9. How are type I talar neck fractures treated?

10. How are type II fractures treated?

ANSWERS

3. An impaction fracture with interlocking of the articular surfaces of the talus and navicular; capsule interposition of the talonavicular joint; transverse fibers of the cruciate ligament or extensor digitorum brevis muscle.

4. An interposed posterior tibial tendon or interlocked fracture of the talus and navicular.

ANSWERS

5. Medial subtalar dislocations are treated by longitudinal anteromedial incision over the prominent head and neck of the talus and manipulation or release of interposed structures. Lateral dislocations are treated by longitudinal incision over the medial aspect of the talar head to get access to the posterior tibial tendon. After reduction, a short leg cast is applied for 3 to 4 weeks. Since the joint is stable after reduction, there is no need for internal fixation.

6. *Type I:* nondisplaced; *type II:* displaced neck fracture with subluxation or dislocation of the subtalar joint; *type III:* displaced neck fracture with dislocation of the body of the talus from both the ankle and subtalar joints.

7. Medial malleolus fracture.

8. Lateral views of the ankle and foot, and anteroposterior (AP) view of the talar neck with the foot in maximal equinus, pronated 15 degrees. The X-ray beam is angled 75 degrees from the horizontal toward the head.

9. In a short leg cast for 8 to 12 weeks, nonweightbearing for 4 to 6 weeks and then partial weightbearing.

10. Closed reduction. Gentle traction is applied and the foot is plantar flexed to reduce the head fragment to the body and correct varus or valgus malalignment. Radiographs of the talar neck should be obtained to assess reduction. With anatomic reduction the foot is immobilized in equinus in a short leg cast for 1 month. The foot should gradually be brought out of equinus provided the reduction is maintained. The foot should not bear weight for 3 months. Fifty percent of the time closed reduction is not successful. Open reduction through a longitudinal anteromedial incision over the talar neck just medial to the anterior tibial tendon allows direct access to the fracture site. Posterior and anterolateral approaches have also been used. Kirschner wires or lag screws stabilize the fracture. A short leg nonweightbearing cast is used for 8 to 12 weeks.

QUESTIONS

11. How are type III talar neck fractures treated?

12. If signs of avascular necrosis of the talar body without collapse are present, how is the patient treated?

13. What is the rate of avascular necrosis for each type of talar neck fracture?

14. When should Hawkin's sign be sought on radiograph?

15. What is the treatment for failed talar neck fractures that are painful and demonstrate arthritic changes?

16. How should talar head fractures be treated?

17. The hindfoot comprises what bones?

18. The midfoot comprises what bones?

19. The forefoot comprises what bones?

20. What is the midtarsal joint?

ANSWERS

11. Open reduction and internal fixation (closed reduction is almost always unattainable) through posteromedial or anteromedial exposures. If the medial malleolus is fractured, this will aid in reduction. If the malleolus is intact, keep the deltoid ligament attachment to the talus intact since this may carry the blood supply to the talar body. To gain exposure, the medial malleolus may be osteotomized. A transverse Steinmann pin through the calcaneus can help open the space to allow replacement of the talar body beneath the tibia. Lag screws or Kirschner wires are used for fixation.

12. This is controversial. After union of the fracture, weightbearing in a patellar tendon weightbearing cast or double upright ankle-foot orthosis to protect the talar body from collapse until revascularization occurs (which may be 2 years).

13. Type I—0% to 13%; type II—20% to 50%; type III—83% to 100%.

14. Six to 8 weeks after fracture.

15. Blair fusion (tibial–talar neck fusion) or tibiocalcaneal fusion.

16. Nondisplaced fractures are treated in a short leg cast for 6 weeks, and arch support for 6 months. Displaced fractures are treated by open reduction and internal fixation.

17. Calcaneus and talus.

18. Navicular, cuboid, and three cuneiforms.

19. Metatarsals and phalanges.

20. Chopart's joint (the junction of the hind and midfoot), the confluence of the talonavicular and calcaneocuboid joints.

QUESTIONS

21. What are the four muscular layers of the plantar foot (from superficial to deep)?

22. Identify the structures on this cross section through the forefoot at the base of the metatarsals.

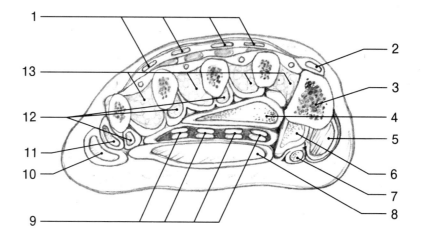

23. Describe the modified Lange-Hansen classification of ankle fractures.

24. Describe the Danis-Weber classification of ankle fractures.

ANSWERS

21. (1) Abductor digiti minimi, flexor digitorum brevis, abductor hallucis; (2) flexor hallucis longus, flexor digitorum longus, quadratus plantae, lumbricals; (3) flexor digiti minimi, adductor hallucis, flexor hallucis brevis; (4) interossei, peroneus longus, tibialis posterior.

22. *1*, extensor digitorum longus; *2*, extensor hallucis longus; *3*, first metatarsal; *4*, adductor hallucis; *5*, abductor hallucis; *6*, flexor hallucis brevis; *7*, flexor hallucis longus; *8*, flexor digitorum brevis; *9*, flexor digitorum longus and lumbricals; *10*, abductor digiti minimi; *11*, flexor digiti minimi brevis; *12*, plantar interossei; *13*, dorsal interossei.

ANSWERS

23. The classification is based on the position of the foot at the time of injury and the direction of force applied. The ankle injuries are described in stages of increasing severity. *Progressive supination-adduction:* transverse fibular fracture at or below the level of the ankle joint, oblique medial malleolus fracture. *Supination-eversion (external rotation): 1*—rupture of the anteroinferior tibiofibular ligament; *2*—spiral or oblique fibula fracture; *3*—posterior tibial lip fracture or tear of the posterior tibiofibular ligament; *4*—medial malleolus fracture or deltoid tear. *Pronation-abduction: 1*—avulsion of the medial malleolus or deltoid tear; *2*—disruption of syndesmosis (but not the interosseous ligament) and posterior tibial lip fracture; *3*—oblique supramalleolar fracture of the fibula. *Pronation-eversion (external rotation): 1*—avulsion of the medial malleolus or deltoid. *2*—syndesmosis tear, tear of the interosseous ligament; *3*—spiral fibula fracture 7 to 8 cm proximal to the tip of the fibula; *4*—posterior tibial lip fracture. *Pronation-dorsiflexion: 1*—medial malleolus fracture; *2*—anterior tibial lip fracture; *3*—intraarticular distal tibia fracture; *4*—supramalleolar fracture of the fibula.

24. The Danis-Weber classification is based upon the type of fibula fracture. *Type A*—internal rotation and adduction—is a transverse fibula fracture at or below the joint line, with a possible shear fracture of the medial malleolus. *Type B*—external rotation—is an oblique fibula fracture arising from the joint line with rupture of the inferior tibiofibular ligament and medial damage. *Type C* is divided into *C1*—abduction—an oblique medial-to-lateral fibula fracture above a ruptured inferior tibiofibular ligament, and *C2*—abduction and external rotation—a short oblique fracture 7 to 8 cm proximal to the distal fibula with extensive syndesmotic rupture. Type C injuries may be associated with deltoid ruptures or with medial or posterior malleolar fractures.

QUESTIONS

25. Draw Böhler's angle. What is the normal range for Böhler's angle?

26. What are the types of extraarticular calcaneal fractures? What are the intraarticular types?

27. What other injuries are associated with calcaneal fractures?

28. Where are the fracture lines in calcaneal body fractures?

29. How are calcaneal body fractures treated?

ANSWERS

25. Böhler's angle is formed by the intersection of a line drawn from the most cephalic point on the tuberosity to the highest part of the posterior facet with a line from the latter to the most cephalic part of the anterior process of the calcaneus. The normal range for Böhler's angle is 25 to 40 degrees.

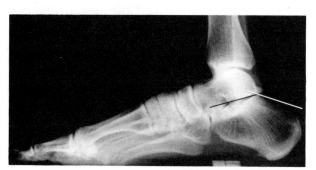

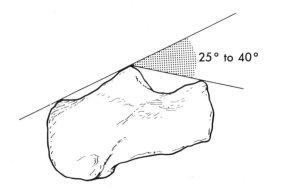

25° to 40°

ANSWERS

26. Extraarticular types are anterior process, tuberosity (break or avulsion), medial process, sustentaculum tali, and body fractures. Intraarticular types are nondisplaced, joint depression, comminuted, and tongue fractures.

27. Thoracolumbar spinal fractures are associated in 10% of calcaneal body fractures. Other injuries of the lower extremity are common. Since bilateral injuries frequently occur, X-ray films of the opposite foot are recommended. Comparison views are useful if no injury is present. Ankle films and thoracolumbar spine films are recommended in all calcaneal fractures.

28. Vertically or obliquely behind the posterior facet. These are, by definition, nonarticular fractures.

29. Elevation, bed rest in a bulky compression dressing for 48 to 72 hours, followed by active range-of-motion, exercises and a touch-down weightbearing cast for 4 to 6 weeks. Young patients with heel widening may benefit from closed reduction using palm pressure to mold the heel into a narrow contour.

QUESTIONS

30. What acts like a wedge, producing intraarticular calcaneal fractures?

31. What are the two main fracture fragments produced by the primary fracture line in intraarticular calcaneal fractures?

32. What are the two patterns of secondary intraarticular calcaneal fracture lines?

33. Where does the secondary fracture line propagate in tongue fractures?

34. How are fractures of the anterior process of the calcaneus treated?

35. How should compression fractures of the anterior process of the calcaneus (intraarticular calcaneocuboid joint) be treated?

36. How are calcaneal tuberosity avulsion fractures treated?

ANSWERS

30. Lateral process of the talus.

31. Anteromedial and posterolateral fragments (see Figure).

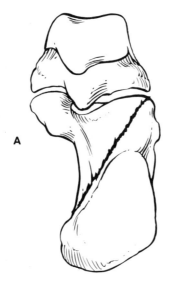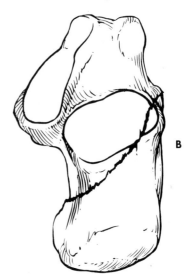

ANSWERS

32. Tongue type and joint depression type.

33. The secondary fracture line runs posteriorly from the apex of the primary fracture line (at the crucial angle). The majority of the posterior facet is in this dorsal tuberosity fragment (see Figure).

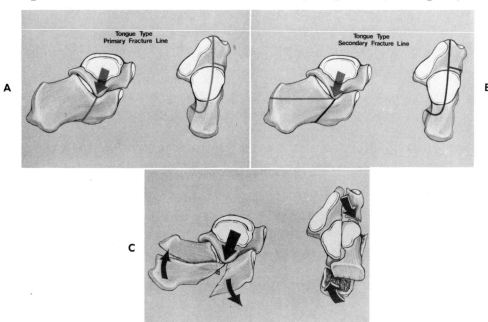

34. Short leg cast for 4 weeks.

35. If large and displaced fragments are present, open reduction and internal fixation.

36. These usually occur in elderly osteoporotic women secondary to a fall. Patients present with calcaneal gait. Undisplaced fractures receive a short leg cast in 5 to 10 degrees of equinus for 6 weeks with partial weightbearing as tolerated. Displaced fractures are treated by open reduction and internal fixation with pins, screws, or wires. A touch-down weightbearing cast is applied for 6 to 8 weeks.

QUESTIONS

37. How should posterior tibial lip fractures in the ankle be treated?

38. How should anterior tibial lip fractures be treated?

39. Which ligament in the ankle prevents excessive ankle inversion in a neutral position?

40. Which ankle ligament prevents excessive inversion in plantar flexion?

41. How are ankle sprains evaluated radiographically?

42. How are complete tears of the anterior talofibular and calcaneofibular ligaments treated?

43. How often does nonunion occur in medial malleolus fractures treated by closed means?

44. How should malunion of an ankle fracture with a talus shifted in the mortise be treated?

45. How often is os trigonum seen in normal feet?

46. What does the lateral process of the talus articulate with?

ANSWERS

37. With fractures involving more than 20% to 25% of the articular surface, open reduction and internal fixation is recommended.

38. With a displaced major fragment, open reduction and internal fixation. If severely comminuted, early range-of-motion exercises using a calcaneal traction pin.

39. Calcaneofibular ligament.

40. The anterior talofibular ligament.

41. Standard views: AP, lateral, and mortise views. Additional studies: AP view neutral and plantar flexion stress radiographs, lateral anterior drawer, and arthrogram.

42. This is controversial, but many repair them and hold in a cast or cast brace for 3 to 4 weeks. Others treat in a long leg cast for 6 weeks.

43. Nonunion occurs in 10% to 15% of cases.

44. If not repaired early, posttraumatic arthritis will occur. Reconstruction should be performed with osteotomy through the fracture sites, repositioning of malleoli, and open reduction and internal fixation. If posttraumatic arthritis is already present, ankle fusion is done.

45. In 50% of cases.

46. With the posterior calcaneal facet and the distal end of the fibula.

QUESTIONS

47. Identify the labeled structures of the medial foot and ankle.

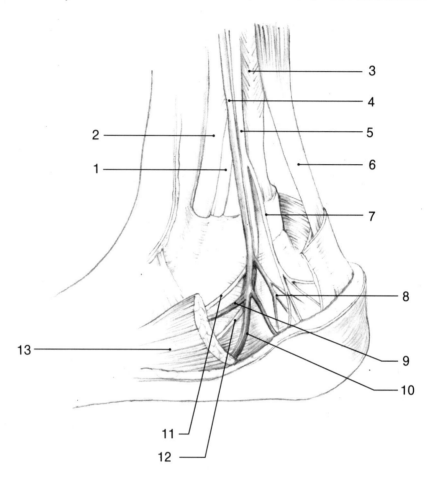

48. What is the blood supply to the talus?

49. Where are fractures of the sustentaculum tali symptomatic?

50. How are nondisplaced fractures of the sustentaculum treated?

51. How are displaced sustentaculum tali fractures treated?

52. How often is the dorsalis pedis artery absent or very small?

ANSWERS

47. *1*, flexor digitorum longus; *2*, tibialis posterior; *3*, flexor hallucis longus; *4*, posterior tibial artery; *5*, tibial nerve; *6*, tendo Achilles; *7*, calcaneal branch of tibial nerve; *8*, calcaneal branches of posterior tibial artery; *9*, medial plantar artery; *10*, lateral plantar artery; *11*, medial plantar nerve; *12*, lateral plantar nerve; *13*, abductor hallucis.

48. The peroneal artery, with branches to the posterior process and a branch which becomes the artery of the sinus tarsi; the anterior tibial artery (dorsalis pedis), with branches to the talar neck and branches to form the artery of the sinus tarsi; the posterior tibial artery to the artery of the tarsal canal, with a deltoid branch to the medial surface of the talar body.

49. Just below the medial malleolus. Pain is worse with foot inversion. Hyperextension of the great toe puts tension on the flexor hallucis longus as it passes under the sustentaculum, which worsens pain at the fracture site. The fracture is best seen on the axial view.

50. Cast immobilization.

51. Closed reduction with direct manipulation of the sustentaculum fragment just below the medial malleolus with foot inversion and plantar flexion followed by a cast for 6 weeks.

52. In 12% of cases.

QUESTIONS

53. Identify the labeled structures on the dorsum of the foot and ankle.

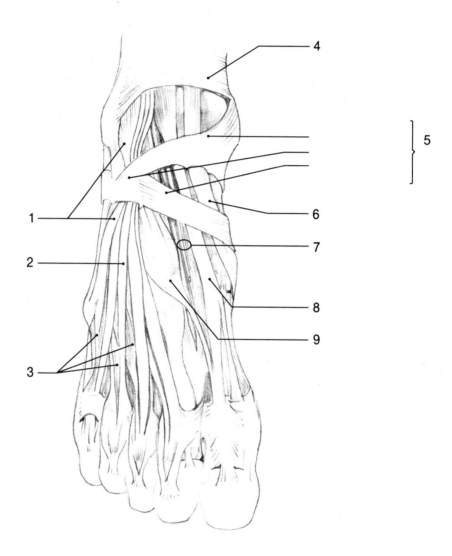

54. What is the recommended treatment for stress reactions of the foot?

55. How should stress fractures of the foot be treated?

56. How should Charcot joints of the foot and ankle be treated?

57. How can one distinguish a Charcot joint from an infection in an adult diabetes patient?

ANSWERS

53. *1*, peroneus tertius; *2*, extensor digitorum longus; *3*, extensor digitorum brevis; *4*, superior extensor retinaculum; *5*, inferior extensor retinaculum (superomedial band, stem, inferomedial band); *6*, tibialis anterior; *7*, neurovascular bundle (dorsalis pedis artery and vein and deep peroneal nerve); *8*, extensor hallucis longus; *9*, extensor hallucis brevis.

54. Stress reactions present with localized pain, swelling, and tenderness, usually within several days of onset of symptoms. Radiographs are negative. The pain is secondary to active remodeling of the bone to the newly applied stresses. The bone scan can be positive as early as 2 days after the pain begins. Complete fracture can be avoided by stress protection until symptoms resolve, usually in 1 to 2 weeks.

55. Immobilization in a short leg walking cast for 4 to 6 weeks.

56. In a cast until the x-ray film shows evidence of healing.

57. Admit the patient to hospital. Place on bed rest with foot elevation and splinting without immediate antibiotics. After 2 to 3 days a Charcot joint will improve, whereas an infection will progress.

QUESTIONS

58. A 32-year-old window washer fell one story from a scaffold, sustaining a "crack" through the tibial plafond which is minimally displaced. How would you treat this patient?

59. How would you treat a comminuted tibial plafond fracture with displacement?

60. Describe the treatment for acute subluxation of the peroneal tendons.

61. What distinguishes an accessory navicular (os tibiale externum) from a navicular tuberosity fracture?

62. How are dorsal lip fractures of the navicular treated?

63. What structure is responsible for avulsion fractures of the navicular tuberosity?

64. How are navicular tuberosity fractures treated?

65. Describe the treatment of navicular body fractures—nondisplaced fractures, large displaced fragments, and comminuted displaced fragments.

ANSWERS

58. With any articular fracture, one should strive toward restoration of the joint surface. Manipulation and casting may be satisfactory treatment. If satisfactory position cannot be obtained through closed reduction, then open reduction with internal fixation is advised.

ANSWERS

59. The options include: (1) Open reduction and internal fixation (ORIF) with compression plating and bone grafting; (2) restoration of fibular length and limited ORIF of plafond with external fixation of the tibia to the calcaneus or talus; (3) if the plafond is too badly comminuted to reconstruct, primary arthrodesis should be performed.

60. Place in plantar flexion in a slightly inverted below-the-knee cast for 6 weeks. If this is not effective in alleviating the problem, then a lateral slip of the Achilles tendon can be detached proximally, left attached distally, and brought in front of the peroneal tendons, and attached to the lateral malleolus. This reconstructs the superior peroneal retinaculum. Another alternative is deepening the peroneal groove on the posterior aspect of the lateral malleolus.

61. The accessory navicular is usually smooth and regular, whereas the fracture has a rough, irregular edge. In addition, the os tibiale externum is bilateral 90% of the time.

62. One should search for a concomitant injury, particularly to the lateral ligaments of the ankle. Chip fractures can be treated with rest and compression dressing. Patients that have fragments larger than just a flake may benefit from immobilization in a short leg walking cast. If there is concomitant injury to the midtarsal joint, then immobilization in a short leg cast is appropriate. Large fragments involving the articular surface should be internally fixed.

63. The tibialis posterior tendon.

64. Most authors advocate symptomatic treatment. If the patient has minimal pain, an Ace bandage wrap and crutches may be used until the pain subsides. For more severe pain, cast immobilization has been recommended. In late cases in which symptomatic nonunion develops, the nonunion fragment may be excised with reattachment of the tibialis posterior tendon.

65. Nondisplaced fractures are treated in an equinus cast for 4 to 6 weeks; large displaced fragments are treated with open reduction and internal fixation; and comminuted displaced fragments with open reduction and internal fixation with bone grafting.

QUESTIONS

66. A 35-year-old runner presents with spontaneous onset of vague pain in the dorsal medial aspect of the foot. The patient noted no injury. On physical examination there is no swelling or discoloration noted. The patient is tender over the tarsal navicular. Radiographs of the foot are normal. What is this patient's most likely diagnosis and how should it be confirmed and treated?

67. What injuries are associated with "nutcracker" fracture of the cuboid?

68. Describe the treatment of a displaced cuboid fracture.

69. How should chip fractures of the cuboid be treated?

70. How are cuneiform fractures treated?

71. Describe the treatment of undisplaced metatarsal shaft fractures.

72. Describe the treatment options of displaced metatarsal shaft fractures.

73. Describe the treatment of metatarsal neck fractures.

74. What is a Jones fracture?

ANSWERS

66. This patient most likely has a stress fracture of the navicular. Bone scan is helpful in identifying this problem as well as tomograms. For nondisplaced fractures, a short leg nonweightbearing cast for 6 to 8 weeks is recommended. With displaced fractures, open reduction and internal fixation should be performed.

ANSWERS

67. Nutcracker cuboid results from a compression of the cuboid between the calcaneus and fourth and fifth metatarsals. These may be associated with tarsometatarsal or midtarsal dislocations.

68. If there is residual displacement of the articular surface of the cuboid, then open reduction and internal fixation should be considered using bone graft, Kirschner wires, or screws. Minimally displaced fractures can be treated in a cast for 4 to 6 weeks.

69. First, rule out injury to the medial aspect of the midtarsal joint. Oblique radiographs of the foot are helpful in delineating this. Injuries with associated midtarsal sprain should be treated in a short leg walking cast for 4 to 6 weeks. Avulsion fractures without midtarsal involvement should be treated symptomatically with either a cast or an Ace bandage wrap.

70. These are rarely displaced and can usually be treated symptomatically.

71. Treatment options range from adhesive taping and a hard-soled shoe to a short leg cast. They usually take 3 to 5 weeks to heal.

72. Treatment is controversial. Closed reduction should be attempted and if satisfactory position is obtained, then treat in a cast for 3 to 6 weeks. Some advocate closed reduction with percutaneous pinning and open reduction and internal fixation following reduction.

73. If nondisplaced, a well-molded short leg walking cast or a hard-soled shoe. If reduction is necessary, then again, a well-molded short leg walking cast followed by a hard-soled shoe is advocated. If reduction cannot be obtained or maintained, then open reduction and internal fixation should be performed.

74. A Jones fracture is a fracture of the proximal fifth metatarsal diaphyseal-metaphyseal junction. This is not the more commonly seen avulsion fracture of the base of the tuberosity.

QUESTIONS

75. How does the Jones fracture differ from an avulsion fracture at the base of the fifth metatarsal?

76. In a child, how do you distinguish an avulsion fracture at the base of the metatarsal from an accessory ossification center?

77. What is the os vesalianum?

78. What is the os peroneum?

79. What is the treatment of acute fifth metatarsal metaphyseal-diaphyseal fractures.

80. What is the treatment of a stress fracture at the metaphyseal-diaphyseal junction of the fifth metatarsal.

81. Describe the treatment of an extraarticular fifth metatarsal base fracture.

82. Describe the treatment of intraarticular fifth metatarsal base fractures.

ANSWERS

75. The avulsion fracture of the base of the metatarsal usually results from the pull of the peroneus brevis tendon and is not usually problematic with regard to healing or becoming asymptomatic. The Jones fracture, on the other hand, has a higher incidence of painful nonunion and may originate as a stress fracture.

76. The orientation of the apophyseal line is parallel to the shaft of the metatarsal and it does not extend proximally into the joint. Fracture lines tend to be oriented more transversely across the metatarsal base.

77. An ossicle in the peroneus brevis tendon where it is seen at the tip of the fifth metatarsal base.

78. A sesamoid in the peroneus longus adjacent to the cuboid.

79. Short leg walking cast for 4 to 8 weeks. Comminuted fractures may require pinning.

80. Patients with low-demand life styles can be treated in a short leg walking cast. High-performance athletes would benefit from open reduction and internal fixation with a lag screw.

81. Symptomatic treatment is appropriate with crutch ambulation and foot support with taping or a firm-soled shoe until the patient feels able to ambulate without support. Patients with displaced fractures sometimes feel better with a period of short leg cast immobilization.

82. Closed treatment is advocated except in high-performance athletes who may benefit from early open reduction and internal fixation. Symptomatic avulsion fractures that have not united can be excised with advancement of the peroneus brevis tendon.

QUESTIONS

83. A 22-year-old ROTC cadet returned from his 2-week summer camp with severe bilateral foot pain. Minimal swelling is noted. There is pain over the second and third metatarsals bilaterally. His activity level has been much higher during his training camp than usual, with 20-mile marches and daily 2-mile runs. What tests should be ordered? What is the most likely diagnosis?

84. Describe the treatment of a displaced great toe proximal phalanx fracture.

85. Describe the treatment of nondisplaced great toe proximal phalanx fractures.

86. Describe the treatment of toe phalangeal fractures other than the great toe.

87. Which sesamoid is more frequently fractured in the great toe?

88. What other conditions can mimic a sesamoid fracture radiographically?

ANSWERS

83. This patient has stress fractures of the metatarsal shafts. They are frequently associated with intensive training, particularly in new recruits. Radiographs of the foot—AP, lateral, and oblique—will diagnose stress fractures 10 to 14 days after they have developed. In this patient's case, the studies may be negative depending upon when, during his training, he developed his stress fractures. They may also be negative if the patient has stress reactions rather than stress fractures. In the aforementioned cases a bone scan is diagnostic. However, with this history, bone scanning is probably unnecessary. The patient should be treated based upon the degree of symptomatology. Minimal pain warrants taping and supportive footwear and a decrease in activities. The patient's activities are limited for 4 to 6 weeks until fracture healing is evident on radiograph and clinical examination. A short leg walking cast is used for more symptomatic patients. Serial radiographs confirm the diagnosis.

84. Closed reduction under local anesthesia with taping to the second digit and a short leg walking cast with a toeplate. If the reduction cannot be obtained or maintained, then open reduction and internal fixation is performed.

85. Short leg walking cast with a toeplate or a hard-soled shoe.

86. Most of these fractures can be treated with closed reduction and taping.

87. The medial sesamoid.

88. Bipartite or multipartite sesamoid and osteochondritis dissecans of the sesamoid. Bipartite sesamoids have smooth margins whereas fractures demonstrate irregular fracture lines. Bipartite sesamoids also are usually larger than a single sesamoid. Bipartite sesamoids are present bilaterally in only 25% of feet. Osteochondritis dissecans of the sesamoid is characterized by fragmentation and irregularity of the sesamoid. These frequently do not have a history of trauma.

QUESTIONS

89. Describe the treatment of acute fractures of a sesamoid.

90. Describe the treatment of total dislocation of the talus.

91. Avulsion or margin fractures of the talonavicular or calcaneocuboid joint are associated with what injuries?

92. What is a Lisfranc fracture-dislocation?

93. What are the three major types of tarsometatarsal dislocation?

94. What is the keystone of the tarsometatarsal joints?

95. Which fractures are most commonly associated with tarsometatarsal dislocations?

96. Describe the treatment of Lisfranc fracture-dislocations.

ANSWERS

89. Some form of padding is placed proximally on the first metatarsal to relieve pressure at the metatarsophalangeal (MTP) joint and on the sesamoid. The leg is placed in a short leg cast or a hard-soled shoe. This type of treatment may be carried on for 4 to 6 months. If pain persists, then excision of the sesamoid is considered.

ANSWERS

90. One attempt at closed reduction can be performed, but this is usually unsuccessful. Open reduction and internal fixation is usually needed. An incision over the talus with the distraction of the calcaneus and tibia through traction pins usually secures reduction. A long leg cast is applied for 4 to 6 weeks followed by a short leg cast and patellar tendon weightbearing brace. In open wounds, which occur in 75% of talar dislocations, thorough debridement is followed by reduction of the talus. Delayed closure is advisable. If the talus is devoid of soft tissue attachment, it can be removed from the wound to facilitate thorough debridement of the open injury. In an open injury with severe contamination of the talus precluding its reduction, a delayed tibiocalcaneal fusion should be planned.

91. Tarsal injuries (sprains, fracture-subluxation, and fracture-dislocation).

92. A fracture-dislocation of the tarsometatarsal joint.

93. (1) Total incongruity of the tarsometatarsal joints with all the joints displaced in the same plane; (2) partial incongruity; one or more of the joints are still reduced; (3) divergent tarsometatarsal dislocations consisting of one or more of the joints displaced in different directions (e.g., the great toe metatarsal is displaced medially while the four lesser toe metatarsals are displaced laterally).

94. The second metatarsal base articulation with the second cuneiform. The metatarsal is recessed between the medial and lateral cuneiforms and therefore articulates with all three. It is rare to see tarsometatarsal dislocations without a fracture of the base of the second metatarsal.

95. Fractures of the base of the second metatarsal and compression fractures of the cuboid.

96. Closed reduction and percutaneous pinning can be performed if anatomic reduction is obtained. In the absence of anatomic reduction, open reduction and internal fixation with Kirschner wires is advocated. Large Kirschner wires across the first and fifth tarsometatarsal joints can stabilize the reduction. The patient is placed in a cast for 6 to 8 weeks after which the pins are removed.

QUESTIONS

97. What are the two types of great toe MTP dislocations?

98. How are dorsal dislocations of the great toe MTP joint treated?

99. Describe the treatment of interphalangeal joint dislocations of the foot.

100. What are the upper limits of the intermetatarsal and MTP angles of the great toe in hallux valgus deformity?

101. What accounts for the medial prominence in hallux valgus?

102. What are the clinical mainfestations of a mild hallux valgus deformity?

103. What are the clinical and radiographic findings in moderate hallux valgus deformity?

104. Describe the clinical and radiographic appearance of a severe hallux valgus deformity.

ANSWERS

97. Type 1 is dorsal dislocation; the sesamoids are not fractured or separated. In type 2A, a rupture of the intersesamoid ligament is present. In type 2B, a transverse fracture of one or both sesamoids is present. Type 1 injuries are difficult to reduce closed; type 2 injuries are easily reduced.

98. Closed reduction is attempted for both type 1 and type 2 dislocations. If closed reduction is successful, a cast with a dorsal block toeplate is applied for 2 to 3 weeks. Then a hard-soled shoe is used. If closed reduction is not obtained after two attempts, an open reduction through a dorsal incision between the first and second metatarsal heads is performed. The adductor hallucis may be detached from the fibular sesamoid and the deep transverse metatarsal ligament to facilitate reduction. These structures are then reattached to the fibular sesamoid after reduction. Postreduction treatment is similar to closed reduction.

ANSWERS

99. These usually reduce closed and are treated with buddy taping and hard-soled shoe ambulation. They are typically stable following reduction. Unstable joints should be stabilized with Kirschner wires for 3 weeks.

100. An intermetatarsal angle greater than 9 degrees and an MTP angle greater than 15 degrees are considered abnormal.

101. Several factors contribute to this deformity. Displacement of the proximal phalanx in a lateral direction uncovers the medial aspect of the metatarsal head, which makes it appear more prominent. In addition, there is hypertrophy of the soft tissues overlying the medial metatarsal head and the bone here may hypertrophy up to 3 to 5 mm. The medial deviation of the first metatarsal also contributes.

102. There is minimal metatarsus primus varus, the MTP joint is congruent, and there is very little valgus deformity (MTP angle <20 degrees). There is, however, a painful, medial prominence of the metatarsal head. The sesamoids are in anatomic position on radiographs.

103. Radiographs demonstrate an MTP angle of 20 to 40 degrees with loss of congruence of the MTP joint. There is nearly complete displacement of the lateral sesamoid from beneath the metatarsal head. The hallux is pronated.

104. Radiographs demonstrate total dislocation of the lateral sesamoid into the intermetatarsal space. The MTP angle is greater than 40 degrees, and there is significant incongruence of the MTP joint. There is marked lateral deviation of the great toe with associated pronation of the hallux. Significant metatarsus primus varus may also be present.

QUESTIONS

105. What is the most common cause of failure of McBride bunionectomy?

106. What type of operation should be recommended for a patient with hallux valgus with an intermetatarsal angle of 25 degrees and an MTP angle of 30 degrees?

107. What are the major deformities in hallux valgus that should be evaluated in planning an approach to surgical correction?

108. What are contraindications to a chevron osteotomy in hallux valgus?

109. What are the indications for a Keller bunionectomy?

110. What is the major complication noted in the Keller procedure?

111. What is the Akin procedure?

112. What are the major problems with an Akin procedure?

ANSWERS

105. Insufficient reefing of the medial capsule or inadequate release of the contracted lateral tissues of the MTP joint. The presence of an untreated significant metatarsus primus varus will also result in failure. Attenuated medial capsular structures which could not hold sutures and improper postoperative dressings are other causes.

ANSWERS

106. An intermetatarsal angle greater than 15 degrees usually requires a proximal metatarsal osteotomy for correction. In addition, an exostosis excision with medial capsular repair, adductor release, division of the transverse metatarsal ligament, and capsulotomy of a contracted lateral MTP joint capsule should be performed. The adductor is transferred to the first metatarsal.

107. Valgus deformity of the MTP joint, the bump over the hallux metatarsal head, pronation of the hallux, subluxation of the sesamoids, and metatarsus primus varus.

108. An MTP angle greater than 35 degrees, intermetatarsal angle greater than 15 degrees, incongruent MTP joint, or significant pronation of the hallux.

109. The Keller procedure consists of resections of the medial metatarsal head and the base of the proximal phalanx. The procedure has largely fallen out of use except for very specific narrow indications. Elderly patients with severe hallux valgus who are poor operative candidates and who have minimal demands on their feet with minimal ambulatory expectations are candidates. Other options should be sought for treatment of MTP arthritis, such as cheilectomy or arthrodesis. A Keller procedure is contraindicated in patients with short first metatarsals. A Keller operation in this situation is likely to lead to transference of major weightbearing forces to the second metatarsal with associated metatarsalgia.

110. Metatarsalgia of the second and third metatarsal heads. One may also find a cockup deformity of the great toe as a result of excessive proximal phalanx resection.

111. A closing wedge osteotomy of the base of the proximal phalanx with associated medial bump excision and capsulorrhaphy.

112. Malunion of the osteotomy is the major complication. Avascular necrosis is also possible if there is significant soft tissue stripping of the proximal phalanx fragment.

QUESTIONS

113. What is the recommended position for MTP joint arthrodesis with regard to dorsiflexion or plantar flexion and varus or valgus angulation?

114. What is the treatment of choice for adolescent hallux valgus deformity?

115. A 55-year-old woman presents with hallux valgus associated with hypermobility of the first metatarsal cuneiform joint. What is your approach to treating this patient?

116. A 60-year-old man has developed severe hallux valgus associated with spasticity from a stroke he sustained 1 year ago. What is the most likely cause of this problem and how should it be treated?

117. A patient has had a first metatarsal osteotomy, which has healed in a dorsiflexed position. What will the patient complain about following this complication?

118. What complication results from excess medial metatarsal head excision in bunion surgery?

119. Following a chevron osteotomy of the distal hallux metatarsal, the patient developed avascular necrosis with painful collapse of the metatarsal head. What is your salvage for this situation?

120. What causes the postsurgical cockup deformity of the first MTP joint?

ANSWERS

113. Because the first metatarsal is normally in 15 degrees of plantar flexion, the MTP joint should be fused in 30 degrees of dorsiflexion to obtain a final angle of 15 degrees of dorsiflexion of the great toe relative to the ground. Fifteen degrees of valgus angulation should be incorporated into the fusion.

ANSWERS

114. Accommodative shoewear should be tried initially. If this does not alleviate symptoms, surgery may be considered. This condition is usually associated with metatarsus primus varus and a soft tissue procedure alone is inadequate for correction. A soft tissue procedure combined with an osteotomy of the metatarsal is usually necessary.

115. Initially, conservative care. If this is unsuccessful, then metatarsal cuneiform arthrodesis in a corrected position should be performed.

116. This usually develops from spastic equinus deformity such that the patient rolls off the medial border of the foot to compensate, producing the hallux valgus deformity. The underlying equinus deformity should be corrected prior to the bunion operation; otherwise the deformity is likely to recur. Arthrodesis of the MTP joint is a fairly reliable procedure.

117. Painful metatarsalgia from weight transfer to the other metatarsal heads.

118. Frequently a hallux varus deformity develops with an associated unstable MTP joint and medial subluxation of the tibial sesamoid. Overly generous resection of the medial metatarsal head can also produce incongruence of the MTP joint with subsequent degenerative changes.

119. MTP joint arthrodesis, sometimes using an interposition graft to prevent collapse, is helpful.

120. This is usually the result of loss of function of the flexor hallucis brevis (FHB) muscle as it inserts into the base of the proximal phalanx. This deformity is often seen associated with a hallux varus deformity, which is the result of medial displacement of the FHB with the intact medial sesamoid following a lateral sesamoid excision. The displaced FHB is ineffective in producing MTP flexion. If both sesamoids have been excised, then this deformity is likely to be caused by the complete loss of short flexor function. In addition, this can be seen after the Keller procedure in which the FHB has been released.

QUESTIONS

121. Describe the treatment for the MTP cockup deformity.

122. A 70-year-old woman has developed an intractable plantar keratosis beneath the great toe MTP joint following a McBride bunionectomy. The lateral sesamoid was excised during this procedure. What is the cause of her plantar keratosis and how should it be treated?

123. List factors that can produce hallux varus deformity.

124. Which toe is most frequently affected in mallet toe deformity?

125. What is the most common cause of hammer toe deformity?

126. What is a clawtoe deformity and how does it differ from a hammer toe?

127. What is the relationship of the interossei tendons and lumbricals relative to the transverse metatarsal ligament in the foot?

128. The intrinsic muscles of the foot are responsible for flexing or extending which joints?

ANSWERS

121. The extensor hallucis longus (EHL) is transferred to the neck of the metatarsal with arthrodesis of the interphalangeal joint. This procedure thereby rebalances the tendons acting across the MTP joint. The EHL helps to dorsiflex the metatarsal while the interphalangeal arthrodesis allows the flexor hallucis longus to function more efficiently across the MTP joint.

122. The medial sesamoid comes to lie between the plantar skin and the midportion of the metatarsal head. This develops because the intersesamoidal ridge, which helps stabilize the sesamoids, has attenuated as a result of longstanding hallux valgus deformity. This allows the medial sesamoid to assume a prominent position. The initial treatment would consist of metatarsal head pressure relief with metatarsal bars, pads, or molded orthoses. If this is unsuccessful, shaving the plantar half of the sesamoid may produce relief.

ANSWERS

with metatarsal bars, pads, or molded orthoses. If this is unsuccessful, shaving the plantar half of the sesamoid may produce relief. One should not remove the sesamoid in the face of a previous excision of a lateral medial sesamoid since this may lead to the cockup deformity of the first MTP joint.

123. In general, hallux varus is rare and is primarily iatrogenic. The surgical factors include overcorrection through excessive capsular plication, medial displacement of the medial sesamoid, excessive medial metatarsal head excision, aggressive postoperative immobilization in a varus position, overpull of the abductor hallucis in association with insufficient lateral support of the MTP joint, excessive lateral correction of the first metatarsal osteotomy, and overcorrection in osteotomy of the medially displaced proximal phalanx.

124. Mallet toe is a flexion deformity at the distal interphalangeal joint. It occurs most frequently in the second toe, which is usually the longest toe of the foot. The cause is pressure against the end of the shoe.

125. Hammer toe deformity can be caused by neuromuscular diseases such as Friedreich's ataxia, Charcot-Marie-Tooth disease, cerebral palsy, multiple sclerosis, compartmental syndrome of the deep posterior compartment, myelodysplasia, disc disease, diabetes, and leprosy. It is most frequently seen in patients with ill-fitting shoes.

126. A clawtoe deformity consists of flexion of the interphalangeal joints with hyperextension at the MTP joints. Hammer toe, in contrast, has no involvement of the MTP joints. Causes of clawtoe are similar to those of hammer toe.

127. The lumbricals are located plantar to the transverse metatarsal ligament whereas the interossei tendons are dorsal.

128. The intrinsics of the foot have a function analogous to the intrinsic muscles in the hand in that they flex the MTP joints and extend the interphalangeal joints.

QUESTIONS

129. What is the major structure in the foot which resists dorsiflexion at the MTP joints?

130. In the treatment of hammer toe deformity, what other factors need to be considered?

131. How should young patients with hammer toes be treated?

132. Describe the DuVries arthroplasty for hammer toe deformity.

133. A patient with hammer toe deformity also has some hyperextension at the MTP joints. What type of approach should be taken toward correction of the MTP deformity?

134. What is the cause of flexible hammer toe deformity?

135. Describe the treatment of mallet toe deformity.

136. A 45-year-old woman with claw deformity of the toes has metatarsalgia. There are no other significant foot problems noted on examination. Her neuromuscular examination is likewise normal. Clawing of the toes resolves with ankle plantar flexion. With ankle dorsiflexion the clawing returns. How should this patient be managed?

137. How is a fixed claw deformity corrected?

ANSWERS

129. The plantar pad, which is a confluence of the plantar aponeurosis and plantar joint capsule.

ANSWERS

130. The tautness of the flexor digitorum longus tendon. If it is tight in the adjacent toe, it will need to be released in the deformed toe to prevent recurrence. If there is MTP hyperextension in a standing position, this too must be corrected at the time of hammer toe surgery or the toe will tend to stick up in the air. Concomitant hallux valgus may narrow the toe box, crowding the toes into the hammer toe position. This should be corrected as well.

131. Conservative care consists of passive stretching of the digits and accommodative shoewear. Local padding may be used. A metatarsal bar may be helpful. In severe resistant cases, extradepth shoes with Plastazote liners may help.

132. This is a resection of the proximal phalanx head.

133. In mild cases, an extensor tenotomy at the same time as correction of the hammer toe is helpful. For more advanced cases, a dorsal capsulotomy with Kirschner wire fixation for 2 to 3 weeks may be appropriate. For dislocations of the MTP joint, an MTP arthroplasty should be performed.

134. Contracture of the FDL tendon. It can be corrected by transfer of the FDL to the EDL tendon over the midportion of the proximal phalanx, thereby changing its function to reinforce the intrinsic function, i.e., MTP flexion and interphalangeal joint extension.

135. Mallet toe deformity is a flexion deformity at the distal interphalangeal joint of a toe. For flexible deformities, release of the FDL tendon is recommended. For a flexion contracture, however, FDL release as well as middle phalanx head resection are required.

136. Conservative care. This consists of accommodative footwear with a metatarsal bar or pad. Surgical options include extensor tenotomies and MTP joint capsulotomies associated with transfer of the FDL to the extensor mechanism, similar to flexible hammer toe correction.

137. Excision of the proximal phalanx head with release of the dorsal contractures of the MTP joints, and release of the flexor tendons with provisional Kirschner wire fixation.

QUESTIONS

138. Atraumatic dorsal subluxation of the base of the proximal phalanx of the second toe is a common problem. What would be a surgical approach to this problem?

139. Describe your treatment for atraumatic unreducible dorsal dislocation of the second toe MTP joint without a hammer toe deformity.

140. What is the surgical treatment for a complete fixed dislocation of the second MTP joint with associated hammer toe deformity?

141. A 50-year-old laborer has had a painful small toe for the past 20 years which is becoming more symptomatic. The small toe is noted to be cocked up with callosities over its dorsal surface. Radiographs demonstrate the proximal phalanx to be sitting at a right angle to the axis of the small toe metatarsal. What is the treatment of choice for this problem?

142. What is the surgical treatment for a symptomatic externally rotated fifth toe which overlaps the fourth toe?

143. What is hallux rigidis?

144. A 16-year-old boy has had problems with great toe pain, particularly when running. On physical examination there is swelling about the MTP joint without any angular deformity. Plantar flexion is satisfactory but he has no dorsiflexion of the toe. Radiographs demonstrate an osteochondritic defect in the metatarsal head. What is this patient's problem and how should it be treated?

145. What is the conservative management for adult hallux rigidis?

ANSWERS

138. Transection of the extensor tendon, collateral ligaments, and dorsal capsule with reduction of the joint and maintenance of the toe in a plantar-flexed position for about 6 weeks.

ANSWERS

139. The surgical approach is similar to that in subluxation, the only difference being that a portion of the articular surface of the metatarsal head is removed to allow reduction of the base of the proximal phalanx. In addition, a Kirschner wire is used to hold the reduction for about 3 weeks.

140. The surgical technique is the same as for the complete dislocation without hammer toe, with the addition of excision of the proximal phalanx head, release of the FDL, and Kirschner wire fixation from the tip of the toe into the metatarsal head.

141. Excision of the proximal phalanx with or without syndactylization.

142. Removal of the proximal phalanx with syndactylization of the fourth toe is a successful technique. Another is the DuVries correction: release of the MTP dorsal medial capsule, medial collateral ligament, and extensor tendon. Another is transfer of the EDL of the fifth toe into the abductor digiti quinti tendon.

143. Degenerative joint disease of the MTP joint of the great toe. It is usually associated with bony proliferation in the dorsal aspect of the joint. The plantar aspect is usually spared.

144. This patient has a congenital or juvenile hallux rigidis. Conservative care includes rest and immobilization. In the adolescent patient, wedge resection of the dorsal aspect of the proximal phalanx has been shown to be helpful in restoring motion and relieving pain. Excision of the osteochondritic defect may also be considered.

145. Accommodative shoewear consisting of a hard-soled or rocker-bottom shoe with an adequate toe box to avoid pressure on the MTP joint of the great toe. Nonsteroidal anti-inflammatory drugs, intra-articular steroid injections, and occasionally a short leg walking cast for 1 month may be beneficial.

QUESTIONS

146. What are the surgical treatment options for hallux rigidis in adults?

147. A 33-year-old motorcycle enthusiast has had persistent midfoot pain following a Lisfranc fracture-dislocation sustained 3 years ago. He had an early closed reduction and pinning. Despite this he has developed flatfoot with abduction of the forefoot. Radiographs demonstrate metatarsal cuneiform degenerative arthritis. What are his treatment options?

148. The previous patient's brother, also a motorcycle enthusiast, crashed his bike 3 years ago and while in the office with his brother, asks if you could look at his injured foot as well. He has posttraumatic arthritis of the talonavicular joint which is bothering him a great deal. He requests treatment for this problem. What do you recommend?

149. What is your initial approach to a rheumatoid patient with metatarsalgia?

150. A rheumatoid patient has had great toe MTP arthritis with deformity unresponsive to conservative care. What is your surgical approach to this problem?

151. A 47-year-old woman with longstanding rheumatoid arthritis has had bilateral hindfoot pain and deformity unresponsive to orthotic treatment. The ankle joint is not affected. The patient has good range of motion and no pain. There is severe hindfoot valgus. When the hindfoot valgus is corrected, the forefoot assumes a more plantigrade position. What is the recommended treatment for this patient?

152. Where does one usually see corns and calluses on the foot?

153. A 50-year-old man has developed a painful callosity over the lateral aspect of the small toe. This area is reddened and tender with thickened skin. Describe your treatment of this lesion.

154. What is the most frequent cause of corns and calluses over the central toes?

ANSWERS

146. Dorsal cheilectomy or MTP arthrodesis.

147. Conservative care would consist of a rigid orthosis or a rocker-bottom shoe. If these modifications are not helpful, then an arthrodesis of the metatarsal cuneiform joints that are involved in the degenerative process should be performed with correction of the abnormal foot alignment.

148. Initially, a padded longitudinal arch support or an AFO are helpful. Ultimately, he will probably require a talonavicular arthrodesis.

149. Metatarsal arch supports, and soft-soled or rocker-bottom shoes. If hammer toes are present, then an extradepth shoe with Plastazote lining may be necessary.

150. Arthrodesis of the MTP joint is probably the best option. Resection arthroplasty is also an option.

151. Subtalar arthrodesis.

152. These are usually located over periarticular areas, specifically near condylar prominences. They are rarely seen over the shafts of long bones. They are the result of pressure from the shoe and underlying bone acting on the skin.

153. This is a very characteristic site for a corn which develops over the head of the proximal phalanx. Conservative care consists of shoe stretching to accommodate the foot, or change in shoewear to a shoe with a wider toe box. Operative treatment consists of condylar excision with or without excision of the base of the middle phalanx.

154. These are usually secondary to hammer or mallet toe deformities. Surgical correction of the underlying condition usually leads to resolution of the corns and calluses dorsally.

QUESTIONS

155. What produces a soft corn between the fourth and fifth toes?

156. What is the surgical treatment for the soft corn between the fourth and fifth toes?

157. What are calluses?

158. What should one evaluate when looking at the potential causes of plantar keratoses?

159. Describe the conservative treatment of plantar keratoses.

160. What is the most common cause of intractable plantar keratosis of the great toe MTP joint?

161. How should an intractable plantar keratosis due to a prominent medial sesamoid be treated?

162. A plantar-flexed first metatarsal produces what type of intractable plantar keratosis?

163. What is the surgical treatment for this condition?

164. Why is it important to differentiate small discrete plantar keratoses from diffuse plantar keratoses in the central three toes?

ANSWERS

155. This is a result of pressure of the base of the fourth proximal phalanx against the medial aspect of the head of the proximal phalanx of the fifth toe. The lesion itself is the same as a corn elsewhere in the foot in that it is the result of excessive pressure. The reason it is termed *soft corn* is because the hyperkeratotic skin is softened by the moisture between the toes.

ANSWERS

156. Medial condylectomy of the proximal phalanx of the fifth toe.

157. These are essentially the same as corns, the only difference being that they occur on the plantar aspect of the foot. Symptomatic plantar calluses are known as intractable plantar keratosis.

158. Hindfoot and forefoot varus or valgus angulation may produce excessive weightbearing on the forefoot, which leads to keratoses. Bony problems such as a plantar-flexed metatarsal, enlarged sesamoid, or a particularly long metatarsal may lead to plantar keratosis. Finally, ill-fitting shoewear such as high-heeled pointed shoes can produce excessive pressure.

159. Low-heeled accommodative shoewear with metatarsal support.

160. A localized keratosis most frequently occurs plantar to the medial sesamoid. This can be due to either medial sesamoid enlargement or displacement to a more central position overlying the metatarsal head, thereby producing excessive localized pressure.

161. Conservative measures previously described for plantar keratosis are applicable here. Surgically, excision of the plantar half of the sesamoid is considered more desirable than total sesamoid excision.

162. This usually produces a diffuse plantar keratosis which is associated with a forefoot valgus deformity and Charcot-Marie-Tooth disease.

163. Osteotomy at the base of the first metatarsal with correction of the plantar flexion. Excessive correction, however, can lead to a transfer of weight to the lateral metatarsal heads. Caution should be exercised not to overcorrect.

164. The causes and thus the treatment are different.

QUESTIONS

165. What causes small discrete plantar keratoses?

166. What is the surgical treatment of a discrete plantar keratotic lesion under the metatarsal head?

167. What is the cause of large, diffuse plantar keratoses over the central three toes?

168. What is the preferred treatment for the large diffuse plantar keratosis under the metatarsal head?

169. What is the current opinion of excision of the metatarsal head for intractable plantar keratosis?

170. What is a tailor's bunion?

171. What are the causes of tailor's bunions?

172. Describe the treatment of tailor's bunion.

173. Where are foot interdigital neuromas most frequently seen?

174. Describe the demographic characteristics of the population with interdigital neuromas.

ANSWERS

165. An enlarged fibular condylar projection from the metatarsal head. Conservative treatment of this lesion consists of trimming of the callus, and accommodative shoewear with an appropriate metatarsal pad.

ANSWERS

166. Condylectomy and arthroplasty of the metatarsal head.

167. This results from plantar-flexed or relatively long metatarsals. This type of lesion is usually about 1.5 cm across and lacks a central keratotic core.

168. Corrective metatarsal osteotomy.

169. This is a bad procedure. It produces transfer lesions (transfer of the intractable plantar keratosis to adjacent submetatarsal head areas) and shortening of the toe.

170. Tailor's bunion, also known as a bunionette, develops at the small toe MTP joint. It is similar to classic hallux valgus except that the bump is on the lateral aspect of the foot and the phalanges angulate toward the great toe.

171. Soft tissue hypertrophy over the lateral aspect of the metatarsal head, congenital enlargement of the metatarsal head, or lateral angulation of the fifth toe metatarsal, singly or in combination.

172. Conservative care is appropriate for mild and moderate cases, and consists of accommodative shoewear. Surgical treatment in severe cases depends upon the cause. If a wide metatarsal head is implicated, then the lateral condyle is excised. If the cause is a laterally deviated plantar-flexed metatarsal, then a fifth toe metatarsal osteotomy should be performed.

173. In the third or second intermetatarsal space. Neuromas of the first and fourth spaces are rare.

174. These are seen more frequently in women than men, with a female-male ratio of 4:1 to 10:1. Average age of patients is the mid-fifties. Most lesions are unilateral.

QUESTIONS

175.   What are the characteristic signs and symptoms of interdigital neuroma?

176.   Describe conservative treatment for interdigital neuroma of the foot.

177.   Failing conservative care, what surgery is performed for interdigital neuroma?

178.   Where are lateral talar dome osteochondritis dissecans lesions located in the AP plane?

179.   Where are the medial talar dome lesions in the AP plane in osteochondritis dissecans?

180.   What is the recommended treatment for undisplaced osteochondritis dissecans of the talar dome?

181.   How is a completely detached osteochondral fragment treated in osteochondritis dissecans of the lateral talar dome that remains in its crater?

182.   What is the surgical approach to a detached osteochondral lesion of the medial talar dome?

183.   In osteochondritis dissecans of the talar dome, is the medial or lateral lesion more likely to have displaced fragments and loose bodies?

184.   What is the common deformity in cavovarus feet?

ANSWERS

175. The primary symptom is pain in the plantar aspect of the foot between the metatarsal heads that is aggravated by activity and relieved by rest. Physical findings consist of plantar tenderness between the metatarsal heads to palpation. Sometimes one can palpate the neuroma. There should be an absence of MTP joint pain with manipulation.

176. Sensible footwear: low heels, wide toe box, a comfortable soft-soled shoe. Sometimes a metatarsal pad proximal to the involved site will distribute the weight over a wider area and relieve symptoms.

177. Excision of the neuroma.

178. The middle one third of the lateral talar dome.

179. The posterior one third of the medial talar dome.

180. A short period of immobilization will usually allow these to heal.

181. Excision with curettage and possibly drilling the base of the lesion. This can be performed arthroscopically or through an anterolateral approach.

182. If the osteochondral fragment is still in its crater, there is a good possibility that this will heal with cast immobilization. If the osteochondral fragment is loose in the joint, then the crater will require curettage and possibly drilling with excision of the loose fragment. A transmalleolar osteotomy may be needed for treatment, although some operating arthroscopists may be able to manage this without a formal arthrotomy.

183. The lateral lesion.

184. A pronated forefoot secondary to plantar-flexed first ray, which causes compensatory hindfoot varus deformity. With growth this may become a structural rigid deformity.

QUESTIONS

185. Describe Coleman's lateral block test.

186. In a cavovarus foot, if the hindfoot is rigid, what surgery is recommended?

187. If the hindfoot is supple in a cavovarus foot, what surgery is usually corrective?

188. Describe the deformity present in metatarsus adductus.

189. A 25-year-old motorcycle enthusiast crashed his three-wheeler, sustaining an injury to his right ankle. He has swelling and tenderness along the medial malleolus as well as the lateral aspect of the distal two thirds of the leg. Ankle radiographs demonstrate a transverse medial malleolar fracture which is displaced 3 mm. What radiographs should be obtained?

190. What is a Maisonneuve fracture?

191. Describe the treatment for a Maisonneuve fracture.

ANSWERS

185. A block is placed so as to allow the plantar-flexed first ray to hang free and thus negate the tripod effect. A supple hindfoot will assume its normal valgus position. With a rigid hindfoot, the varus heel position is maintained.

ANSWERS

186. Plantar medial release: radical plantar release and medial tarsal release.

187. Radical plantar release: release of the abductor hallucis, plantar intrinsics, plantar calcaneonavicular (Spring) ligament, and calcaneonavicular portion of the bifurcate ligament.

188. Forefoot adduction and slight varus. The lateral border of the foot is convex with a dorsal and lateral prominence at the base of the fifth metatarsal and cuboid. Moderate to severe heel valgus is present. No equinus is present. Radiograph shows the first metatarsal to be more sharply angulated than the fifth.

189. AP and lateral films of the leg should be obtained to rule out a proximal fibula fracture. It is likely that this patient has a Maisonneuve fracture.

190. An injury resulting from an external rotation force to the ankle with transmission of the force through the interosseous membrane, which exits through a proximal fibular fracture. This injury may occur with a medial malleolus avulsion fracture or deltoid ligament rupture, rupture of the anterior talofibular ligament or avulsion of its insertion; rupture of the interosseous ligament; rupture of the posterior tibiofibular ligament or an avulsion fracture from the posterior tibia; and a fracture of the proximal one third of the fibula.

191. Examination under anesthesia is advised to evaluate the degree of instability. In unstable injuries, repair of the deltoid ligament and open reduction and internal reduction of the medial malleolus is performed with repair of anteroinferior tibiofibular ligaments and placement of a syndesmotic screw. The proximal fibular fracture requires no fixation. The patient is then placed in a short leg non-weightbearing cast for 6 weeks. Injuries that are thought to be stable can be treated with long leg cast immobilization. If closed treatment is elected, patients must be followed frequently with radiographic evaluation for displacement of the mortise. This often occurs after swelling subsides and the cast no longer fits well.

CHAPTER 11

Biomechanics

Thomas Otto, M.D.

QUESTIONS

1. What is biomechanics?

2. What is the *Système International d'Unités* (SI units)?

3. What are the four base SI units used in the study of biomechanics?

4. What is a pascal (Pa)?

5. What is a joule (J)?

6. Define the following terms: *abduction, adduction, varus, valgus.*

7. What is meant by the term *abiotrophy?*

8. What is the normal periodicity of collagen fiber?

9. What is meant by the term *density?*

10. What is the Donnan osmotic pressure?

ANSWERS

1. Biomechanics is the study of mechanical motion as it relates to biological systems.

2. The SI is the modernized metric system adopted by the General Conference of Weights and Measures in 1960. It is the international language of mechanics and biomechanics.

3. The meter (m), the kilogram (kg), the second (s), and the kelvin (K).

4. A pascal is the pressure that is produced by a force of 1 newton applied over an area of 1 square meter, i.e., 1 Pa = 1 N/m². A pascal is the international unit of pressure and stress.

5. A joule is the unit of work done by the force of 1 newton moving an object through a distance of 1 meter in the direction of the force, i.e., 1 J = 1 Nm.

6. *Abduction* refers to movement away from the anatomic midline. *Adduction* refers to movement toward the anatomic midline. *Valgus* refers to angulation with the distalmost part away from the midline. *Varus* refers to angulation with the distalmost part toward the midline.

7. *Abiotrophy* refers to a degeneration or failure of microscopic or macroscopic structure of a body tissue or part. This term may also refer to conditions that result from some inborn defect which are not evident until sometime after birth. Huntington's chorea, for example, is an abiotrophic disease process.

8. The normal periodicity of collagen fiber is 640 Angström units.

9. Density is the mass per unit volume.

10. Donnan osmotic pressure refers to the pressure that is generated across a semipermeable membrane from a solution of lesser solute concentration to one of greater solute concentration.

QUESTIONS

11. What is meant by the term *dynamics?*

12. What are the four mechanisms of metallic corrosion as applied to orthopedic surgery?

13. What are the three classes of metal alloys used in orthopedic implants?

14. As it applies to implant materials or bone, define the term *strength.*

15. As it applies to implant materials or bone, define the term *rigidity.*

16. What is the theoretical disadvantage of a fracture fixation implant with too much rigidity?

17. What is the trade name of polyglycolic acid suture? What is the trade name of polyglactin 910?

18. After 2 weeks in vivo, what is the approximate strength of polyglactin 910 suture?

19. Comparing silk, polyester, nylon, and polypropylene, which appears to be the most nonreactive and the one retaining the greatest strength for the longest period of time?

20. What is the biomechanical effect of excessive femoral component flexion in total knee arthroplasty?

21. Of the three metal alloys commonly used in orthopedic surgery, which is most susceptible to corrosion?

22. What is passivity?

ANSWERS

11. *Dynamics* refers to the study of forces acting on a body in motion.

12. (1) General corrosion, (2) galvanic corrosion, (3) localized corrosion, and (4) stress corrosion.

13. (1) Cobalt chrome alloys, (2) stainless steel alloys, and (3) titanium alloys.

14. *Strength* is the resistance of a material to an applied load.

15. *Rigidity* is the resistance of a material to deformation, i.e., rigidity = load/deformation.

16. The theoretical and observed response to too much fracture rigidity is osteoporosis about the fracture site. This is believed to result from a suppression of the normal physiologic bending stimulus to bone.

17. Polyglycolic acid suture is also known as Dexon suture. Polyglactin 910 is also known as Vicryl.

18. Fifty percent.

19. Monofilament polypropylene (Prolene) suture.

20. Excessive femoral component flexion is the most common technical error in the sagittal plane. Excessive flexion of the femoral component causes a relative hyperextension of the femoral component in full extension. This places an abnormal load on the anterior portion of the tibial component.

21. Stainless steel.

22. Passivity is the process or theory by which each of the three metal alloys is protected by a so-called protective film from the surrounding corrosive environment in which it lies.

QUESTIONS

23. Give an example of galvanic corrosion.

24. Give an example of crevice corrosion.

25. What are the two systemic effects of orthopedic implant materials?

26. What are the two biomechanical requirements of a fracture fixation device?

27. What two mechanical terms are used to describe the performance of an implant?

28. Describe a load-sharing system.

29. Doubling the thickness of a bone plate does what to its bending strength?

30. Doubling the width of a bone plate does what to its bending strength?

31. Compare the torsional stiffness of a slotted and an unslotted intramedullary rod.

ANSWERS

23. The term implies that dissimilar metals become, in effect, a battery (galvanic cell). Galvanic corrosion may occur when 316L stainless steel alloy comes in contact with either chrome cobalt alloy or titanium alloy. Galvanic corrosion apparently does not occur when cobalt chrome alloy and titanium alloy come in contact.

ANSWERS

24. Crevice corrosion is a localized corrosion in which an area of the implant surface is minimally exposed to the surrounding physiologic environment. There is an apparent influx of the corrosive chloride ion because of the localized depletion of oxygen and localized increase in the metallic and hydrogen ion concentration. An example of this is the corrosion frequently seen between the head of a screw and its contact point with a bone plate.

25. Toxicity and allergic reaction. Allergic reactions have been reported to cobalt chrome and nickel.

26. First, that it maintain the alignment and apposition of the fractured bone. Second, that it be able to transmit forces through the device or bone fragments to optimize fracture healing.

27. *Strength* and *cross-sectional area* of the implant. Strength is a function of the yield strength. Stiffness is a function of the elastic modulus multiplied by the cross-sectional area of the plate.

28. Load sharing refers to the equal or unequal distribution of load through two adjacent materials. An example is a fractured radius internally fixed with a compression bone plate. The compressive load is shared by both the radius and the bone plate. When an axial compressive load is applied to the bone plate system, the bone and plate share the load in a manner proportional to the relative stiffnesses of the two materials.

29. Bending strength is proportional to the thickness of a plate squared. Therefore, doubling the thickness increases bend strength by a factor of 4.

30. Bending strength is directly proportional to the width of a plate. Therefore, doubling the width increases the bend strength by a factor of 2.

31. Torsional stiffness is greater for an unslotted intramedullary rod.

QUESTIONS

32. One of the requirements of a successful total hip arthroplasty is to accomplish load transfer from the prosthesis to the femur. What are the three mechanisms by which this occurs?

33. What is a surface load transfer system?

34. What is Young's modulus?

35. What is ductility?

36. What is the biomechanical function and result of the metal backing of a tibial component in an unconstrained total knee arthroplasty system?

37. What is the biomechanical function of a stem attached to a tibial tray in a total knee arthroplasty system?

38. What is the most common technical error in primary total knee arthroplasty surgery?

39. What is the yield strength of a material?

40. Of the three classes of metallic implants, which has the lowest modulus of elasticity?

41. What does the process of cold-working 316L stainless steel do to tensile strength, stiffness, and its fatigue strength?

ANSWERS

32. It is possible to apply a direct load to the femoral neck area by the use of a collar. Second, by use of a tapered femoral stem, it is possible to create a compressive load between the stem-cement or stem-bone interface. Third, adhesions between the prosthesis and bone or prosthesis-cement or cement-bone interfaces will allow transfer through shear mechanisms. This has been termed an *intramedullary load transfer system*.

ANSWERS

33. A surface load transfer system refers to a joint arthroplasty or portion thereof in which the load is transferred directly from the prosthetic system to the underlying cancellous or cortical bone. The femoral component of a total knee, the tibial component of a total knee, and the acetabular component of a total hip arthroplasty all represent surface load transfer systems.

34. Young's modulus is the ratio of stress to strain at any point in the elastic region of a load deformation curve. This is also known as the modulus of elasticity and is an expression of a material's stiffness.

35. Ductility is that quality of a material that allows deformity prior to failure under load.

36. The metal backing effectively increases the stiffness of the ultra-high-density polyethylene at the prosthesis-cement and cement-bone interfaces. This results in a more even distribution of load across the upper tibial surface.

37. A tibial stem reduces shear forces at the prosthesis-bone interface, as well as distributing angulatory load through the upper tibia.

38. Malalignment of the leg into varus or valgus angulation. This results in a medial or lateral shifting of the mechanical axis of weightbearing, placing excessive loads in either the medial or the lateral compartment.

39. Yield strength refers to the stress at which a material takes on permanent deformity on a stress-strain curve.

40. Titanium has the lowest modulus of elasticity and therefore is the least stiff.

41. Tensile strength is almost doubled. The ductility is markedly diminished, and the fatigue strength is moderately increased.

QUESTIONS

42. What is a super alloy?

43. What is the chemical composition of ceramic material used in orthopedic implants?

44. What mechanical changes in tibial component design have reduced the negative effects of cold flow on polyethylene?

Use the following diagram to answer questions 45 through 48.

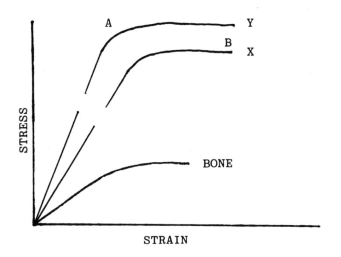

45. In the above stress-strain curve, compare the stiffness of materials *X* and *Y*.

46. What does point *A* refer to?

47. What does point *B* refer to?

48. Assuming *X* and *Y* represent orthopedic biometals, which metal would share the load more evenly with bone?

49. What is the instantaneous center of rotation or "motion?"

50. What is strain?

ANSWERS

42. A metal alloy is considered to be a super alloy if its tensile strength is greater than 1,000 megapascals (MPa).

43. Ceramic is made of aluminum oxide (Al_2O_3).

44. Cold flow effects have been minimized by applying a metal backing to the component to encapsulate its base, as well as using a polyethylene component of at least 10 mm in thickness.

45. The modulus of elasticity for material Y is greater. Therefore, it is stiffer than material X.

46. Point A is the yield point, i.e., the point at which a material can no longer retain its elasticity and undergoes plastic deformation.

47. Point B is the failure point, i.e., the point at which the material fractures.

48. Metal X. The modulus of elasticity is smaller for metal X than for metal Y, and therefore better suited for load sharing.

49. The instantaneous center of motion is the point in space existing at an instant in time about which all other points on the object rotate.

50. Strain is a measure of deformation, or potential energy, or the amount of work a deformed body is capable of doing in returning to its undeformed state. The unit is a change in size or shape of a body.

QUESTIONS

51. What is stress?

52. What is the endurance limit?

53. At what age does lamellar bone begin to form?

54. At what age has lamellar bone fully matured?

55. What is the biomechanical function of lamellar bone formation?

56. Compare the relative stiffness of cancellous bone to cortical bone.

57. What is the ultimate strength of bone in compression or tension?

58. What biomechanical factors govern the shape of a fracture of human bone?

59. Load applied in torque results in what type of fracture?

60. Load applied in tension results in what type of fracture?

61. Load applied in bending creates what type of fracture?

62. Load applied in axial compression results in what type of fracture?

ANSWERS

51. Stress is the intensity or load per unit area that develops at a point in response to an externally applied force. The unit used to describe stress is force per unit area.

ANSWERS

52. The endurance limit is the maximum stress level under which no fracture can be obtained, regardless of the number of loading cycles applied.

53. Lamellar bone begins to form at about 1 year of age.

54. Lamellar bone does not fully develop and mature until the third decade of life.

55. Lamellar bone increases the stiffness (modulus of elasticity) and the yield strength of bone. There is a corresponding increase in brittleness.

56. Cancellous bone has one fifth to one tenth of the stiffness of cortical bone in axial compression.

57. One megapascal (MPa).

58. The shape of a fracture depends upon the inherent qualities of the bone fractured, the externally applied load, and the amount of energy released. Therefore, fractures of immature bone, cancellous bone, and cortical bone will vary with similar exogenous loads.

59. Spiral fracture.

60. Tension typically causes an avulsion or transverse fracture.

61. Typically, a bending load causes a short oblique fracture.

62. Impaction fracture.

QUESTIONS

63. Briefly describe the anatomy of the three bony arches in the hand.

64. Describe the equiangular spiral.

65. Which joint of a finger ray maintains the greatest degree of flexion?

66. What biomechanical function do flexor tendon pulleys perform?

67. What biomechanical effect takes place with loss of the flexor pulley system?

68. Biomechanically, what are the two most important pulleys in the flexor tendon sheath?

69. Prehensile kinetics refers to movements of the hand in which objects are brought or held within the longitudinal arches of the hand. What are the two types of prehensile movement?

70. Efficient prehensile function depends on what basic hand requirements?

71. How does the relative strength of extrinsic finger flexion compare with extrinsic finger extension?

72. Functional wrist motion requires how much flexion and extension arc?

ANSWERS

63. There are two transverse arches and one longitudinal arch. There is a proximal transverse arch which is centered over the distal carpal row. There is a distal transverse arch which is centered over the head of the third metacarpal. There is a longitudinal arch comprised proximally of the carpal bones and distally of the four digital rays.

ANSWERS

64. The equiangular spiral, or logarithmic spiral, is the complex biomechanical movement or sweep of fingers in flexion to full extension. The equiangular spiral motion of finger flexion and extension allows for limitless positions for the function of grasping.

65. The proximal interphalangeal joint flexes to an average of 110 degrees, while the metacarpophalangeal joint and the distal interphalangeal joint flex to an average of 90 degrees.

66. In combination, the five annular (A) and three cruciform pulleys keep the flexor tendon close to the skeletal plane of the finger ray, therefore maintaining a relatively constant moment arm.

67. Biomechanically, this creates a bowstring effect during flexion of the finger, increasing the moment arm and therefore increasing the tendon excursion requirement. From a practical standpoint, this creates a weakness in flexion of one or more joints in the finger ray.

68. The A2 and the A4 pulleys.

69. Power grip and precision grip.

70. (1), Relatively mobile first carpometacarpal and fourth and fifth metacarpophalangeal joints, and relatively rigid second and third carpometacarpal joints; (2), well-balanced extrinsic and intrinsic muscle function; (3), adequate sensory function.

71. Extrinsic finger flexion is more than twice the force of extrinsic finger extension.

72. Sixty-five degrees.

QUESTIONS

73. What is the biomechanical function of articular cartilage in a typical diarthrodial joint?

74. Articular cartilage has been described as a *biphasic material*. What is meant by that term?

75. What is the biomechanical effect of immobilization on ligament tensile strength?

76. What are the effects of maturation and of aging on the tensile strength of tendon and ligament?

77. What is the rate of growth of regenerating nerve fibers?

78. What are the effects of stretching of a muscle tendon complex as a part of physical training?

79. What is the fundamental chemical occurrence during muscle fatigue?

80. What are the three main muscle fiber types?

81. Endurance training is associated with a relative increase in what fiber types?

82. What is the mean range of motion of the tibiofemoral joint in the sagittal plane during normal walking?

83. What is considered a minimum range of motion at the tibiofemoral joint for normal activities of daily living?

ANSWERS

73. First, to increase the load of area distribution. Second, to provide a wear-resistant surface by reducing friction.

74. The biphasic nature of articular cartilage consists of a 25% collagen proteoglycan solid matrix and a 75% interstitial fluid. The complex chemical interaction of the matrix and fluid portions allows for significant mobility and permeability of the fluid segment, rendering unique properties to articular cartilage.

75. Immobilization has been found to decrease the tensile strength of ligaments.

76. Maturation, i.e., growth up to the age of 20 years, is associated with a gradual increase in the quantity and quality of collagen molecule cross-links that is associated with a gradual increase in tensile strength. Aging is associated with a decrease in the tensile strength of collagen.

77. The maximum rate of growth is 1 mm/day.

78. Stretching increases muscle and ligament flexibility and elasticity. It has also been shown to allow the musculotendinous unit to store more energy.

79. Muscle fatigue occurs when adenosine triphosphate (ATP) breakdown exceeds ATP synthesis.

80. Type 1, or slow-twitch muscle fibers, and type 2A, fast-twitch oxidative, and type 2B, fast-twitch glycolytic, muscle fibers.

81. Type 1 and 2A fibers.

82. The mean range is 0 to 67 degrees.

83. The range of motion should be from full extension to at least 117 degrees.

QUESTIONS

84. What is meant by the screw home mechanism of tibiofemoral motion?

85. What are the three types of joint surface motion?

86. What is the biomechanical function of the patella?

87. What is the best lag screw position for interfragmentary fixation?

88. When a dynamic compression plate is applied without prebending and compression is exerted across a transverse fracture site, where is that compressive load applied?

89. What is the optimal site for prebending a dynamic compression plate?

90. What are the three theoretical functions of the grooves on the undersurface of a limited contact dynamic compression plate (LC-DCP)?

91. What is the metal composition of an LC-DCP?

92. What is the shaft diameter of a 6.5 AO cancellous bone screw?

93. What is the core diameter of a 6.5 AO cancellous bone screw?

94. What properties of bone are important in determining whether it fractures?

95. What is fatigue failure?

ANSWERS

84. With the knee held in full flexion, the tibia is in a relative position of internal rotation. As the knee is brought into full extension, the tibia is in a relative position of external rotation. The screw home mechanism appears to increase the stability of the knee joint in full extension.

85. Rotation, rolling, and gliding (translational) motion.

86. The patella allows for a wider distribution of forces on the distal femur. In addition, it effectively lengthens the lever arm of the quadriceps muscle through knee range of motion. It also prevents tendon-joint contact in flexion.

87. The best position is at right angles to the fracture plane.

88. The great majority of the compressive load is applied to the near cortex beneath the plate.

89. Prebending a dynamic compression plate is done between those screw holes immediately spanning the fracture site.

90. (1), To improve circulation about the fracture site; (2), to allow bone formation beneath the plate at the fracture site; (3), they result in a more even distribution of plate stiffness.

91. Titanium.

92. 4.5 mm.

93. 3.0 mm.

94. Energy-absorbing capacity, modulus of elasticity, fatigue strength, and density.

95. When a material is subjected to repeated or cyclic stresses that are lower than the ultimate tensile strength of the material, it leads to material failure.

QUESTIONS

96. Bone has resistance to both compression and tension stress. What components of bone are responsible for each of these properties?

97. What is the pitch of a screw?

98. What is the lead for a screw?

99. What is the main determinant of the tensile strength of a screw?

100. Describe the effect on breaking strength of drilling holes in bones. How do holes fill in with time?

101. What is fretting corrosion?

102. What four factors influence nonunion rates in tibia fractures?

103. How are muscles best strengthened?

104. How is endurance achieved?

105. What makes up vitallium?

106. Which has the least amount of corrosion and tissue reaction—titanium, vitallium, or stainless steel?

107. Rank these metals according to ultimate strength (point of metal failure): stainless steel, titanium, cast cobalt chrome, wrought cobalt-chrome.

ANSWERS

96. Collagen resists tension forces. Mineral matrix resists compression. (Bone is a viscoelastic material.)

ANSWERS

97. The distance between threads.

98. The distance through which a screw advances in one turn.

99. The root diameter of the screw—the minimum diameter between the threads.

100. Insertion of screws into a bone immediately reduces the breaking strength of bone. The size of the hole has little effect on the breaking strength, provided it is less than 20% of the diameter of the bone. When this size is exceeded, the degree of weakening is proportional to the size of the hole. Screw holes are usually filled after screw removal with woven bone in 6 to 8 weeks. The forearms and lower extremities are protected for 6 weeks after screw removal with short arm casts for the forearms and nonweightbearing crutch ambulation for the lower extremities.

101. Sites of metal-metal contact causing abrasion of the metal surfaces causing removal of the protective oxide coating.

102. (1) The degree of initial displacement, (2) comminution, (3) soft tissue wound, and (4) infection.

103. Contraction at maximum power daily without overloading.

104. Repetitive exercise stopping short of fatigue.

105. Cobalt-chrome-molybdenum.

106. Titanium.

107. From highest to lowest: wrought cobalt chrome, cast cobalt chrome, stainless steel, titanium.

QUESTIONS

108. Rank the above metals according to yield strength (point of permanent metal deformation).

109. A _____ material breaks before any plastic deformation takes place.

110. A _____ material has a plastic behavior before it breaks.

111. What is the key factor in biocompatibility of metallic materials?

112. Why is a low modulus of elasticity desirable in internal fixation plates?

113. Where have fractured stems most commonly occurred in total hip arthroplasty?

114. What three clinical factors are associated with stem failure?

115. Metallic analysis done on polished cross sections have indicated the presence of what specific problem in almost every case of stem fracture?

116. What is the best range of pore size for bony ingrowth?

117. What sterilization process has deleterious effects on ultra-high— molecular weight polyethylene (**UHMWPE**)?

118. What mixing techniques reduce the strength of polymethylmethacrylate (**PMMA**)?

119. How long does it take PMMA to achieve ultimate strength?

120. True or false? Polymers and acrylic bone cement are viscoelastic materials.

ANSWERS

108. From highest to lowest: cast cobalt chrome, titanium, wrought cobalt chrome, stainless steel.

109. Brittle.

110. Ductile.

111. Corrosion resistance.

112. This may decrease stress shielding which results in cortical osteoporosis.

113. Middle one third of the stem.

114. (1) Loosening, (2) lack of support at the level of the femoral calcar, (3) varus position.

115. Microstructural defects.

116. The best range is 175 to 450 μm. With less than 30 μm, no bone growth takes place.

117. Radiation sterilization. Radiation causes many free radical fragments which oxidize.

118. Rapid beating while mixing decreases strength 10%. Mixing for 2½ minutes decreases strength 11%. Insertion of cement with decreased viscosity results in greater cement strength. Low viscosity prevents laminations which significantly weaken the polymerized cement mass. Pressurized insertion will also increase compressive and tensile strength.

119. Twenty-four hours.

120. True.

QUESTIONS

121. True or false? Viscoelastic materials are stiffer and stronger at high strain rates than at low strain rates.

122. How strong is PMMA compared to bone?

123. What is the net effect of PMMA polymerization regarding cement volume?

124. Using the following diagram, if total body weight is equal to 50 kg and distance a = 15 cm and distance b = 3 cm, calculate the value of P (joint reaction force).

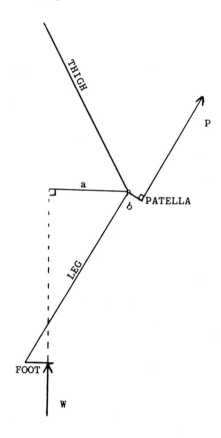

ANSWERS

121. True.

122. PMMA is half as strong as compact bone. If cement is not tightly packed between the bone and the components and gaps or spaces are left between the surfaces, cement will break because it is subjected to shear and tension rather than compression.

123. It contracts by 3% to 7%.

124. $P = 250$ kg.

QUESTIONS

Use the following diagram for questions 125 through 127.

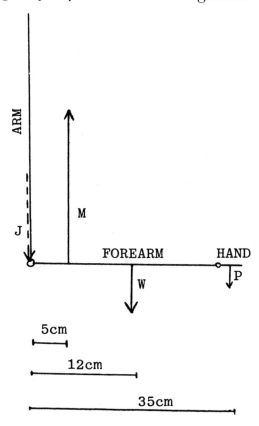

125. Given the following values, calculate the value for *M* (force produced through elbow flexors): *W* (gravitational force of forearm) = 20 N; *P* (force produced by weight held in hand) = 10 N

126. Calculate the joint reaction force (*J*) given the same values.

127. What happens to the value for *J* when *P* is increased to 30 N?

ANSWERS

125. M = 118 N. This is calculated by using the equilibrium equation for moments (*M*): $\Sigma M = 0$.

126. *J* = 88 N. The joint reaction force is calculated by using the equilibrium equation for forces (*F*): $\Sigma F = 0$.

127. *J* = 208 N.

CHAPTER 12

Tumors

Douglas McDonald, M.D.

QUESTIONS

1. How common are bone tumors?

2. How do patients with neoplasms of bone or soft tissue present?

3. What are other ways new patients present with skeletal neoplasms?

4. What is the role of trauma in development of tumors?

5. Does the duration of a patient's symptoms give any clue to the diagnosis?

6. How is the pain from a neoplasm usually described?

7. What physical finding is probably the most helpful in evaluating a neoplasm?

ANSWERS

1. Primary, benign and malignant, tumors of the skeleton are uncommon and make up less than 1% of the benign and malignant lesions of the body.

2. The clinical presentation varies depending on the location, but most patients, up to 90%, will present with pain or a mass.

3. Occasionally, pathologic fracture may be the first sign of a tumor, particularly in patients with metastatic disease. Lesions near the axial skeleton may present primarily with neurologic dysfunction and occasionally patients will present with a deformity.

4. There is no good evidence to suggest that trauma is a direct cause of tumors, although many patients will link the onset of their symptoms to a traumatic event. It seems more likely that a traumatic event draws attention to a preexisting lesion, perhaps making it symptomatic at an earlier point in time.

5. It is generally not helpful. Certainly a lesion that has been present for many years is more likely to be benign, but this is not universal. The symptom progression in a chondrosarcoma, for example, may be indolent and in certain soft tissue lesions, particularly synovial sarcoma, the patient may notice a mass for years prior to diagnosis. For most aggressive benign and malignant neoplasms, symptoms will develop over a few months and usually within a year. Extremely rapid development of pain or a mass in the range of days to weeks suggests an acute inflammatory process.

6. Most patients describe their pain as deep, aching, or boring, often accentuated at night. Importantly, the pain is usually slowly progressive.

7. The presence of a soft tissue mass in association with a bone lesion is helpful as it generally denotes an aggressive and probably malignant tumor.

QUESTIONS

8. What two clinical features are most helpful in establishing a diagnosis?

9. How is the location of the lesion helpful in establishing the diagnosis?

10. The radiographic evaluation of a patient with skeletal neoplasm involves what four modalities?

ANSWERS

8. The age of the patient and location of the lesion. Many lesions of bone and soft tissue tend to occur in well-recognized age groups. For example, solitary bone cysts, aneurysmal bone cysts, osteochondromas, and Ewing's sarcoma are examples of lesions which occur almost exclusively in young persons, usually prior to skeletal maturity. Osteosarcoma generally occurs in the second or third decade of life. Giant cell tumors are rare prior to skeletal maturity. Chondrosarcoma and malignant fibrous histiocytoma are lesions of adulthood, while metastatic carcinoma and myeloma are rare before age 45.

9. Although many lesions are metaphyseal in origin in long bones, some lesions, particularly giant cell tumor and chondroblastoma, almost always involve the epiphyseal region and subchondral bone. Ewing sarcoma and adamantinoma have a predilection for a diaphyseal portion of bone, and some lesions, such as enchondroma, have a distinct distribution to the small bones of the hand and feet.

10. Plain radiograph, computed tomography (CT), magnetic resonance imaging (MRI), and technetium 99m bone scanning are the most helpful imaging modalities. Other modalities, such as ultrasound, angiography, myelography, and other radionucleotide studies, such as gallium scanning, have limited roles and are only used in specific circumstances.

QUESTIONS

11. Of the primary imaging techniques, which gives the most information with regard to the character of a lesion?

12. For further evaluation of a lesion, which is better, CT or MRI?

13. What are the strengths of the CT scan?

14. What specific lesion in the skeleton is therefore best imaged with a CT scan?

ANSWERS

11. The plain radiograph. For many lesions of bone it may be diagnostic and, if not, will usually establish a reasonable differential diagnosis (see Figure). For primary soft tissue lesions, it will usually confirm the absence of bone involvement. (AP radiograph of the distal femur in a 15-year-old girl. There is an obvious destructive lesion present with areas of sclerosis and lysis. In this age and location, the most likely diagnosis is osteosarcoma.)

ANSWERS

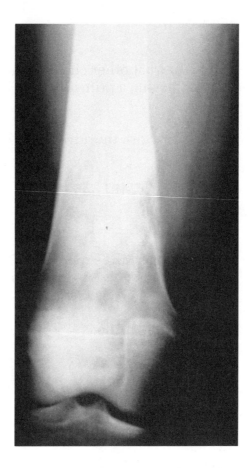

12. This is an unfair question, since each has strengths and weaknesses and they are used to gain different information. It should be remembered that on the whole CT and MRI are competitive examinations and not complementary. It is unusual that the evaluation of a lesion will require both.

13. CT is superior to MRI in demonstrating calcification, periosteal reaction, and endosteal thinning.

14. The clearest example of the use of CT over MRI is when one considers an osteoid osteoma on the basis of the plain film. The identification of a radiolucent nidus buried within sclerotic bone usually confirms the diagnosis.

QUESTIONS

15. In what other circumstances may CT be preferable to MRI in imaging a primary lesion?

16. What are the advantages of MRI?

17. Why is MRI helpful in determining the intraosseous extent of a lesion?

18. Why is MRI superior to CT in illustrating soft tissue lesions or the extraosseous extent of a bone lesion?

19. What role does ^{99m}Tc bone scanning have in the evaluation of bone lesions?

20. Do all lesions of bone need further imaging with either CT, MRI, or bone scanning?

21. What lesions require further staging?

22. What tests are helpful in evaluating for potential systemic disease?

ANSWERS

15. Lesions located in the flat bones of the pelvis, scapula, ribs, or spinal vertebrae may be better imaged with CT. Unlike the appendicular skeleton, lesions occurring in the flat bones are less well characterized on plain film because they may be difficult to see in their entirety or because of overlapping structures. CT is therefore invaluable because it can analyze in the axial plane and provide information regarding extent and type of bony involvement and provide an analysis of the matrix of the lesion.

16. MRI is superior to CT in determining the intraosseous and extraosseous extent of a lesion, but gives less information with regard to the character or histologic diagnosis.

ANSWERS

17. Most bone tumors, benign or malignant, will have a low signal on T1-weighted images. Using coronal or sagittal imaging, the intramedullary extent is seen in clear contrast to the high signal generated by normal marrow fat.

18. Many soft tissue masses are of similar density to muscle and other normal soft tissue structures. CT images therefore give less information regarding the exact soft tissue extent of a mass. The sole exception may be an intramuscular lipoma where, because of the differing densities, the distinction is easy. With MRI, most soft tissue masses, whether benign or malignant, will have a high signal on T2-weighted images. Since the signal for muscle, cortical bone, nerves, and vessels remains low on T2-weighted images, a clearer picture of its relationship to these structures is seen. In addition, since MRI can image in coronal and sagittal planes, a better appreciation of the caudocephalad extent is gained.

19. Prior to MRI, bone scanning was helpful in determining the local extent of a lesion. However, since MRI is superior in this regard, bone scanning is now used primarily to determine whether the lesion is solitary or whether there are other bony lesions. Another use of the bone scan may be to gain some appreciation of a lesion's biologic activity. Lesions which radiographically appear nonaggressive and have a completely negative bone scan are most assuredly benign and probably asymptomatic.

20. No. Many benign tumors do not need further staging. Nonossifying fibromas and asymptomatic fibrous dysplasia are examples of lesions which may be discovered incidentally and require no further workup. Other lesions which are well characterized by plain films and are clearly benign, such as solitary bone cysts or osteochondromas, may be treated without further staging.

21. All potentially malignant lesions and some benign, but aggressive lesions, such as giant cell tumor, may require further imaging. For malignant lesions this also should include an evaluation for potential systemic disease.

22. Since most sarcomas of bone and soft tissue metastasize preferentially to the lung, a plain chest film as well as a CT scan of the chest is needed. Technetium 99m bone scanning is also helpful as some sarcomas will metastasize to other bones.

QUESTIONS

23. Are laboratory tests helpful in the evaluation of a patient with a primary bone or soft tissue lesion?

24. A 15-year-old girl presents with pain and a mass on the distal portion of her right femur. The plain films show an obvious destructive lesion with mixed areas of lysis and sclerosis of bone and new bone formation in the soft tissues. If your differential diagnosis includes osteosarcoma as the most likely lesion, how would you proceed with her workup?

25. What completes the staging process?

26. Is there a "best" way to do a biopsy?

ANSWERS

23. For most lesions, benign or malignant, most laboratory tests are usually negative. Serum alkaline phosphatase can be elevated in many patients with bone destruction, but it is generally nonspecific. An elevated white blood cell count or sedimentation rate may suggest the presence of an inflammatory process, although occasionally patients with round cell neoplasms, such as Ewing sarcoma, may also develop slight elevation of these values. In evaluating patients with metastatic disease or myeloma, however, the laboratory tests can be very helpful. Tumor-specific antigens, such as prostatic-specific antigen, are elevated in patients with metastatic prostate cancer and patients with myeloma may have an abnormal serum protein electrophoresis, hypercalcemia, or proteinuria.

24. Since the patient's age, location, and plain films characterize the lesion well, further local staging need only include MRI, since it will give the most information regarding the anatomic extent (see Figure). Coronal or sagittal T1-weighted images should include the entire femur to aid in identification of any skip lesions. Systemic staging should include a chest film, chest CT, and ^{99m}Tc bone scan. (Coronal T1-weighted MRI of the distal femur in a patient with osteosarcoma. A clear appreciation of the intramedullary extent of the lesion is noted as well as appreciation of its extraosseous extent.)

ANSWERS

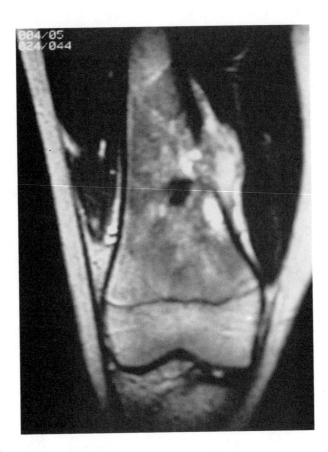

25. Biopsy.

26. The best way to do a biopsy depends upon the specific goals. The primary goal of the biopsy is obviously to provide a histologic diagnosis. However, if tissue is needed to provide histologic confirmation in a patient with probable metastatic carcinoma, a needle aspirate and cytologic examination may be sufficient, with little morbidity. Similarly, in a patient with an obvious osteosarcoma around the knee, sufficient tissue may be obtained with a core needle biopsy to confirm the diagnosis. This has less potential of infection or hematoma which could contaminate multiple tissue planes. It also results in a smaller biopsy tract that would have to be removed at definitive surgery. These are all potential advantages in a candidate for limb salvage.

QUESTIONS

27. What other biopsy techniques are there?

28. When is an open biopsy preferred over a needle biopsy?

29. What principles should be adhered to with regard to the placement of the biopsy incision in patients who are candidates for limb salvage?

30. In a bone lesion that contains a soft tissue extension, which part of the lesion should be biopsied?

31. Why do a frozen section at the time of biopsy?

32. What staging system is used most commonly for musculoskeletal tumors?

33. What are the components of the staging system?

34. How are tumors of bone and soft tissue classified?

ANSWERS

27. The alternative to a needle biopsy (either fine needle for cytology or a core needle for histology) is to do an open biopsy. These may be incisional or excisional. An excisional biopsy implies the removal of the entire tumor as part of the biopsy and generally is only reserved for small or superficial lesions. An incisional biopsy creates a direct path from the skin to the lesion without contamination of other tissue planes around the lesion. This is preferred for most malignant lesions, as this biopsy tract can then be excised en bloc with the lesion at definitive surgery.

28. If there is any potential of diagnostic difficulty, needle biopsies may not provide sufficient tissue for diagnosis. This may be true for many aggressive and potentially malignant-appearing lesions. The second reason may be where a greater amount of tissue is needed to subcharacterize the lesion, as in the case of lymphoma.

ANSWERS

29. The placement of the biopsy incision and tract is critical and should be done with a clear view of the incisions required for ultimate surgical resection. On extremities, biopsy incisions should be longitudinal and placed so that they may be incised en bloc with the specimen.

30. The extraosseous component. This generally provides the most rapidly growing and viable tissue that can be immediately cut with a frozen-section technique.

31. Most important, it provides information regarding the adequacy of the specimen. Occasionally surrounding tissue which appears grossly to be neoplasm may simply be inflammatory or fibrotic and not representative of the true tumor. In addition, many malignant lesions have large amounts of necrosis within them and a frozen section can determine whether the tissue obtained is viable. Furthermore, sufficient information may be gained from the frozen section alone to proceed with therapy. This includes inflammatory lesions and many benign lesions, such as giant cell tumor or aneurysmal bone cyst.

32. The staging system developed by Enneking and members of the Musculoskeletal Tumor Society.

33. The system stages lesions on the basis of their histologic grade and anatomic extent. Stage I lesions are low grade histologically and if confined to an anatomic compartment are stage I-A. If extraanatomic involvement is noted, they are stage I-B. Stage II lesions are high grade histologically and either A or B depending on their compartmental extent. Stage III lesions have regional or distal metastasis, regardless of their histologic grade or compartmental extent.

34. Tumors are first characterized as being either primary lesions of bone or soft tissue or metastatic. Primary tumors are then classified based upon their presumed cell of origin or differentiation and their malignant potential.

QUESTIONS

35. Which is more common, the primary tumors of bone or metastatic tumors?

36. What are the basic categories of primary bone tumors?

37. What is the most common primary malignancy of bone?

38. Of the primary benign bone lesions, which occurs most frequently?

39. Describe the radiographic characteristics of osteochondroma.

40. Which bones are the most frequently affected by osteochondromas?

41. Do osteochondromas ever become malignant?

42. Is it possible to predict if an osteochondroma is likely to become malignant?

43. Where do most enchondromas occur?

44. Describe the radiographic appearance of an enchondroma.

ANSWERS

35. Metastatic lesions are far more common than primary tumors.

36. Most classification systems subdivide the tumors into basic categories depending on the type of differentiation shown by the tumor cells and type of intercellular material produced. The important categories are bone-forming tumors, cartilage-forming tumors, marrow element tumors, vascular tumors, other connective tissue tumors, and neural or notochordal element tumors. Some tumors, such as giant cell tumor, arise from an unknown cell, and other lesions, such as solitary bone cysts, are classified as tumor-like lesions.

ANSWERS

37. Overall, myeloma is the most common, with osteosarcoma being the second most common primary bone malignancy.

38. As a group, the benign cartilage lesions are the most common with osteochondromas making up a majority of the lesions.

39. Radiographically, osteochondromas are seen as an exostosis on a bone. They may be either sessile or pedunculated and are characterized by direct continuity of trabecular bone from the medullary cavity out into the lesion.

40. As with most bone tumors, osteochondromas occur near the rapidly growing end of a bone. Therefore, most will occur around the knee in the lower extremity and around the proximal humerus in the upper extremity.

41. Malignant transformation in solitary osteochondromas is very rare. However, in patients with multiple hereditary osteochondromas, malignant transformation is estimated to occur in approximately 10% of patients.

42. Not really, although lesions of large size in a more proximal location probably have greater potential for malignant transformation. Certainly the development of pain or a lesion that is growing in size after skeletal maturity should raise the suspicion of malignancy.

43. Over 40% of enchondromas will occur in the hands or feet, usually in the phalanges.

44. When located in the small bones of the hand or feet, the lesions are generally radiolucent and have a variable amount of mottled or stippled calcification within them. When located in other bones, the amount of calcification may vary greatly and occasionally the lesions resemble bone infarcts.

QUESTIONS

45. What are the multiple forms of chondromas?

46. What is the relative risk of malignant transformation in patients with enchondromas?

47. What benign cartilage tumor characteristically involves the epiphysis of a skeletally immature patient?

48. What are the radiographic features of chondroblastoma?

49. Of the benign bone tumors, which is best characterized by CT scan?

50. Describe the histologic features of osteoid osteoma.

51. How are osteoid osteoma and osteoblastoma differentiated?

52. When arising in the spine, in what portion of the vertebra are osteoid osteomas and osteoblastomas located?

53. In a 14-year-old boy with painful scoliosis, what diagnosis should be considered?

54. Describe the radiographic appearance of giant cell tumor.

ANSWERS

45. Some patients simply have multiple enchondromas. A specific syndrome associated with multiple enchondromas is called Ollier's disease. This is characterized by more widespread skeletal involvement and a tendency toward unilaterality with the lesions appearing radiographically as a metaphyseal streak extending up to the physis. The involved extremity is usually short as well. Maffucci's syndrome is a disorder characterized by multiple enchondromas associated with angiomas of soft tissue.

ANSWERS

46. As with osteochondromas, malignant transformation of a solitary enchondroma is exceedingly rare. However, in patients with multiple enchondromas, malignant transformation may occur in up to a third of patients.

47. Chondroblastoma.

48. Chondroblastomas are generally radiolucent lesions with well-defined margins. Mottled areas of calcification may be present within the lesion.

49. Osteoid osteoma.

50. Histologically, an osteoid osteoma is characterized by a nidus of well-differentiated osteoblasts and loosely arranged osteoid trabeculae. The margin of the nidus is well demarcated from the surrounding sclerotic and reactive bone.

51. Histologically they are considered to be the same lesion and the distinction is made primarily on the basis of size. Lesions less than 1.5 cm are called osteoid osteomas and larger lesions are called osteoblastomas. Another name for osteoblastoma is giant osteoid osteoma.

52. Both tend to characteristically involve the posterior elements. Osteoid osteomas can be located in the lamina, pedicles, near the facet joints, or in the pars interarticularis. They are not seen in the vertebral body. Similarly, when located in the spine, osteoblastomas typically involve the posterior elements, although they can extend anteriorly. In addition, they may involve adjacent vertebrae.

53. Osteoid osteoma. Scoliosis is present in approximately 70% of patients with spinal osteoid osteomas with the nidus located on the concave side of the deformity.

54. When occurring in a long bone, giant cell tumors are purely lytic lesions, often eccentric, and extend directly up to the subchondral bone. The overlying cortex may be thin and expanded and occasionally there may be apparent soft tissue extension.

QUESTIONS

55. What is the peak age incidence of giant cell tumors?

56. Besides the long bones, what other locations are frequent sites of giant cell tumors?

57. Describe the histologic appearance of giant cell tumors

58. What are "malignant" giant cell tumors?

59. What other lesions are often included in the radiographic differential diagnosis of giant cell tumors?

60. What is the peak age incidence of myeloma?

61. What is the apparent proliferating cell in myeloma?

62. What laboratory studies are helpful in the evaluation of a patient with suspected myeloma?

63. Do all patients with myeloma of bone have these abnormal laboratory findings?

ANSWERS

55. Almost all giant cell tumors occur in the skeletally mature patient with a peak incidence in the third decade. Giant cell tumors in the skeletally immature are very unusual.

56. Giant cell tumors can occur in the bones of the pelvis, particularly the ilium near the sacroiliac joint. In addition, giant cell tumors can occur in the spine, usually in the vertebral body, and have a distinct predilection for the sacrum.

ANSWERS

57. The typical appearance shows two apparent cell populations. The basic proliferating cell is small with a round, oval-shaped nucleus and ill-defined cytoplasmic borders. An abundance of multinucleated giant cells are also present, with the nuclei of the giant cell tumors being very similar to the nuclei of the small cells. There is no significant matrix production.

58. Malignancy in giant cell tumors is seen in two conditions. The most common cause is secondary malignant transformation, usually after therapeutic radiation of a benign giant cell tumor. On rare occasions one may find areas of high-grade sarcoma juxtaposed with apparent benign giant cell tumors without any previous treatment. In either case, the malignant portion represents high-grade sarcoma with little resemblance in appearance or behavior to routine giant cell tumors.

59. Most commonly, aneurysmal bone cyst and chondroblastoma (as other radiolytic lesions in a relatively similar age group) may occur in the differential diagnosis. Occasionally telangiectatic osteosarcoma may resemble an aggressive giant cell tumor.

60. Myeloma, either as a solitary lesion or multiple myeloma, has a peak incidence in the sixth and seventh decades of life. It is particularly rare prior to the fifth decade.

61. The plasma cell.

62. Most patients will have anemia with hypercalcemia and Bence Jones proteinuria is seen in approximately one half of patients. The erythrocyte sedimentation rate is generally elevated. Serum protein electrophoresis will show elevations in various globulin fractions in approximately three fourths of patients. A monoclonal gamma globulin spike is the characteristic finding.

63. No. Patients with so-called 'solitary' myeloma lesions have a single bone lesion with no other apparent evidence of myeloma. Many of these patients, however, develop systemic signs within a few years.

QUESTIONS

64. What is the typical radiographic appearance of myeloma?

65. Is ^{99m}Tc bone scanning an effective way to screen for skeletal myeloma lesions?

66. What are the common sites of occurrence of osteosarcoma?

67. What histologic features must be present to classify a lesion as an osteosarcoma?

68. Are all osteosarcomas basically alike?

69. What are some of the variants or subtypes of osteosarcoma?

70. How does one distinguish parosteal from periosteal osteosarcoma?

71. What are secondary osteosarcomas?

ANSWERS

64. Classically, one sees radiolytic punched-out lesions with no surrounding bony reaction. Occasionally, expansile lesions are seen, as well as lesions showing a more diffuse permeative pattern of bone loss, usually in the flat bones of the pelvis or vertebral bodies. On rare occasions a sclerosing type of myeloma is seen.

65. No. A positive bone scan is estimated to be present only in approximately one half of the lesions. This is one instance where a skeletal survey is more helpful than bone scanning in the identification of other bony lesions.

ANSWERS

66. Like many bony tumors, they tend to be metaphyseal in origin and generally occur at sites of rapid skeletal growth. Approximately one half of all lesions occur around the knee with the distal femur being the most common site by far. Other relatively common sites include the proximal femur, proximal humerus, and para-acetabular lesions of the ilium. The lesions are particularly rare distal to the wrist and ankle.

67. There must be a proliferating population of malignant cells that produce osteoid.

68. No. Osteosarcoma is an inhomogeneous disease with subtypes of varying malignant potential which require different treatments and have different prognoses.

69. Of the primary lesions, the conventional intramedullary lesions are the most common and have been subdivided into osteoblastic, chondroblastic, and fibroblastic types, depending upon their predominant histologic pattern. In addition, a telangiectatic variant has been described. All of these are high-grade lesions with a similar prognosis. An important subset of osteosarcomas includes the surface lesions. These include the parosteal, the periosteal, and the high-grade surface variants. Finally, a low-grade intramedullary lesion has been described which radiographically mimics fibrous dysplasia.

70. Radiographically, parosteal lesions are generally heavily ossified and typically occur in the posterior aspect of the distal femur. The periosteal lesions generally show much less ossification. Histologically, the parosteal lesion has a prominent component of regularly arranged trabeculae. The space between these apparently normal-appearing trabeculae is filled, however, with a proliferation of atypical cells. The periosteal lesion characteristically will have areas of chondroid differentiation in addition to osteoid matrix, and normal-appearing trabeculae are absent. In general, the periosteal lesion is of a higher grade than the parosteal, but not as malignant as conventional osteosarcoma.

71. These generally refer to lesions that have arisen at the site of a preexisting lesion, as in Paget's disease or fibrous dysplasia, or after radiation to a primary lesion. In addition, the high-grade portion of a dedifferentiated chondrosarcoma may appear histologically as an osteosarcoma.

QUESTIONS

72. How do chondrosarcomas differ from osteosarcomas in terms of their age distribution and localization?

73. How are chondrosarcomas subdivided?

74. What radiographic appearance is characteristic for cartilaginous lesions, particularly chondrosarcomas?

ANSWERS

72. Chondrosarcomas are tumors of adulthood and older age with a peak distribution in the fifth and sixth decades. Osteosarcoma has a clear peak distribution in the second decade. In addition, whereas most osteosarcomas occur around the knee, chondrosarcomas tend to be more frequent in the proximal limb girdles, including the pelvis and proximal femur, as well as around the shoulder, both in the proximal humerus and the scapula.

73. Chondrosarcomas can be divided into primary lesions, secondary lesions (which occur at the site of a previous osteochondroma or enchondroma), and dedifferentiated subtypes which represent the occurrence of a high-grade sarcoma juxtaposed with areas of more conventional chondrosarcoma. In addition, two rare variants, the clear cell chondrosarcoma and the mesenchymal chondrosarcoma, have been described.

ANSWERS

74. The punctate, mottled densities due to calcification of a chondroid matrix are a characteristic finding (see Figure). (Lateral radiograph of the diaphyseal portion of the tibia in a 53-year-old man. This pattern of mineralization with the slight surrounding radiolucency, as well as slight endosteal scalloping, is consistent with the calcified chondroid matrix seen in an enchondroma. The patient is entirely asymptomatic and the lesion shows only mild uptake on a ^{99m}Tc scan.)

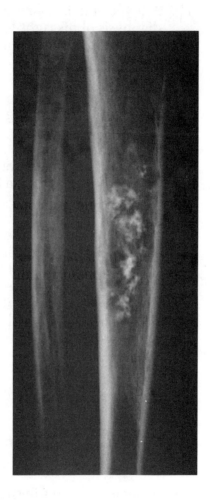

QUESTIONS

75. In general, are chondrosarcomas of a higher grade or lower grade than the typical osteosarcoma?

76. What histologic features are used to determine the grade of a tumor?

77. A 6-year-old boy presents with permeative destruction of the diaphysis of his right femur with associated periosteal reaction and apparent soft tissue mass. What lesion should be considered in the differential diagnosis?

78. What is the cell of origin in Ewing tumor?

79. What histochemical stain has been advocated in helping to differentiate Ewing sarcoma from other round cell tumors?

80. A 65-year-old man presents with pain in his lower back and sacrum, no definite neurologic dysfunction, and with a presacral mass present on rectal examination. Plain films show ill-defined lytic destruction of the sacrum and the CT scan definitely shows destruction of terminal sacral bone in the presence of an anterior mass. This clinical and radiographic description is characteristic of which tumor?

81. Is there any other tumor that should be considered?

82. Other than the sacrum, where else do chordomas occur?

83. Mucous vacuoles in the cytoplasm of chordoma cells is a characteristic finding in chordoma. These cells are called what?

ANSWERS

75. Lower grade. Approximately 90% of chondrosarcomas are grades I and II (based on Broder's method, which grades lesions numerically from I to IV). Conventional osteosarcomas are either grade III or IV.

ANSWERS

76. There are a number of criteria used, but important are the degree of cellularity and the amount of cellular atypia. Cellular atypia includes variation in size and shape, nuclear atypia in number of nuclei or shape, as well as the presence of abnormal number and pattern of mytotic activity. Other features are the presence of abnormal matrix production and areas of cellular necrosis.

77. Ewing sarcoma.

78. Unknown. The most likely source is a pluripotent mesenchymal stem cell. It is suggested that this malignant stem cell can actually differentiate into other tumors as well, which in part explains the histologic similarity of Ewing sarcoma, neuroblastoma, peripheral neuroectodermal tumor of bone, mesenchymal chondrosarcoma, and even the so-called small cell osteosarcoma.

79. Most typical Ewing sarcomas will stain positive for glycogen, although this is not absolutely specific. Other immunohistochemical stains and markers can also help separate tissue with neural differentiation or lymphocytic differentiation from the typical Ewing tumor.

80. Chordoma.

81. Probably not. In this age group a midline mass in the terminal end of the sacrum should represent chordoma. Lytic destruction of the sacrum is also seen in giant cell tumors, but they generally occur in younger patients and they are usually eccentric in the upper sacral segments. Metastatic lesions to the sacrum are distinctly unusual.

82. Sacrococcygeal chordomas account for approximately one half of the lesions with approximately 35% occurring at the cranial end of the spinal column in the spheno-occipital area. The remainder occur within the spinal vertebrae, usually in the cervical area.

83. Physaliferous cells.

QUESTIONS

84. Adamantinoma of long bones has been described histologically as containing two types of cellular tissue. What are these two types?

85. Which bone is involved with over 90% of adamantinomas?

86. What are two types of bone cysts that are generally considered tumor-like lesions?

87. How does one distinguish the solitary bone cyst from the aneurysmal bone cyst based on their radiographic appearance?

88. What is the difference between an active and a latent solitary bone cyst?

89. What is inside a solitary bone cyst?

90. On a histologic basis, how do aneurysmal bone cysts differ from solitary cysts?

91. What are fibrous cortical defects?

92. What is the characteristic radiographic appearance of fibrous cortical defects?

93. What is the natural history of fibrous cortical defects?

ANSWERS

84. Although considerable cellular variation is present in adamantinoma, the tumors generally will have circumscribed masses of epithelial-type cells surrounded by more fibrous or spindle-celled tissue.

85. The diaphysis of the tibia.

ANSWERS

86. The solitary bone cyst, also called a simple or unicameral bone cyst, and the aneurysmal bone cyst.

87. Solitary cysts appear as a fusiform widening of the metaphysis in a skeletally immature patient. The cortex may be thinned, but is usually not expanded. The apparent widening of the bone is secondary to failure of metaphyseal remodeling. Aneurysmal bone cysts, in addition to the apparent lytic lesion seen within the bone, will show cortical thinning and expansion. This is sometimes described as a balloon-like expansion of the cortex. In addition, the lesions are often eccentric.

88. An active cyst abuts the growth physis, whereas a latent cyst has "moved away" from the growth physis.

89. Occasionally the cyst may be empty, but it is usually filled with a clear or yellowish-brown fluid. There is generally a thin lining of fibrous tissue in the inner surface of the cyst wall. It may have ridges, which accounts for the apparent trabeculated appearance on the plain film.

90. The inside of an aneurysmal bone cyst usually contains multiple blood-filled spaces. It often contains more solid, fleshy tissue. Histologically, aneurysmal bone cysts are characterized by the presence of cavernous spaces filled with blood. The walls of the spaces lack the normal features of blood vessels and show varying amounts of fibrous tissue, giant cells, and even osteoid.

91. Proliferations of benign fibrous tissue, generally eccentrically located in the metaphyseal portion of long bones in the skeletally immature. Other names for histologically identical lesions include fibroma, nonossifying fibroma, and metaphyseal fibrous defect.

92. Lesions are characteristically eccentrically located in a cortical bone and have a thinning of the overlying cortex with a well-demarcated skeletal line of sclerosis along the inner margin.

93. In their classic form, they are almost exclusively seen in childhood and adolescence, and generally resolve spontaneously. For this reason, many authors believe that they represent a failure of proper ossification rather than a true neoplasm.

QUESTIONS

94. In addition to fibrous cortical defects, what other benign fibrous lesion is probably the result of abnormal bone development rather than a neoplasm?

95. Describe the radiographic features of fibrous dysplasia.

96. What histologic features are typical for fibrous dysplasia?

97. Is there an age and skeletal distribution for eosinophilic granulomas?

98. Describe the radiographic appearance of a solitary eosinophilic granuloma.

99. What are the multiple forms of histiocytosis?

100. What is the histologic appearance of an eosinophilic granuloma?

101. Do all bone tumors require treatment?

ANSWERS

94. Fibrous dysplasia.

95. The radiographic appearance of fibrous dysplasia can be somewhat variable, but generally fairly well-defined zones of rarefaction are seen surrounded by a narrow rim of sclerotic bone. Typically, these zones of rarefaction will have a ground-glass appearance. Expansion and thinning of cortical bone can occur and, depending upon the extent of the process, bony deformity. Multiple bone lesions can also occur.

ANSWERS

96. An abundant fibroblastic proliferation which surrounds rather bizarre and immature woven bone trabeculae. It is said these trabeculae take the shape of letters of the alphabet, particularly an "O" or a "U." Metaplastic chondroid tissue and osteoid are occasionally present.

97. Yes. Most commonly they arise in children and young adults, with the most frequent anatomic sites being the femur and skull.

98. Radiographically, eosinophilic granulomas generally appear as round, slightly ovoid, lytic lesions which are fairly well defined. A periosteal reaction may be present. When located in a vertebral body, the body can be partly or completely collapsed, producing a so-called vertebra plana.

99. Hand-Schüller-Christian disease and Letterer-Siwe disease. Hand-Schüller-Christian disease classically refers to the triad of skull lesions, exophthalmos, and diabetes insipidus. This generally has a rather chronic evolution and occurs in children over the age of 3 years. Letterer-Siwe disease is believed to represent a more acute manifestation of histiocytosis and generally has an age of onset of less than 3 years. In addition to bone lesions, clinical findings are recurrent bacteremia, diffuse lymphadenopathy, and skin lesions. The disease is commonly fatal.

100. Although the histologic appearance of eosinophilic granuloma varies, sections should show a mixture of pale-staining histiocytic cells, along with a variable number of eosinophilic leukocytes, lymphocytes, plasma cells, and neutrophils. The histiocytic cells typically have a large, ovoid, indented nucleus and well-defined cytoplasmic borders.

101. No. Certain nonprogressive, benign conditions, such as fibrous dysplasia or benign fibrous cortical defects, may not need specific treatment or can simply be followed radiographically. Treatment is generally indicated for symptomatic lesions or for lesions that are known to progress and become symptomatic. Certainly, all malignant lesions require treatment.

QUESTIONS

102. How are surgical margins defined?

103. What sort of margin is achieved by an amputation?

104. How does one decide what surgical treatment is appropriate?

105. What are the indications for treatment of an osteochondroma?

106. Do osteoid osteomas require removal?

107. What sort of surgical margin is required for effective treatment of an osteoid osteoma?

108. What is appropriate treatment for a giant cell tumor?

109. How does one do an aggressive surgical curettage?

ANSWERS

102. Margins are defined as intralesional, marginal, wide, or radical. An intralesional margin is achieved when the lesion is removed by actually entering the tumor, as occurs with curettage. A marginal margin implies removal of the lesion through its pseudocapsule or reactive zone, as occurs when a lesion is shelled out. A wide margin implies complete removal of the lesion, including a surrounding cuff of normal tissue beyond the reactive zone of the tumor. A radical margin requires removal of the entire anatomic compartment(s) that the lesion occupies.

103. The term *amputation* tells you nothing about the margin achieved. One could conceivably amputate directly through the middle of a tumor and therefore end up with an intralesional margin. For a distal femoral tumor, a midthigh amputation, provided it was through entirely normal tissue, would result in a wide surgical margin, since the entire compartment, i.e., the femur, was not removed. In general, radical margins can usually only be achieved by amputation.

ANSWERS

104. Surgical treatment corresponds roughly to the stage of the tumor, i.e., its histologic aggressiveness and anatomic extent. Many benign lesions can be treated with a lesional margin through aggressive curettage. Marginal excision may be warranted for some lesions. The minimal amount of surgery required for most malignant lesions would be a wide margin.

105. Removal is usually indicated for symptomatic lesions. Symptoms usually arise from pressure on nearby structures, such as nerves or tendons. It is also reasonable to remove large lesions for cosmetic reasons. Any growth or enlargement after skeletal maturity warrants removal.

106. Yes. Most symptomatic lesions require removal before the symptoms resolve. There are isolated reports of osteoid osteomas resolving spontaneously, or with long-term anti-inflammatory medication. However, histologic confirmation of the diagnosis is obviously lacking.

107. Complete removal of the nidus is required. Theoretically, this should be able to be accomplished with aggressive lesional surgery. Localization of the nidus, however, can be difficult. En bloc excision of the nidus and some of the surrounding reactive bone is often suggested as the treatment of choice. Not all reactive bone need be removed.

108. This is controversial, but most surgeons agree that complete surgical removal through an aggressive curettage, supplemented with some surgical adjunct, is appropriate.

109. The lesion should be approached through a wide cortical window, so that the entire tumor cavity can be visualized. The tumor is removed with a series of curettes and the margin of removal extended beyond the apparent cavity by use of a motorized burr.

QUESTIONS

110. What are surgical adjuncts?

111. What local recurrence rate is generally reported after treatment of a giant cell tumor?

112. If the local recurrence rate for giant cell tumors is dramatically lower after wide en bloc excision, why isn't this the recommended treatment of choice?

113. Are surgical adjuncts used for any other tumors?

114. Is there any role for radiation in the treatment of giant cell tumors?

115. What is the recommended treatment for a chondrosarcoma?

116. Is there a role for chemotherapy or radiotherapy?

117. What is the overall survival for patients with chondrosarcoma?

ANSWERS

110. The use of additional methods, usually either chemical or thermal cautery, to provide further cytotoxic effect in a tumor cavity. Chemical agents commonly used include phenol, hydrogen peroxide, and alcohol. Thermal cautery can be achieved with liquid nitrogen, as in cryosurgery or, when the polymethylmethacrylate cementation technique is employed, the heat of polymerization of the cement is believed to provide an additional cytotoxic effect.

ANSWERS

111. The incidence of local recurrence is most closely correlated with the degree of surgical removal. For curettage alone, recurrence rates of approximately 30% to 40% have been reported. With a technique of aggressive curettage and surgical adjuncts, the recurrence rate can probably be lowered to less than 20%. If an en bloc resection is done, or a wide margin achieved, the recurrence rate should be 1% to 2%.

112. Owing to the tumor's propensity for extension directly into subchondral bone, a wide margin necessitates removal of the patient's own articular cartilage surface. This results in a significant functional deficit. Preserving the patient's own articular cartilage is paramount to achieving a maximal long-term functional result.

113. Yes. They are occasionally used for aneurysmal bone cysts, and benign cartilage lesions, such as enchondromas, chondroblastomas, or chondromyxoid fibromas. Less commonly adjuncts are used for benign bone-forming tumors, such as osteoid osteoma and osteoblastoma.

114. The risk of malignant transformation has led most surgeons away from its use as a primary treatment modality. For large lesions of the pelvis, sacrum, or spine, which cannot be effectively removed surgically, there is still a role for radiation treatment.

115. Complete surgical removal with a wide surgical margin. This can be done either through amputation or limb-sparing resection.

116. No. Chondrosarcomas are relatively radioresistant and chemoresistant tumors.

117. This is somewhat dependent on the grade of the lesion. With high-grade (grade **III**) lesions, overall survival may be as low as 40%. This may in part be due to the ineffectiveness of current chemotherapy. For lower-grade lesions, survival may be closer to 70% to 80%.

QUESTIONS

118. How often do local recurrences arise after surgical treatment for chondrosarcoma?

119. Are there any variants of chondrosarcoma that have a differing prognosis?

120. What is the recommended treatment for conventional high-grade osteosarcoma of bone?

121. What is considered appropriate surgical management for conventional osteosarcoma?

122. What is the rationale for limb salvage for osteosarcoma?

123. Is the local recurrence rate after limb salvage for osteosarcoma comparable to amputation?

124. Are the functional results obtained with limb salvage better than amputation and prosthetic fitting?

ANSWERS

118. If adequate wide margins can be achieved, the local recurrence rate should be relatively low (approximately 10%). However, owing to the often large size of some of these tumors and their locations in anatomically difficult areas, such as proximal limb girdles, wide surgical margins may be difficult to obtain. The tumors are notorious for their implantability and actual recurrence rates are closer to 30%. Since the tumors are relatively slow-growing, these recurrences can also occur late, even many years after the initial treatment.

119. The so-called dedifferentiated chondrosarcoma carries a very poor prognosis with 5-year survival of less than 20%. Another variant with a poor prognosis is mesenchymal chondrosarcoma. Although rare, it represents a high-grade tumor with significant potential to metastasize.

ANSWERS

120. Surgery plus chemotherapy.

121. Historically, these tumors are treated with ablative surgery of the affected limb, either with a wide or a radical margin. In the last 10 to 20 years, there has been a great deal of enthusiasm for limb-sparing resection of the lesion with a wide margin.

122. If a limb-sparing resection can be done that achieves a rate of local recurrence and patient survival comparable with that of amputation, but which provides a superior functional result, then limb salvage represents a viable option.

123. In the hands of experienced tumor surgeons, a local recurrence rate of approximately 5% occurs after a limb-sparing resection with a wide surgical margin. This is only a few percentage points higher than that achieved with an amputation and wide margin. This small difference does not have a significant effect on overall patient survival.

124. That depends on the level of amputation required. For a lesion of the distal tibia, for example, it would be difficult for an extensive limb-sparing resection and reconstruction, with its inherent problems at that location, to have a functional result that was significantly better than a below-knee amputation and prosthetic fitting. Conversely, for lesions of the proximal femur or pelvis, a hip disarticulation or hemipelvectomy results in such significant functional loss that almost any reconstruction that preserves some limb function would be an improvement. For most lesions that occur around the knee, either in the distal femur or proximal tibia, surgical management with an amputation requires at least a midthigh level. Most limb-sparing reconstructions about the knee result in a functional level superior to an above-knee prosthesis.

QUESTIONS

125. What factors have led to the increased use of limb salvage for osteosarcoma?

126. What is the role of chemotherapy in osteosarcoma?

127. What are the specific chemotherapeutic agents found to be most effective for osteosarcoma?

128. What is neoadjuvant chemotherapy?

129. What are the advantages of preoperative or neoadjuvant treatment?

130. How much necrosis is considered a good response to preoperative chemotherapy?

131. What are the disadvantages of neoadjuvant chemotherapy?

ANSWERS

125. A better understanding of tumor biology and surgical margins required for control; significant advancements in imaging techniques, particularly the use of CT, and more recently, MRI; better reconstructive techniques and materials; and the development of effective adjuvant chemotherapy.

126. Chemotherapy is now an accepted adjunct to surgical removal for all patients with high-grade conventional osteosarcoma. It improves long-term survival, in some groups of patients up to 60% to 80%, compared with the historical controls of 20% to 40% seen with surgical treatment alone.

ANSWERS

127. Methotrexate, cisplatin, and doxorubicin (Adriamycin) have been found to be the most effective agents. Newer agents, particularly ifosfamide, are also showing promising results.

128. A treatment regimen in which chemotherapy is initiated after histologic diagnosis, but before definitive surgical removal of the tumor. Depending on the specific protocol, surgical resection is done approximately 6 to 15 weeks after initiation of treatment. Chemotherapy is then resumed as maintenance treatment.

129. There are a number of potential advantages, including, perhaps, earlier treatment of micrometastatic disease, which is believed to be present in the majority of patients at the time of diagnosis. Pretreatment may, through maturation of the margins of the lesion or possible shrinkage, make a patient a candidate for limb salvage when previously an amputation would be needed. Most important, it provides an in vivo test of the agents used. Measurement of tumor necrosis after definitive resection has been used as a prognostic indicator, as well as a means of directing further chemotherapy.

130. Although a subjective assessment, most authors suggest that a good response requires over 90% necrosis.

131. The primary disadvantage is a delay in definitive treatment in the event that the patient does not respond to the agents used. Fortunately, it has been the experience of most institutions that most patients do respond, at least in part, and that neoadjuvant use has not led to adverse effect on survival or increased incidence of pulmonary metastasis. Another potential disadvantage is that preoperative chemotherapy may be associated with an increased incidence of complications, particularly wound healing and infection, at the time of surgical treatment, due to the immunocompromised condition of the patient.

QUESTIONS

132. Given the apparent effectiveness of chemotherapy and limb salvage for the management of osteosarcoma, what are the indications for amputation?

133. After resection for malignant neoplasm of a major segment of the bony skeleton that involves a joint, what is the basic reconstructive goal?

134. In considering bony resections about the knee, what are the basic methods by which an arthroplasty can be created?

135. What are the advantages and disadvantages of an endoprosthesis?

136. What are the advantages and disadvantages of an osteoarticular allograft?

137. What are the basic methods by which a stable arthrodesis can be created?

138. What soft tissue structure around the knee and leg is felt to be essential for an effective arthroplasty?

139. In the upper extremity, what structures need to be present before reconstruction about the shoulder will result in functional abduction?

ANSWERS

132. Amputation may be indicated for distal lower extremity lesions, where the results of amputation and prosthetic fitting are quite good; for very large lesions that have compromised important neurovascular structures; for lesions associated with pathologic fracture, which has contaminated multiple tissue compartments; for local recurrence after a previous attempt at limb salvage; and possibly for lesions in the very young, in whom the anticipated leg length discrepancy at adulthood after limb salvage becomes too great.

ANSWERS

133. The restoration of skeletal continuity, either by creation of a functional arthroplasty or a stable arthrodesis.

134. An endoprosthesis, an osteoarticular allograft, or an allograft-prosthesis composite.

135. The advantages are that they are technically easier, have less operative time, are associated with fewer early complications, and allow for an earlier return of function. The disadvantages include failure to reconstruct bone stock and potential for long-term mechanical failure and loosening.

136. The advantages include a potential restoration of bone stock, the creation of a biologic arthroplasty with potential for soft tissue attachment, and ability to customize the reconstruction intraoperatively. The disadvantages are that they are technically more demanding and usually require a longer operative time, are associated with a higher rate of early complications, including infection and nonunion, and require a long period of protective weightbearing and casting, thus a delay in functional return. There is also the potential for late complications, including fracture, joint instability, and cartilage degeneration.

137. They can be done with autogenous bone grafts, either as local grafts from around the resection site, or as iliac crest or fibular grafts combined with internal fixation, or they can be done with large fragment allografts combined with internal fixation.

138. A functional extensor mechanism.

139. In addition to restoration of skeletal continuity, functional abduction requires the restoration of rotator cuff, as well as deltoid action.

QUESTIONS

140. Is there a role for thoracotomy in attempting to excise pulmonary metastasis in a patient with osteosarcoma?

141. The management of Ewing sarcoma generally includes what therapeutic modalities?

142. Should all Ewing sarcoma primaries be resected?

143. If radiation is used as the sole means of local treatment, what dose is generally employed?

144. What are the potential side effects from radiotherapy for Ewing sarcoma?

145. If surgery is used as a means of local control, can radiation be avoided altogether?

146. Is preoperative neoadjuvant chemotherapy used for Ewing sarcoma?

147. What specific chemotherapeutic agents are used in the treatment of Ewing sarcoma?

148. What is the primary treatment for myeloma?

ANSWERS

140. An aggressive approach to resection of pulmonary disease has proved beneficial for a number of patients. This is most effective when the amount of pulmonary disease is minimal, usually less than four to five nodules. Even multiple thoracotomies to eradicate pulmonary disease may be justified, in combination with systemic chemotherapy. If a patient has multiple bilateral pulmonary nodules (usually more than 10–15), however, then it is unlikely that an aggressive approach will result in a significant change in prognosis.

ANSWERS

141. Ewing sarcoma often requires the combination of not only surgery and chemotherapy but the addition of radiotherapy to the treatment regimen, because it is generally considered a radiosensitive tumor. In fact, a more traditional approach to treatment would utilize radiation alone for the primary lesion and chemotherapy as systemic treatment. More recently, however, a number of investigators have found that the addition of a wide surgical margin of the primary lesion leads to not only improved local control but improved survival.

142. This is somewhat controversial. Certainly, lesions in relatively expendable bones, or lesions in extremities where an adequate surgical margin as well as an effective method of reconstruction is available, should be considered candidates for resection. Large lesions of the pelvis or spine, however, may not be amenable to resection and consideration should be given to radiotherapy as the primary method of treatment.

143. From 6,000 to 7,000 cGy.

144. Joint stiffness or ankylosis, or both; leg length inequality, secondary to arrest of growing physes; and the possibility of radiation-induced sarcomas in patients that survive their Ewing sarcoma.

145. Generally, if an adequate surgical margin can be attained, radiation can be avoided. However, if a marginal margin is obtained, or any contaminated margin, radiotherapy should be used as an adjunct to surgical resection. If used as an adjunt, a lower dose can be delivered, generally in the range of 4,000 to 5,000 cGy.

146. Yes. Treatment is begun after histologic diagnosis. A striking volumetric reduction in the size of the soft tissue component of the tumor is often seen prior to surgical resection.

147. Vincristine, cyclophosphamide, Adriamycin, and dactinomycin. Newer agents, particularly ifosfamide and etoposide, are also being studied.

148. Chemotherapy for the systemic disease, and occasionally radiation for symptomatic lesions not responding to chemotherapy.

QUESTIONS

149. What is the role of surgery for myeloma?

150. Can chordoma of the sacrum be treated effectively with surgery alone?

151. What neurologic dysfunction arises from sacrifice of sacral nerve roots?

152. Is there a role for radiation in the management of chordoma?

153. What is the recommended treatment for adamantinoma?

154. What role does surgery have in the management of a patient with metastatic carcinoma to the skeleton?

155. Are there any criteria that can be used to decide whether a specific lesion is at risk for pathologic fracture?

156. Is the histologic classification of soft tumors simpler or more complex than for bone tumors?

157. What other differences are there between bone and soft tissue tumors when it comes to histologic diagnosis and classification?

ANSWERS

149. Surgery may be required to make a histologic diagnosis, or for the management of fractures or impending pathologic fractures. In addition, there may be an argument for more aggressive surgical management in the patient with solitary myeloma. A final indication occurs in patients with myeloma of the spine with neurologic compromise. For these patients, neurologic decompression and spinal stabilization may be indicated.

ANSWERS

150. Yes, but it requires an en bloc resection of the tumor with wide margins. This almost universally requires sacrifice of terminal sacral nerve roots as the resection level can usually be done no lower than the interval between the S2–3 foramen.

151. If the nerve roots up to S3 can be preserved, at least on one side, patients will usually have minimal alteration in their bowel and bladder function. If both S3 roots are sacrificed, patients will usually have adequate bowel and bladder function, not requiring catherization, but they may need to employ some external stimulation maneuvers to empty their bladder.

152. Chordomas have an unpredictable response and radiation is generally reserved for unresectable lesions or lesions resected with less than a wide margin.

153. Wide resection and intercalary reconstruction of the tibial shaft. Radiation and chemotherapy are not used.

154. Surgery is generally indicated for occasional tissue diagnosis and in the management of fracture or impending pathologic fractures.

155. Lesions that occupy over 50% of the diameter of a weightbearing bone are said to be at increased risk of pathologic fracture. Prophylactic fixation may also be indicated in patients who have failed to get relief of symptoms from radiotherapy. It must be recognized, however, that prophylactic fixation is something that should be individualized for each patient, taking into consideration the specific location of the lesion, the patient's overall medical condition, and anticipated life expectancy.

156. More complex. Whereas the World Health Organization (WHO) classification of bone tumors contains seven major tumor categories, the WHO classification of soft tissue tumors contains 16 tumor categories with a number of lesions of uncertain histogenesis that cannot be completely classified.

157. Most bone tumors can be diagnosed with good-quality hematoxylin-eosin stains. The diagnosis and appropriate classification of soft tissue tumors, however, often requires the use of special immunohistochemistry stains and occasionally electron microscopy.

QUESTIONS

158. Are soft tissue sarcomas more or less common than bone sarcomas?

159. Is there any relationship between age and the incidence of various histologic types of soft tissue sarcomas?

160. Is there any relationship of tumor location to histologic types?

161. Other than age and location, are there any other clinical features that are helpful in determining the cause of a soft tissue mass?

162. An adult patient presents with a deep-seated mass in the thigh. How do you proceed with the evaluation?

ANSWERS

158. More common, but, they are still relatively rare compared with other types of cancer, particularly lung, breast, and colon cancer, and probably represent only about 1% of all cancers.

159. Yes. Rhabdomyosarcoma, for example, occurs almost exclusively in patients under the age of 30 with a peak incidence in the first and second decades. Synovial sarcoma is another tumor which usually occurs in a younger adult. Liposarcomas and particulary the malignant fibrous histiocytoma rarely occur in patients less than 20 years old and have a peak incidence in patients over 40 years of age.

160. Yes. Although tumors can occur in virtually any location, most malignant fibrous histiocytomas and liposarcomas, for example, will occur proximal to the knee and elbow, while synovial sarcoma is noted for its tendency to also occur distally in the extremities.

ANSWERS

161. On examination, most soft tissue sarcomas are firm, slightly mobile (not affixed to bone), and may have some surrounding edema and erythema. Physical findings that suggest a particular diagnosis include pulsation (or bruit) suggesting a vascular lesion or transillumination in the presence of a benign cystic lesion. In addition, most lipomas are soft and nontender and many nerve sheath tumors will be freely mobile in a transverse direction, yet relatively fixed in a longitudinal direction.

162. First, it is prudent that all deep-seated masses in adults be considered potentially cancerous until proved otherwise. This implies that the lesions be appropriately staged prior to biopsy and treatment. Plain films are necessary to determine the presence of bone involvement, followed by MRI, which gives the most information regarding histology and extent (see Figure). (Axial T1-weighted MRI showing a large soft tissue mass in the buttock of a 59-year-old man. Most soft tissue sarcomas, regardless of their histologic diagnosis, will have an inhomogeneous low signal on T1-weighted images.)

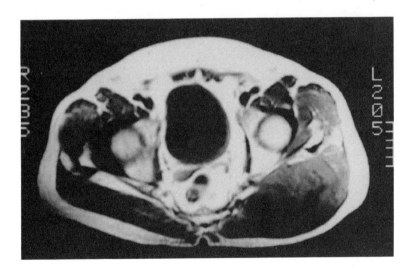

QUESTIONS

163. Are there any deep-seated soft tissue masses that can be diagnosed with certainty by radiographic studies?

164. In general, what is the recommended local treatment for soft tissue sarcomas of the extremities?

165. What is the role of chemotherapy for soft tissue sarcomas of the extremities?

ANSWERS

163. Yes. Benign lipomas have a characteristic appearance on both CT and MRI. On CT scan an intramuscular lipoma has a relatively uniform low-density appearance. With MRI, lipomas maintain their fat signal on both T1- and T2-weighted images (see Figure). (Axial T1-weighted MRI in the thigh of a 52-year-old man. This is a fairly uniform high signal [due to fat] and is typical for an intramuscular lipoma. A few internal septa are noted.)

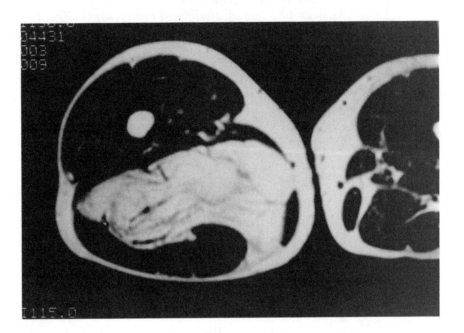

164. Subcutaneous or small intracompartmental tumors can be adequately treated with a wide surgical excision, including the biopsy tract and any surrounding contaminated tissue. For deep-seated lesions of larger size, particularly if extracompartmental, wide excision alone may not be enough. Usually adjuvant therapy in the form of radiation or chemotherapy, or both, are necessary to prevent local recurrence. As with bone sarcomas, amputation or radical excision may be necessary.

165. For certain histologic subtypes, particularly rhabdomyosarcoma, chemotherapy is an established part of the treatment protocol. For other lesions, its role in preventing local recurrence or altering survival is less clear. Many investigational protocols are currently underway.

FIGURE
CREDITS

Chapter 1
Answer 120 from Reckling FW, Reckling JB, Mohn HP: *Orthopedic Anatomy and Surgical Approaches.* St. Louis, Mosby-Year Book, 1990, p 425.

Chapter 2
Answer 8 from Canale ST, Beaty JH: *Operative Pediatric Orthopaedics.* St Louis, Mosby-Year Book, 1990, p 97.
Answer 48 from Canale and Beaty, *Operative,* p 747.
Answer 111 from Canale and Beaty, *Operative,* p 725.
Answer 191 from Canale and Beaty, *Operative,* p 901.

Chapter 3
Answer 135 from Crenshaw AH: *Campbell's Operative Orthopaedics,* ed 8. St Louis, Mosby-Year Book, 1991, p 1194.

Chapter 6
Question 198 from Reckling et al., *Orthopedic,* p 44.

Chapter 7
Question 12 from *AAOS Instructional Course,* vol 24. St Louis, Mosby-Year Book, 1975, p 207.
Question 24 from Reckling et al, *Orthopedic,* p 120.
Question 26 from Green DP: *Operative Hand Surgery,* ed 2. Philadelphia, WB Saunders, 1988, p 1332.
Question 28 from Reckling et al, *Orthopedic,* p 123.
Question 35 from Green, *Operative Hand,* p 2393.
Answer 139 from Milford L: *The Hand,* ed 3. St Louis, Mosby-Year Book, 1988, p 313.
Question 154 from Reckling et al, *Orthopedic,* p 120.

Chapter 8
Answer 9 from Crenshaw, *Campbell's,* pp 827,830.
Answer 125 from Browner BD, Jupiter JB, Levine AM, et al: *Skeletal Trauma,* Philadelphia, WB Saunders, 1991, p 1491.
Answer 127 from Browner, *Skeletal,* p 900.
Answer 131 from Browner, *Skeletal,* pp 902, 903.
Question 166 from Reckling et al, *Orthopedic,* p 319.
Question 167 from Reckling et al, *Orthopedic,* p 327.
Question 168 from Reckling et al, *Orthopedic,* p 320.
Question 169 from Reckling et al, *Orthopedic,* p 318.
Question 170 from Reckling et al, *Orthopedic,* p 325.
Question 171 from Reckling et al, *Orthopedic,* p 407.
Question 172 from Reckling et al, *Orthopedic,* p 396.
Question 173 from Reckling et al, *Orthopedic,* p 404.

FIGURE CREDITS

Chapter 10
Question 1 from Reckling et al, *Orthopedic,* p 433.
Question 22 from Reckling et al, *Orthopedic,* p 735.
Answer 25 from Crenshaw, *Campbell's,* p 2906.
Answer 31 from Mann RA: *Surgery of the Foot,* ed 5. St Louis, Mosby-Year Book, 1986, p 629.
Answer 33 from Mann, *Surgery,* p 627.
Question 47 from Reckling et al, *Orthopedic,* p 440.
Question 53 from Reckling et al, *Orthopedic,* p 431.

INDEX